INTERNATIONAL REVIEW OF
Experimental Pathology

VOLUME 16

EDITORIAL ADVISORY BOARD

K. M. BRINKHOUS
Chapel Hill, North Carolina

H. HARRIS
Oxford, England

T. O. CASPERSSON
Stockholm, Sweden

P. KOTIN
Denver, Colorado

P. DUSTIN
Brussels, Belgium

M. G. P. STOKER
London, England

E. FARBER
Toronto, Canada

B. THORELL
Stockholm, Sweden

D. W. FAWCETT
Boston, Massachusetts

H. U. ZOLLINGER
Basel, Switzerland

J. L. GOWANS
Oxford, England

CONTRIBUTORS TO THIS VOLUME

RAMZI COTRAN
JUDAH FOLKMAN
J. A. FRAZIER
ROBERT C. GALLO
FINN HARDT
FARID LOUIS
GEORGE W. MITCHELL, JR.
BENOY B. PAUL

L. N. PAYNE
PAULA K. F. POSKITT
P. C. POWELL
PAUL RANLØV
MARVIN S. REITZ, JR.
TAPIO RYTÖMAA
ANTHONY J. SBARRA
RATNAM J. SELVARAJ

JAN M. ZGLICZYNSKI

INTERNATIONAL REVIEW OF
Experimental Pathology

EDITED BY

G. W. RICHTER
*University of Rochester
School of Medicine and Dentistry
Rochester, New York*

M. A. EPSTEIN
*University of Bristol
Medical School
Bristol, England*

VOLUME 16—1976

ACADEMIC PRESS
NEW YORK   SAN FRANCISCO   LONDON
A Subsidiary of Harcourt Brace Jovanovich, Publishers

64493

COPYRIGHT © 1976, BY ACADEMIC PRESS, INC.
ALL RIGHTS RESERVED.
NO PART OF THIS PUBLICATION MAY BE REPRODUCED OR
TRANSMITTED IN ANY FORM OR BY ANY MEANS, ELECTRONIC
OR MECHANICAL, INCLUDING PHOTOCOPY, RECORDING, OR ANY
INFORMATION STORAGE AND RETRIEVAL SYSTEM, WITHOUT
PERMISSION IN WRITING FROM THE PUBLISHER.

ACADEMIC PRESS, INC.
111 Fifth Avenue, New York, New York 10003

United Kingdom Edition published by
ACADEMIC PRESS, INC. (LONDON) LTD.
24/28 Oval Road, London NW1

LIBRARY OF CONGRESS CATALOG CARD NUMBER: 62-21145

ISBN 0-12-364916-1

PRINTED IN THE UNITED STATES OF AMERICA

Contents

Contributors vii
Contents of Previous Volumes ix

Molecular Probes for Tumor Viruses in Human Cancer

ROBERT C. GALLO AND MARVIN S. REITZ, JR.

I.	Introduction	1
II.	DNA Viruses and Human Normal and Neoplastic Cells	2
III.	RNA Tumor Viruses	7
IV.	Summary	38
	References	38
	Note Added in Proof	58

Pathogenesis of Marek's Disease

L. N. PAYNE, J. A. FRAZIER,
AND P. C. POWELL

I.	Introduction	59
II.	Historical Concepts and Nomenclature	61
III.	Virus–Cell Relationships	62
IV.	Pathology	70
V.	Immunity	126
VI.	Factors Affecting Pathogenesis and Immunity	140
	References	145

The Chalone Concept

TAPIO RYTÖMAA

I.	Introduction	156
II.	Strategy of Growth	157
III.	Chalone Mechanism; Some Theoretical Aspects	162
IV.	Impurities in Chalone Preparations	168
V.	Composition and Effects of Crude Leukocyte Extracts; Some Original Data	173
VI.	Tissue Specificity	179
VII.	Putative Chalone Systems	187
VIII.	Regulation of Growth by Factors Other Than Chalone	189
IX.	Chalones and Cancer	194
X.	Conclusions	198
	References	199

Relation of Vascular Proliferation to Tumor Growth

JUDAH FOLKMAN AND RAMZI COTRAN

I.	Endothelial Turnover and Capillary Regeneration	208
II.	Biology of Tumor Angiogenesis	214
III.	Tumor Angiogenesis Factor	228
IV.	Discussion	230
	References	245

Biochemical, Functional, and Structural Aspects of Phagocytosis

ANTHONY J. SBARRA, RATNAM J. SELVARAJ, BENOY B. PAUL, PAULA K. F. POSKITT, JAN M. ZGLICZYNSKI, GEORGE W. MITCHELL, JR., AND FARID LOUIS

I.	Introduction	249
II.	Production and Maturation	250
III.	Chemotaxis	252
IV.	Recognition Factors	253
V.	Morphological Events during Phagocytosis	254
VI.	Biochemical and Antimicrobial Activities of Different Cells	255
VII.	Alterations and Decreased Resistance to Infections	263
	References	270

Transfer Amyloidosis

FINN HARDT AND POUL RANLØV

I.	Introduction	273
II.	Experimental Amyloidosis	274
III.	Transfer of Experimental Amyloidosis	289
IV.	Transfer of Amyloid-Enhancing Factor (AEF)	315
V.	Conclusions and Summary	329
	References	330

Subject Index 335

Contributors

Numbers in parentheses indicate the pages on which the authors' contributions begin.

RAMZI COTRAN, *Department of Surgery, Children's Hospital Medical Center, Department of Pathology, Peter Bent Brigham Hospital, and Harvard Medical School, Boston, Massachusetts* (207)

JUDAH FOLKMAN, *Department of Surgery, Children's Hospital Medical Center, Department of Pathology, Peter Bent Brigham Hospital, and Harvard Medical School, Boston, Massachusetts* (207)

J. A. FRAZIER, *Houghton Poultry Research Station, Houghton, Huntingdon, Cambs., England* (59)

ROBERT C. GALLO, *Laboratory of Tumor Cell Biology, National Cancer Institute, Bethesda, Maryland* (1)

FINN HARDT,* *University Institute of Pathological Anatomy, Copenhagen, Denmark* (273)

FARID LOUIS, *Department of Medical Research and Laboratories and Department of Pathology, St. Margaret's Hospital, and Department of Obstetrics and Gynecology, Tufts University School of Medicine, Boston, Massachusetts* (249)

GEORGE W. MITCHELL, JR., *Department of Medical Research and Laboratories and Department of Pathology, St. Margaret's Hospital, and Department of Obstetrics and Gynecology, Tufts University School of Medicine, Boston, Massachusetts* (249)

BENOY B. PAUL, *Department of Medical Research and Laboratories and Department of Pathology, St. Margaret's Hospital, and Department of Obstetrics and Gynecology, Tufts University School of Medicine, Boston, Massachusetts* (249)

L. N. PAYNE, *Houghton Poultry Research Station, Houghton, Huntingdon, Cambs., England* (59)

PAULA K. F. POSKITT, *Department of Medical Research and Laboratories and Department of Pathology, St. Margaret's Hospital, and Department of Obstetrics and Gynecology, Tufts University School of Medicine, Boston, Massachusetts* (249)

*Present address: Department of Medicine II, Kommunehospitalet, 1388 Copenhagen K, Denmark.

P. C. POWELL, *Houghton Poultry Research Station, Houghton, Huntingdon, Cambs., England* (59)

POUL RANLØV,* *University Institute of Pathological Anatomy, Copenhagen, Denmark* (273)

MARVIN S. REITZ, JR., *Laboratory of Tumor Cell Biology, National Cancer Institute, Bethesda Maryland* (1)

TAPIO RYTÖMAA, *Second Department of Pathology, University of Helsinki, and Institute of Radiation Protection, Helsinki, Finland* (155)

ANTHONY J. SBARRA, *Department of Medical Research and Laboratories, and Department of Pathology, St. Margaret's Hospital, and Department of Obstetrics and Gynecology, Tufts University School of Medicine, Boston, Massachusetts* (249)

RATNAM J. SELVARAJ, *Department of Medical Research and Laboratories, and Department of Pathology, St. Margaret's Hospital, and Department of Obstetrics and Gynecology, Tufts University School of Medicine, Boston, Massachusetts* (249)

JAN M. ZGLICZYNSKI, *Department of Medical Research and Laboratories, and Department of Pathology, St. Margaret's Hospital, and Department of Obstetrics and Gynecology, Tufts University School of Medicine, Boston, Massachusetts* (249)

*Present address: Department of Medicine B, Frederiksborg Amts Centralsygehus, 3400 Hillerød, Denmark.

Contents of Previous Volumes

Volume 1

Genetic Control of Lymphopoiesis, Plasma Cell Formation, and Antibody Production
G. J. V. NOSSAL

Arteriolar Hyalinosis
PIERRE DUSTIN, JR.

The Ultrastructure of Human and Experimental Glomerular Lesions
SERGIO A. BENCOSME AND B. J. BERGMAN

Common Cold Viruses
D. A. J. TYRRELL

Bone Disease Induced by Radiation
JANET VAUGHAN

Cellular Interactions in Experimental Histogenesis
A. A. MOSCONA

Author Index—Subject Index

Volume 2

The Nucleic Acids of Viruses as Revealed by Their Reactions with Fluorochrome Acridine Orange
HEATHER DONALD MAYOR

Cytochemical Aspects of Experimental Leukemia
B. THORELL

A Lymphoma Syndrome in Tropical Africa With a Note on Histology, Cytology, and Histochemistry
DENIS BURKITT AND D. H. WRIGHT

The Use of Statistics in the Etiological Study of Malignant Neoplasms
JOHANNES CLEMMESEN

Biological Effects of Ionizing Radiations
ARTHUR C. UPTON

Microscopic Morphology of Injured Living Tissue
IAN K. BUCKLEY

Cellular Recognition of Foreign Matter
STEPHEN BOYDEN

Melanin Granules: Their Fine Structure, Formation, and Degradation in Normal and Pathological Tissues
P. DROCHMANS

Author Index—Subject Index

Volume 3

The Use of Labeled Antibodies in Ultrastructural Studies
G. B. PIERCE, JR., J. SRI RAM, AND A. R. MIDGLEY, JR.

The Mode of Reproduction of the Psittacosis-Lymphogranuloma-Trachoma (PLT) Group Viruses
NOBORU HIGASHI

Ultrastructural and Subcellular Pathology of the Liver
JAN W. STEINER, MELVILLE J. PHILLIPS, AND KATSUMI MIYAI

Ultrastructure of the Enamel Organ
ENNIO PANNESE

The Significance of the "Dying Back" Process in Experimental and Human Neurological Disease
J. B. CAVANAGH

Intravascular Clotting: Focal and Systemic
GEORGE D. PENICK AND HAROLD R. ROBERTS

Experimental Production of Malformations of the Limbs by Means of Chemical Substances
BERTHE SALZGEBER AND ETIENNE WOLFF

Teratogenic Effects of Ionizing Radiations on the Embryonic Development of the Higher Vertebrates
JEAN-MICHEL KIRRMANN AND ETIENNE WOLFF

Author Index—Subject Index

Volume 4

Recent Advances in Correlating Structure and Function in Mitochondria
D. F. PARSONS

Ultrastructural Cytochemistry: Principles, Limitations, and Applications
DANTE G. SCARPELLI AND NORBERT M. KANCZAK

Cellular Necrosis in the Liver Induced and Modified by Drugs
A. E. MCLEAN, ELIZABETH MCLEAN, AND J. D. JUDAH

The Constitution and Genesis of Amyloid
ALAN S. COHEN

Complement: Hemolytic Function and Chemical Properties
P. G. KLEIN AND H. J. WELLENSIEK

Author Index—Subject Index

Volume 5

Life-span, Recirculation, and Transformation of Lymphocytes
J. L. GOWANS

Basic Aspects of the Interaction of Oncogenic Viruses with Heterologous Cells
JAN SVOBODA

The Cytopathology of Enteroviral Infection
G. C. GODMAN

Cytopathophysiology of Tissue Cultures Growing under Cellophane Membranes
GEORGE G. ROSE

Use of Freeze-Etching in the Study of Biological Ultrastructure
HANS MOOR

Autoimmune and Immunoproliferative Diseases of NZB/Bl Mice and Hybrids
ROBERT C. MELLORS

Atherosclerosis in Relation to the Structure and Function of the Arterial Intima, with Special Reference to the Endothelium
J. E. FRENCH

Author Index—Subject Index

Volume 6

The Examination of Mineral Deposits in Pathological Tissues by Electron Diffraction
D. F. PARSONS

The Hemostatic Mechanism and Its Defects
R. G. MACFARLANE

The Picorna Viruses: H, RV, and AAV
HELENE W. TOOLAN

The Induction of Cancer by Combinations of Viruses and Other Agents
F. J. C. ROE AND K. E. K. ROWSON

The Biochemical Morphology and Morphogenesis of Hepatomas
ROBERT K. MURRAY, LAMIA KHAIRALLAH, WILLIAM RAGLAND, AND HENRY C. PITOT

Hypersensitivity and Infection in the Pathogenesis of the Rheumatic Diseases
K. W. WALTON

Author Index—Subject Index

Volume 7

The Cell Cycle of Mammalian Cells
RENATO BASERGA AND FRIEDRICH WIEBEL

Sex Chromosome Aneuploidy in Man and Its Frequency, with Special Reference to Mental Subnormality and Criminal Behavior
W. M. COURT BROWN

Partial Cell Irradiation by Ultraviolet and Visible Light: Conventional and Laser Sources
GIULIANA MORENO, MARC LUTZ, AND MARCEL BESSIS

Recent Contributions of Electron Microscopy to the Study of Normal and Pathological Muscle
CLAUDIO PELLEGRINO AND CLARA FRANZINI-ARMSTRONG

Spontaneous Hypertension in Rats
KOZO OKAMOTO

Diabetic Glomerulosclerosis: A Comparison between Human and Experimental Lesions
T. STEEN OLSEN

Structural and Functional Changes of the Endoplasmic Reticulum of Hepatic Parenchymal Cells
EDWARD A. SMUCKLER AND MUFIT ARCASOY

Author Index—Subject Index

Volume 8

The Granulomatous Inflammatory Exudate
W. G. SPECTOR

Inductive Tissue Interactions in Vertebrate Morphogenesis
LAURI SAXEN AND JUHANI KOHANEN

Slow Virus Infections of the Nervous System
E. J. FIELD

Immunological Enhancement
NATHAN KALISS

Author Index—Subject Index

Volume 9

Microtubules in Disk-Shaped Blood Cells
O. BEHNKE

Lysosomes and Storage Diseases
ANNE RESIBOIS, MICHEL TONDEUR, SYLVIA MOCHEL, AND PIERRE DUSTIN

Cell Association and Somatic Cell Hybridization
GEORGES BARSKI

Production Disease in Ruminants under Conditions of Modern Intensive Agriculture
J. M. PAYNE

Tissue Typing in Relation to Transplantation
V. C. JOYSEY

Author Index—Subject Index

Volume 10

Chemical Properties of Basement Membranes
NICHOLAS A. KEFALIDES

Human Lymphocyte Growth *in Vitro:* Morphologic, Biochemical, and Immunologic Significance
STEVEN D. DOUGLAS

Cell Fusion in the Study of Tumor Cells
J. F. WATKINS

Genetic Diseases and Developmental Defects Analyzed in Allophenic Mice
BEATRICE MINTZ, R. PHILIP CUSTER, AND ANDREW J. DONNELLY

The Role of Membranes in the Replication of Animal Viruses
A. C. ALLISON

Feline Leukemia
W. F. H. JARRETT

The Murine Sarcoma Virus (MSV)
JENNIFER J. HARVEY AND JUNE EAST

Studies on the Etiology of Nasopharyngeal Carcinoma
K. SHANMUGARATNAM

Author Index—Subject Index

Volume 11

The Use of Fluorescence Techniques for the Recognition of Mammalian Chromosomes and Chromosome Regions
TORBJÖRN CASPERSSON, JAN LINDSTEN, GÖSTA LOMAKKA, AAGE MØLLER, AND LORE ZECH

Clinical Renal Transplantation
K. A. PORTER

The Effects of Ethanol on the Liver
EMANUEL RUBIN AND CHARLES S. LIEBER

Epstein-Barr Virus in Human Tumor Cells
HARALD ZUR HAUSEN

CONTENTS OF PREVIOUS VOLUMES

The Biology of the Mouse Mammary Tumor Virus
P. BENTVELZEN

Author Index—Subject Index

Volume 12

Pathological Effects of Lead
ROBERT A. GOYER AND BONNIE C. RHYNE

Activities of Specific Cell Constituents in Phagocytosis (Endocytosis)
J. V. SIMSON AND S. S. SPICER

The Endocrine Elements of the Digestive System
JUAN LECHAGO AND SERGIO A. BENCOSME

The Role of Renal Factors in the Pathogenesis of Experimental Hypertension
SIMON KOLETSKY

The Genetic Mucopolysaccharidoses (GMS)
M. DARIA HAUST

Author Index—Subject Index

Volume 13

Localization of Intracellular Antigens by Immunoelectron Microscopy
J. P. KRAEHENBUHL AND J. D. JAMIESON

Spontaneous Autoimmune Diseases of Domestic Animals
ROBERT M. LEWIS

Reactivation of Chick Erythrocyte Nuclei by Somatic Cell Hybridization
N. R. RINGERTZ AND L. BOLUND

In Vitro Hemoglobin Synthesis in the Thalassemia Syndromes
D. J. WEATHERALL AND J. B. CLEGG

Ultrastructural and Functional Correlations of the Parathyroid Gland
SANFORD I. ROTH AND CHARLES C. CAPEN

Author Index—Subject Index

Volume 14

Complex Mitochondrial DNA
DAVID A. CLAYTON AND CHARLES A. SMITH

Detection of Tumor Virus Genomes by Nucleic Acid Hybridization
MEIHAN NONOYAMA

Problems Connected with the Separation of Different Kinds of Cells
THOMAS G. PRETLOW, II, E. EARL WEIR, AND JUDY G. ZETTERGREN

Automated Cytology
MYRON R. MELAMED AND LOUIS A. KAMENTSKY

Subject Index

Volume 15

Amyloid, Amyloidosis, and Amyloidogenesis
GEORGE G. GLENNER AND DAVID L. PAGE

Humoral Host Defense Mechanisms against Tumors
CHOU-CHIK TING AND RONALD B. HERBERMAN

Chemical Carcinogenesis in the Nervous System
P. KLEIHUES, P. L. LANTOS, AND P. N. MAGEE

Morphometry in Experimental Pathology: Methods, Baseline Data, and Applications
HANSPETER ROHR, MARTIN OBERHOLZER, GEORGE BARTSCH, AND MARTIN KELLER

Subject Index

Molecular Probes for Tumor Viruses in Human Cancer

ROBERT C. GALLO and MARVIN S. REITZ, JR.

Laboratory of Tumor Cell Biology, National Cancer Institute, Bethesda, Maryland

I.	Introduction	1
II.	DNA Viruses and Human Normal and Neoplastic Cells	2
	A. Epstein–Barr Virus	2
	B. Other Herpes Viruses	5
III.	RNA Tumor Viruses	7
	A. Primate Type-C RNA Tumor Viruses	10
	B. Studies and Techniques for Investigating the Molecular Relationships of RNA Tumor Viruses to Human Normal and Neoplastic Cells	13
	C. Isolation of Type-C Virus from Human Leukemic Cells	36
IV.	Summary	38
	References	38
	Note Added in Proof	58

I. Introduction

There are now a number of techniques that utilize molecular probes for detecting different components of tumor viruses in animal cells. Listed here are some of the advantages that these techniques offer over other methods that rely on the detection of whole virus particles, such as electron microscopy, which demands budding or complete virions, and biological assays, which rely on infectivity. (1) The presence of virus can be established when the quantity of virus is too low to be detected by morphological or biological approaches. (2) Subviral components can be detected when complete viral particles are not present, as in the case of the murine sarcoma viruses, which transform cells in the absence of virus particle expression. (3) Viruses that fail to show biological activity, such as many endogenous viruses, are easily detected by molecular probes. (4) Molecular techniques can be used to determine the degree of genetic and immunological relatedness between virus and host or between viruses from different species. (5) Finally, they may be useful in determining what portion of the complete viral genome is necessary for the induction and maintenance of neoplasia.

In the light of the nature of what is detectable by these techniques and the nature of tumor viruses themselves, our use herein of several terms should be defined. We use the term "virus" to indicate either an extracellular virion that can reproduce itself and cause a biological change by infection of an appropriate host cell, or else an established set of DNA sequences (the provirus), either integrated into cellular DNA or existing as an episome, that can code for all or part of the viral genome and proteins. By our use of the term here, a virus need not ever have an extracellular existence. By "infection" we mean the establishment within the cell of all or a part of the viral genome in such a way that this genetic information can be replicated and packaged in virions or passed on to daughter cells. "Viruslike particle" we use to indicate particles that biochemically and/or immunologically resemble viruses but for which no biological activity such as infection can be established.

Molecular approaches offer unusual sensitivity, but like most very sensitive assays they require great care and abundant controls. In the past few years they have found extensive application to studies of human cancer, and in this review we will concentrate on and attempt critically to appraise some of these applications. We have concentrated on results that relate to the RNA tumor viruses (especially studies with leukemic cells) because of our interests and limited experience. It should therefore be remembered that this appraisal must be to a degree biased and surely limited by the same interests and experience.

II. DNA Viruses and Human Normal and Neoplastic Cells

A. Epstein–Barr Virus

The earliest successful and widespread use of molecular probes for detecting viral components in human cancer followed the isolation from Burkitt's lymphoma cells of the Epstein–Barr virus (EBV)[1] (77), a herpeslike virus. This

---

[1] The following abbreviations are used in the text: EBV, Epstein–Barr virus; FeLV, feline leukemia virus; FeSV, feline sarcoma virus; RLV, Rauscher leukemia virus; MoLV, moloney leukemia virus; MuLV-AKR, AKR murine leukemia virus; KiSV, Kirsten sarcoma virus; RSV, Rous sarcoma virus; AMV, avian myeloblastosis virus; BEV, baboon endogenous virus; SSV-1, simian sarcoma virus; GaLV, gibbon ape lymphoma virus; MPMV, Mason–Pfizer monkey virus; HLV, human leukemia-associated virus; AML, acute myelogenous leukemia; ALL, acute lymphocytic leukemia; CML, chronic myelogenous leukemia; CLL, chronic

discovery triggered a widespread search for molecular components of this virus in a wide variety of human tumors, and such components have been detected in some tumors by means of immunological and nucleic acid hybridization techniques. Various immunological approaches have shown the presence in Burkitt lymphoma cells of EBV-induced membrane antigen (*199*), EBV early antigen (*168*), EBV nuclear antigen (EBNA) (*219, 273*), and viral capsid antigen (*166*). Their presence appears to be specific to Burkitt lymphoma and nasopharyngeal carcinoma cells (*61*) and to cultured normal cells infected with EBV (*201*). In addition, the virus has been shown by similar approaches to be associated with infectious mononucleosis (*167*) and elevated levels of antibody to EBV have been reported in Hodgkin's disease (*212*).

Various investigators have reported the presence of EBV-specific DNA in various human cell types using labeled viral DNA or complementary RNA as a molecular probe. By hybridization of labeled EBV DNA to cell DNA immobilized on nitrocellulose filters, zur Hausen and colleagues have demonstrated the presence of the EBV genome in biopsies from Burkitt tumors (*391*) and cells cultured from them (*390*), in biopsy specimens from nasopharynageal carcinoma (*391*), and in human lymphoblastoid cell lines (*389*).

In this technique, labeled EBV DNA can form a stable base-paired complex with complementary unlabeled DNA immobilized on the filters, which are then washed to remove uncomplexed DNA. The percentage of original radioactive label retained on the filter is used to calculate the percentage of hybridization and hence to determine the amount of EBV DNA contained in a fixed amount of cellular DNA. A second technique for the detection of EBV DNA in cellular DNA is the use of *Escherichia coli* RNA polymerase to copy purified EBV DNA into highly labeled radioactive complementary RNA. Since this RNA can be prepared to a higher specific activity than EBV DNA labeled *in vivo*, it is a more sensitive molecular probe and can reportedly detect as few as two viral genomes per cell. Positive results with this technique have been achieved with DNA from both Burkitt's lymphoma and nasopharyngeal carcinoma tissue (*251*).

An even more sensitive technique uses measurement of the reassociation rate of double-stranded labeled purified EBV DNA in the absence and in the presence of unlabeled DNA from cells or tissue. The speed of reassociation of duplex EBV DNA from heat-denatured single-stranded DNA is proportional to the concentration of both strands. Therefore, addition of unlabeled EBV-specific DNA from cells to a hybridization mixture increases the apparent reassociation rate of the labeled EBV DNA. The amount of duplex labeled DNA can be measured by

---

lymphocytic leukemia; IgG, immunoglobulin; PHA, phytohemagglutinin; NC 37, human lymphoblastoid cell line from normal person; (A), adenylic acid; (dA), deoxyadenylic acid; (rC), cytidylic acid; (dG), deoxyguanylic acid; (T), thymidylic acid; (U) uridylic acid; $C_0 t$, concentration of DNA multiplied by time of hybridization expressed as mole seconds per liter.

treating the reaction mixture with nucleases which hydrolyze unpaired DNA but are inactive on double-stranded DNA and then measuring the unhydrolyzed labeled DNA by acid precipitation. Alternatively, the reaction mixture may be fractionated by hydroxyapatite chromatography. Single- and double-stranded DNA elutes at different salt concentrations, and the amount of labeled DNA eluting as double-stranded DNA can be used to measure the reassociation rate. A more detailed description of these assays is given below. Measurement of the acceleration of labeled duplex EBV DNA formation can reportedly detect as little as one viral genome equivalent per 30–50 cells and has been used to show the presence of EBV DNA in Burkitt's lymphoma and nasopharyngeal carcinoma (*252*) tissue and in most human lymphoblastoid B-cell lines (*252*). On the other hand, EBV DNA has not been detectable even by this technique in a myeloma cell line (*191*), a few lymphoblastoid cell lines (*235*), and most recently in tumors of the American Burkitt type (*263*).

Using *in situ* techniques, Wolf *et al.* (*378*) have been able to show that in nasopharyngeal carcinoma the epithelial cells, but not the infiltrating lymphoid tissue, have both EBV-specific DNA and antigen. This is particularly interesting because of the presence of EBV in lymphoblastoid cell lines, in a lymphoproliferative disease (infectious mononucleosis), and in lymphoma, indicating a strong tropism of EBV for lymphoid tissue. Consequently, localization of EBV-related molecules to epithelial tissue is unexpected. *In situ* techniques use cytologically fixed microscope specimens, which are then treated with the appropriate molecular probe (often labeled nucleic acid or fluorescing antibody) under appropriate conditions for hybridization or antibody fixation. In the case of ^{3}H-labeled nucleic acid, autoradiography reveals the intracellular location of complementary DNA, while fluorescent antibody reveals the exact location of a specific antigen by fluorescent microscopy. Not only is the intracellular location of given components ascertained, but also the cell type, as noted above, which contains the component in question. The disadvantage of this type of experiment is that it is not highly quantitative and is subject to experimental pitfalls. Partly because of this, the above observation was not fully appreciated initially, but recently Klein and his collaborators, using a different approach, confirmed that EBNA antigen and EBV DNA are present in the epithelial cells of this tumor (*200*).

The detection of DNA from EBV in Burkitt lymphoma cells is taken as evidence that these cells were once infected from without by this virus, the DNA of which subsequently became integrated into the host-cell DNA. These results, indicate that some or all of the EBV genome is present in the cell in question, and hence, at minimum, they tell us whether the potential exists for formation of complete EBV. They do not tell us whether whole virions are present in the cell (or released by the cell) nor whether the genome is being expressed, i.e., whether EBV messenger RNA (mRNA) and subsequently EBV-specific proteins are synthesized. Since EBV DNA is not detected in the majority of normal cells, it is believed that these positive molecular hybridization experiments indicate that a complete virus specifically infected the tumor cells. Such experimental results were one of several lines of investigation that have led to the general belief that EBV is somehow necessarily causatively involved in this disease. The results of the immunological studies suggest that the EBV genome in Burkitt's lymphoma is expressed since proteins specifically associated with the presence of the EBV genome have been found. The results of these and seroepidemiological studies argue then for a causative role for EBV in Burkitt's lymphoma. However, two factors have been used to argue against making a final conclusion that EBV *alone* is sufficient to cause Burkitt lymphoma.

The first factor is the absence of EBV genetic information (263), and low levels or absence of antibody to EBV in American Burkitt lymphoma and in a few cases of African Burkitt lymphoma (272). It can be argued that the disease in America is not the same as the African disease and that in the cases of the few negative African cases the diagnosis was incorrect or the techniques were not sufficiently sensitive. An alternative possibility is that EBV may be a common cofactor, which markedly increases the incidence of the disease, but may not be the *sole* primary mechanism essential for inducing Burkitt lymphoma. It is possible that the detection in Burkitt lymphoma cells of various components related to type-C murine leukemia virus is pertinent to this (see below) (205, 207), but the data for a type-C virus involvement in this disease are not at all conclusive.[2]

The second factor is that the lymphoblasts of many people contain EBV DNA, indicating that infection of lymphoid cells by EBV is common whereas Burkitt's lymphoma is rare. However, this could be a result of variation in the host and in itself is not a good argument against EBV as the causative agent. It would be of benefit if there were available an animal model of a naturally occurring neoplasia of mammals known to be regularly induced by EBV or a related virus.

B. Other Herpes Viruses

What about other human neoplasias and DNA viruses? Molecular probes have also been used in an attempt to link other DNA viruses of the Herpes family with certain other human neoplasias. For instance, Roizman and colleagues have carefully demonstrated the presence of a DNA fragment homologous to about 20% of the genome of herpes simplex-2 by DNA–DNA hybridization in a

---

[2] Consistent with this possibility is the report that Marek's disease, a Hodgkin's disease-like neoplasm of chickens for which a herpeslike virus is the causative agent (54, 55, 326), does not appear without the simultaneous presence of an RNA tumor virus (267). Presumably in most chickens an endogenous type-C virus serves as a cofactor. Although the nature of the interaction is not clear, it may be related to the immunosuppressive properties of these viruses (245).

cervical carcinoma (*87*). Furthermore, this DNA is transcribed into RNA in amounts equivalent to 5% of the viral genome. This work was stimulated by earlier seroepidemiological studies reported by a number of groups, most notably by Nahmias and his colleagues (*185, 241–244*), Rawls *et al.* (*270, 271*) and Aurelian (*8,289*) implicating herpes simplex virus in the etiology of cervical cancer. In the meantime, Hollinshead and Tarro (*170*) and Sabin and Tarro (*292*) described serological evidence supporting herpes simplex viruses as a causative agent in patients with cervical carcinoma and a number of other ectoderm- and entoderm-derived human neoplasias. This was done with an assay measuring a nonvirion herpes antigen. The assay is type specific with respect to herpes simplex type 1 and type 2 (*338*), and the antigens are found specifically in cancers of the lip, oropharynx, nasopharynx, kidney, urinary bladder, prostate, cervix uteri, and vulva, but not in other tumors or normal controls.

The difficulty encountered in drawing conclusions from these results is the possibility that the presence of herpes virus in these tumors represents association rather than causation. Herpes simplex I, of course, is a common infectious agent of the oral region and may remain dormant over a considerable period of time. Hence, its DNA might be detected in a carcinoma of the same region without being the causative agent. It is also possible that the carcinoma may itself lead to a derepression of the integrated herpes genome which has nothing to do etiologically with the neoplasia. One might then, of course, discover herpes-specific RNA and/or proteins in these cells. The same may be said for herpes simplex II and cervical carcinoma. Added to these difficulties are: (a) subsequent reports that herpes DNA is not detected in many cervical cancers (*262*) (there is no clear reported evidence on the incidence of successful detection of this DNA in cervical cancer) and (b) a recent failure by Sabin to confirm his own findings with Tarro (*291*). On the other hand, one should also be cautious about placing too much faith in negative data, and in this respect it is worthy of note that recent studies involving transformation of cells in tissue culture by DNA viruses have shown that only a very small portion of the DNA genome is required to produce transformation (*141,317*). It is possible that this amount of DNA is sufficiently small to have been missed by the molecular hybridization approaches which have been applied to human cancer. Suffice it to say that at the time of this writing there is no strong incontrovertible evidence supplied by "molecular probes" to support the view that either herpes simplex I or II are important causative agents in any human cancer, and in our judgment the strongest presently available arguments for a causative role for a herpes simplex virus in a human cancer are the results of the seroepidemiological studies with cervical cancer and herpes simplex II, but they are not definitive.

Because of our lack of personal experience with the DNA tumor viruses, we will not attempt to describe and evaluate the methodologies employed in the molecular studies. Instead we refer the reader to select papers from some of the prominent invetigators who have described and employed molecular techniques in this area (*61,87,166,168,169,199,219,251,252,273,292,378,389–391*).

III. RNA Tumor Viruses

There is clear evidence that RNA tumor viruses can cause leukemias, lymphomas, and sarcomas in a number of species (*76,89,125,140,146,181,197,198, 238,239,277,278,288,324,381*). They have also been found in many naturally occurring neoplasias of these types (*35,76,125,146,178,181,192,193,194, 209,269,277,288,324,346*), and there is evidence for horizontal transmission under natural conditions as well as strong evidence that the transmitted virus is involved in the cause of the natural disease in some species, particularly cats (*44,56,177,179,180,193,194,278,279*). However, there are factors that make it difficult to prove that these viruses or information derived from and/or related to these viruses are the natural causes of these diseases in some of these species, including man.

It appears that these viruses had their origin from cells in the relatively recent past (*107,133,137,138*). Some appear to have changed considerably, evolving away from the DNA of the host cell. (An alternative to this is that the virus in question originated independent from the host cell, infected the cell, remained with it, and evolved toward the genome of the host cell but retained some differences.) Others have changed very little if at all. Results from molecular hybridization experiments indicate that at best technology can show that the genome of these viruses is identical or nearly identical to nucleotide sequences found in "uninfected" DNA of the species of origin (*132*). These have been called endogenous RNA tumor viruses, but because of semantic confusion and differences of opinion over what truly constitutes an "endogenous" virus, we prefer to call them "Class I" viruses (*107,132,133,137,138*). We believe that at least some of the genetic information related to Class I viruses may be involved in development, possibly in providing selective advantages by some sort of gene shuffling or amplification mechanism, and/or in transmitting information between cells (*99,102*). This information is perhaps expressed in embryonic tissue (*366*), but not in differentiated adult cells. These viruses are characteristically xenotropic, that is, they will not productively infect cells from the species of origin[3] (*25,84,214–216,220,299,351*), and are transmitted with the genes of a parent cell to both daughter cells (see Fig. 1). This process has been called "vertical" transmission of viruses, a term coined by Ludwig Gross (*147*).

Other RNA tumor viruses are transmitted horizontally (one cell to another cell or one animal to another animal). We believe that in this process the potential for genetic change is created not only in the infected cell, but also for the infecting virus (*133,137,138*). In other words, we believe that the acquisition of the capacity to move from one cell or animal to another confers the potential for the greatest genetic change away from the original host cell. We have

---

[3] Although the xenotropic endogenous viruses do not productively infect cells, it has not to our knowledge been excluded that they can establish a provirus within cells of the species of origin.

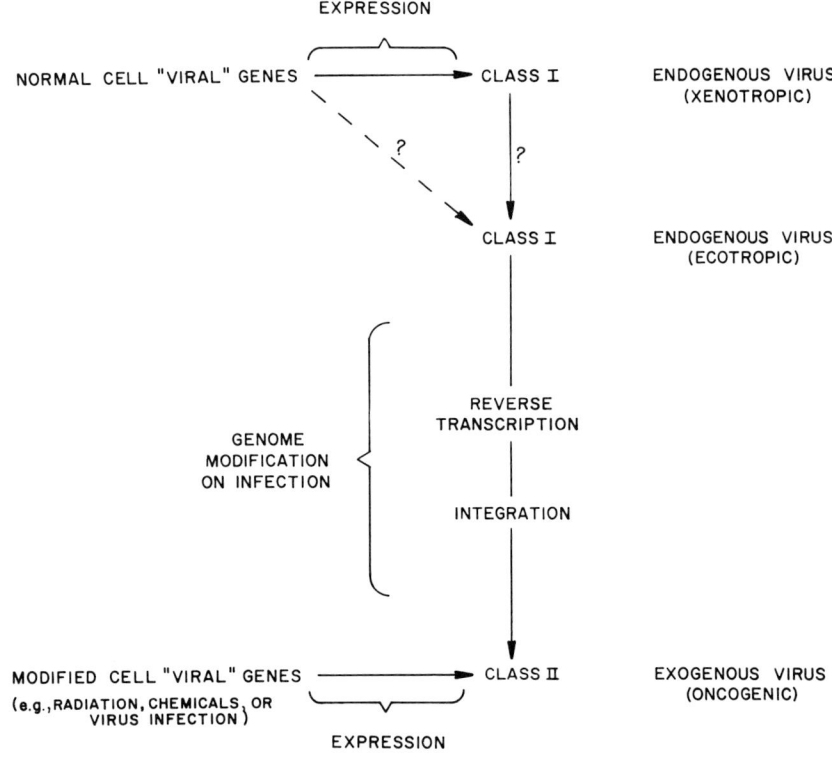

FIG. 1. Proposed mechanism for formation of Class II oncogenic viruses.

proposed that this process of evolution away from the original host results in a virus acquiring oncogenic potential (*102*), perhaps by interfering with the interaction between a cell and its endogenous virus(es). The history of the most oncogenic RNA tumor viruses [Rous sarcoma virus being the classic example (*288*)] has, in fact, generally involved repeated laboratory infection of new cells and animals. These laboratory procedures probably, in effect, force a more rapid and diverse genetic change than is found naturally. Hybridization experiments have shown that these viruses, which we call Class II viruses, are not highly related to DNA from the species of apparent origin (*107,132,133,137,138*). When an RNA tumor virus is isolated from a naturally occurring tumor and its RNA is shown by molecular hybridization to have limited relatedness to the DNA of the animal of origin, it may indicate that this virus originated as an endogenous virus of another species which subsequently infected the species in question. Alternatively, the virus may have originated from the species in question and rapidly evolved by a history of relatively frequent horizontal intraspecies transmission [or possibly by DNA→RNA→DNA pathways within the lifetime of one organism as Temin proposed in the protovirus theory (*343*)] or by laboratory manipulation.

How would this change occur during infection? It is known that during the establishment of infection the genome of the RNA tumor virus is first converted to a DNA (the "provirus") (*128, 150, 151, 359*), catalyzed by the viral DNA polymerase (reverse transcriptase) (*13, 345*). It is possible that errors in the process of transcribing RNA into DNA introduce genetic change into the viral genome. Loeb and his colleagues have, in fact, provided evidence that reverse transcriptase may make more genetic errors than cellular DNA polymerases (*328*), and they have suggested this as a mechanism for carcinogenesis. The greatest change probably occurs as a result of recombination of the proviral DNA with the host cell DNA. Thus, the virus coming out may consist of information derived from the incoming virus combined with host cell information. In any case, there is evidence to suggest that it is horizontal rather than vertical transmission of the viral genome which leads to the most significant genetic change (*107,132−134,137,138*). Thus, it is possible that a Class II virus arises by modification of the genome of a Class I virus. Another possibility should be considered. Class I "viral" genes are endogenous to cells, i.e., DNA of the normal uninfected cell of different vertebrate species contains the complete information for formation of a type-C endogenous virus. Some of these nucleotide sequences may be easily modified ("hot spot") by mutation (chemical or radiation) or by recombination (by infecting viruses) (*102*). If this occurs and the information is subsequently completely expressed (DNA→RNA) than a type-C virus with modified sequences would be the consequence, i.e., a Class II virus (see Fig. 1 for an outline of this).

Many of the frankly oncogenic (Class II) tumor viruses are primarily laboratory "creatures" and are not usually found associated with or thought to cause tumors occurring in nature. Good examples are Rauscher (*269*) and Moloney (*238*) murine leukemia viruses, Harvey (*158*), Moloney (*239*), and Kirsten (*196,198*) sarcoma viruses, and Rous sarcoma virus (*288*). Even as "laboratory viruses" they are still of considerable importance, since they have been isolated for a property of interest, namely oncogenicity. Therefore, these viruses would seem to be splendid models for the study of properties that lead to oncogenesis. Furthermore, there are, in fact, examples of viruses known to be oncogenic for the host of origin which have been found in naturally occurring neoplasias and which contain an RNA genome only minimally related to the host cell DNA. In other words, they are not endogenous vertically transmitted viruses but are typical Class II agents. Good examples are found in both feline and primate systems. Different strains of cat leukemia virus (FeLV) and sarcoma virus (FeSV) are typical Class II viruses and have much less genetic homology to DNA from uninfected cells of the host of origin (~40%) (*134*) than does RD114 virus (*230*), a Class I virus found in the DNA of all cat cells (*16,134,248,290*) and not known to be oncogenic for cats. FeLV and FeSV, in contrast, are oncogenic for cats. FeLV has been shown to be the causative agent of natural leukemias in cats. It has been estimated that most cat leukemia is due to infection by FeLV (*44,177,194,279*). More relevant to cancer in man are the type-C virus isolated in the past few years from primates. In our view, these viruses have provided tools for major progress in the application of molecular probes to human cancer, especially for the leukemias (see below).

A. Primate Type-C RNA Tumor Viruses

The first authentic primate RNA tumor viruses were isolated in the past few years. One was derived from the placenta of a baboon (*165*), but it can be induced from other normal tissues as well (*351*). We refer to this as the baboon endogenous virus (BEV), and it is an excellent example of a Class I virus. This virus has not been shown to transform any cell or to be oncogenic in any animal. The genome of this virus is apparently represented by nucleotide sequences in the DNA of normal baboon tissues (*23*). Since these endogenous viruses, particularly in noninbred animals, have no demonstrable role in neoplasia, finding related components in human tumors may not be telling us anything about the etiology of human neoplasia. Unless proved otherwise, detection of expression of these viruses or of molecules related to molecular components of these viruses in human tumors should in our view be regarded as analogous to the finding of fetal antigens in tumors. Since this virus appears to belong to a class of viruses expressed in embryonic and placental tissue and because of the possibility that such viruses play a role in differentiation and development, their presence in tissue which in growth or other life parameters has regressed to a more embryonic and undifferentiated state is to be expected. Certainly, BEV has been of great use in supporting the notion that endogenous (Class I) virogenes are in primates including man as well as in lower species (*27,28,318*). Predictably, DNA nucleotide sequences found in different primates are related to the genome of BEV in approximate proportion to the phylogenetic relatedness of the baboon to the species in question (*27,28*).

In contrast to this virus, two Class II type-C RNA tumor viruses have also been recently isolated. The simian sarcoma virus (SSV-1), sometimes called the woolly monkey sarcoma virus, was isolated from a spontaneous fibrosarcoma of a New World primate, a woolly monkey (*346*) that was a household pet. This virus is oncogenic when inoculated into some primates (*381*), transforms fibroblasts in tissue culture (*381*), and has been recently shown to cause brain tumors in primates when injected intracerebrally (*378*). The sarcoma virus component is associated with an excess of nontransforming "helper" virus (*380*), a property it shares with other mammalian sarcoma viruses (*156, 159, 172, 173, 298*). So far, this virus or its components have been found only in neoplasias of primates.

A second Class II virus was isolated from an Old World primate, a gibbon ape (*193*). Although it was originally isolated from a lymphosarcoma, similar isolates were also obtained from a lymphoma and a myelogenous leukemia (*192*). The history of this virus is particularly interesting. Gibbon apes were used for malaria research at an Air Force base in Thailand. Some were inoculated with the blood of two people with malaria, and the blood of the inoculated apes were then serially given to other animals. In a colony of 195 animals, 9 developed hematopoietic neoplasms, especially lymphosarcomas and myelogenous leukemias (63,184). Two virus isolates were obtained from these animals. As is true for SSV-1, so far the gibbon ape lymphosarcoma virus (GaLV) or its components have been found mainly in neoplasias of primates. There is also evidence that this virus causes myelogenous leukemia when injected into primates (195). Gibbons within one colony from which one of the GaLV isolates originated were studied for the presence of this virus. Animals that were virus negative had high levels of circulating antibody to GaLV, indicating that these animals had been exposed to the virus. Viremic animals, on the other hand, have low or undetectable levels of circulating antibody to the virus. Some of the viremic animals, but none of the nonviremic animals, have developed hematopoietic neoplasias (195). Thus, GaLV is a naturally occurring, horizontally transmitted oncogenic Class II virus. Recently, four members of one family in Ohio developed a lymphocytic leukemia, an osteosarcoma, and two malignant brain tumors within a short period. It was later learned that the patient developing the first neoplasia (the leukemia) had been bitten and scratched about one year previously by a pet gibbon. This may well be an odd coincidence, but the suspicion of causation by an animal virus with known leukemogenicity in primates must be stronger by virtue of species proximity than that from anecdotes about cat-associated human leukemia cases.

The proteins tested (gs antigen and reverse transcriptase) of SSV-1 and GaLV are immunologically very closely related (130,131,265,312,355). In addition, molecular hybridization experiments (27,311, our unpublished data) have shown that the two viruses are closely related genetically, as much or more so than two groups of murine leukemia viruses (Gross type compared to Friend–Moloney–Rauscher type). This is perplexing in view of the evolutionary divergence and physical distance between New World and Old World primates. There is one known common denominator that should be kept in mind. Both animals of origin were exposed to man. It is possible that the vector for the infecting RNA tumor virus was either human or human-associated. In contrast to the close relatedness of SSV-1 and GaLV, these viruses are not detectably related to the Class I primate type-C virus, BEV (23, 318, our unpublished results). The genome of SSV-1 and GaLV show only slight (about 5–10%) homology to DNA from uninfected normal cells of gibbon or woolly monkey (311). Clearly, these viruses are typical Class II viruses, analogous to FeLV and FeSV, and may very well be important primary causes of naturally occurring primate leukemias, lymphomas, and sarcomas.

Mason-Pfizer monkey virus (MPMV) was isolated from a rhesus monkey adenocarcinoma (53,183); it is of neither type-B or type-C morphology, but is intermediate between the two (203). So far, it has not been shown to be pathologic for any species, and its genome shows little relatedness to DNA

TABLE I
PRIMATE RNA TUMOR VIRUS ISOLATES

Virus	Morphology	Isolated from	Proved to be oncogenic	Components found in normal cells[a]	Genetic relatedness to other viruses
Baboon, endogenous virus	Type C	Baboon placenta, other tissues	No	Yes	RD114 (8%)
Mason–Pfizer monkey virus (MPMV)	Partly type B, partly type C	Rhesus monkey breast adenocarcinoma	No	No	None known
Gibbon ape leukemia virus (GaLV)	Type C	Lymphosarcoma, myelogenous leukemia of gibbon	Yes	No	Highly related to SSV-1
Simian sarcoma virus (SSV-1)	Type C	Fibrosarcoma of woolly monkey	Yes	No	Highly related to GaLV
Human leukemia virus (HL23V-1)	Type C	Peripheral leukocytes of human AML patient HL-23	No	No	Highly related to GaLV, SSV-1
Human leukemia virus (HL23V-2)	Type C	Bone marrow of human AML patient HL-23	No	No	Highly related to GaLV, SSV-1

[a] May be occasionally detected in normal cells, but is not routinely present. For example, GaLV-related proteins have been detected in some gibbon brains (G. Todaro, personal communication), but this is a consequence of infection from without.

from uninfected cells (*306*) or to RNA from other RNA tumor viruses (*234*). MPMV-like viruses have been isolated from several long-term tissue culture cell lines originally obtained from human tissue, especially the HeLa line (*387*), but the significance of these reports is difficult to assess. It is not detectably related to any of the known type-C viruses. For instance, its reverse transcriptase is biochemically (*3*) and immunologically (*312,313*) different from this enzyme in other RNA tumor viruses, and its structural antigens also appear to be unrelated to those of other RNA tumor viruses (*353*). In Table I we have summarized the important properties of the primate type-C viruses, and later we shall show data in human leukemias that make use of molecular probes of these viruses.

Additional viruses considered in this manuscript include Rauscher (RLV) (*269*) and Moloney (MoLV) (*238*) murine leukemia viruses, viruses that cause leukemia in mice and have been isolated only once, and may be, in part, laboratory variants. Kirsten sarcoma virus (KiSV) was isolated from a rat sarcoma induced by inoculation of Kirsten leukemia virus (*197*) into rats (*196,198*); it has also been isolated only once and contains both mouse- and rat-specific nucleotide sequences (*314*). AKR murine leukemia virus (MuLV-AKR) is causally related to leukemia in AKR mice, is a Gross-type MuLV (*7,257*), is easily isolated from viremic AKR mice (*146*), and is more related serologically to naturally occurring or wild-type murine leukemia viruses (*6,157*).

It should be clear from this discussion that a Class I endogenous virus from one species may acquire the potential to infect a different species. A Class I virus of one species may thus become a Class II virus of another species. If the provirus integrates into the gametes of the new species and stays with these species for some period, the viral genome might then evolve toward the genome of the new species, and become a more Class I-like virus for the second species.

We have gone into these considerations in some detail because some of the concepts are new and potentially confusing and because we believe they are important for an adequate estimation of whether a virus in question or components of an RNA "tumor" virus (especially nucleic acid sequences) demonstrated in a tumor cell are important to the disease or are related to derepression of a gene or genes which, though virus-related, are not necessarily involved in the cause of the neoplasia.

B. Studies and Techniques for Investigating the Molecular Relationships of RNA Tumor Viruses to Human Normal and Neoplastic Cells

1. *Intracellular Localization of Virus-Related Cell Components*

Because cells have so many more components than viruses, the first step toward isolation and identification of viruslike components has often been some kind of fractionation into subcellular components. One method that we have employed involves removing nuclei, plasma membrane, and mitochondria by differential centrifugation followed by collection of the high speed (60,000 g, 1 hour) sedimentable fraction, which includes microsomes and membrane fragments. The rationale is that any intracellular particles with the size and shape properties of tumor viruses (~600 S) (316) would be partially purified by this means. This fraction is often then banded to equilibrium in sucrose density gradients, and the density areas of interest are further examined. Again, the 1.15–1.18 gm/ml density area has often been of interest because it is the density of type-C viruses in sucrose (316). Although it may be unreasonable to expect any intracellular viral component to be incorporated into a particle with at least some of the physical attributes of mature extracellular virus, empirically this has often been found to be the case, as noted below. This empirical finding may be due to the fact that this fraction includes membrane fragments. If the virus in question were defective for complete budding and consequent extracellular production but capable of starting to bud, it would fractionate with membrane fragments. A mutant of Moloney sarcoma virus, for example, behaves in such a fashion (382), in that it cannot bud off from the cell membrane at a nonpermissive temperature.

Other subcellular fractionation procedures depend on the type of viral component that is sought (i.e., nuclei for integrated viral DNA, polysomes for viral RNA, membrane fractions for viral structural protein antigens) and are performed according to standard procedures described elsewhere by others. RNA tumor viral components with which we shall concern ourselves in this article include viruslike RNA, i.e., RNA of high molecular weight (45–70 S) which contains poly(A) and viruslike nucleotide sequences; viruslike reverse transcriptase activity; purified reverse transcriptase, immunologically related to reverse transcriptases of known RNA tumor viruses; virus-related nucleotide sequences in cell DNA; extra nucleotide sequences found in neoplastic, but not in normal, cells but not necessarily related to known RNA tumor viruses; and other virus-related proteins (gs antigen, p30, gp70).

2. Detection of 70 S RNA in Human Neoplasias

The genome of RNA tumor virus consists of a large (45–70 S) (4,41,64,69,72, 73,155,176,187,281–283) RNA molecule, which contains a tract of polyadenylic acid (136,143,208,286) at the 3'-OH end (276,329,370) consisting of 150–200 bases (136,329,370). The molecule is predominantly single stranded but can be converted by heat or by other conditions that disrupt hydrogen bonds to a molecule 20–35 S in size (64,70,72,73,155,231). This could be due to either a disassociation to subunits (70,72,73,145) or an unfolding to a less compact molecular form (22). Its size and poly(A) content are similar to those of some of the heterogeneous nuclear RNA of normal cells (60, 74, 75, 171, 182, 233,304,325), but distinguish it from most of the RNA found in the cytoplasm of normal cells. The finding, therefore, of a high molecular weight poly(A)-containing RNA in the cytoplasm of cells or in the media of cultured cells is suggestive of the presence of a fully transcribed and at least partially expressed RNA tumor virus.

One pitfall of this type of study is that the percentage of virus-specific RNA in the cytoplasm is very low (0.04–1%) even in cells producing high titers of virus (23,26,30,80,129,161,211,371,385) so that detection of any 70 S RNA necessitates labeling cells in culture with uridine-^{3}H. Leakage of large heterogenous nuclear RNA from nuclei is nearly impossible to rule out, and care must be taken to avoid aggregation of RNA, which would form high molecular weight artifacts. Even 70 S RNA from intracellular particles of viruslike densities may not represent a viral component, since many subcellular fractions band at or near 1.16 gm/ml. In addition, there is no known reason to expect intracellular viral RNA to be 70 S, since, for the viruses reported on so far, the RNA has been reported to exist primarily in 35 S and 20 S forms (34,80,122,129, 160,161,211,356) and may be converted to 70 S RNA only in mature virions (47,52,67). Detection of 70S RNA from extracellular particles which have the density of virions is of somewhat greater significance, but release of materials from dead or dying cells is also difficult to rule out without demonstration of clear morphology and biological activity. In this case, reliance upon detection of 70 S RNA to show the presence of a virus is hardly necessary.

Much work has relied upon the "simultaneous detection" assay devised by Schlom and Spiegelman (308) partially to circumvent these difficulties. An endogenous DNA polymerase reaction is performed with the particle in question, using labeled deoxyribonucleoside triphosphates. The reaction product–template complex, containing labeled newly synthesized DNA and unlabeled RNA and/or DNA, is banded on a velocity gradient. In a reaction directed by 70 S RNA at least some of the labeled DNA moiety would be hydrogen bonded in a labeled 70 S complex, and positive results constitute a presumptive simultaneous detection of 70 S RNA and reverse transcriptase. Positive results depend in practice on detection of a labeled 70 S complex, which is absent after pretreatment of the complex with heat to disrupt the hydrogen bonding, liberating the labeled DNA and hence not detecting the large RNA. The 70 S complex is also lost after treatment with ribonuclease, owing to hydrolysis of the template. The nascent DNA moiety, even from virions, is small (4–8 S) (340,363,364). The rationale is summarized in Fig. 2. This technique has so far been used to implicate RNA tumor virus involvement in human leukemias (19), lymphomas including Burkitt's (206), breast cancer (9,83,309,310), brain tumors (59), melanomas (12), cancer of the colon and rectum (58), and lung cancer (58). The 70 S RNA apparently involved in the positive simultaneous detection test has also been reported to have a poly(A) tract of 150–200 nucleotides (307), a characteristic of tumor virus RNA. This test in its basic form, however, can have serious pitfalls. Normal cells, human lymphocytes, for example, have en-

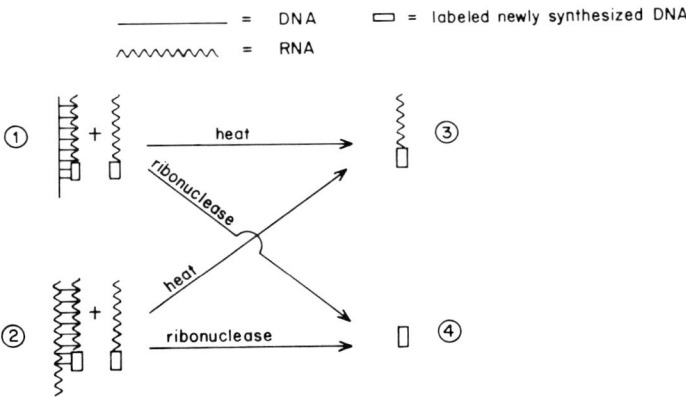

FIG. 2. Size analysis of newly synthesized DNA. Representation of possible labeled complexes formed for a "simultaneous detection" assay. Heat treatment of complexes 1 or 2 gives complex 3, which can be very small (~4 S). RNase treatment of complex 1 or 2 gives complex 4, which is often so small as to not be acid-precipitable. Hydrogen bonds are indicated by short horizontal lines.

dogenous DNA polymerase activities that are directed by DNA but apparently primed by small RNA molecules, which serve as points of initiation for DNA synthesis (86,202,250,275). These are similar to Okazaki pieces (335,336) in *E. coli* DNA synthesis. The product of this reaction is a high molecular weight complex with unlabeled (template) DNA hydrogen bonded to unlabeled (primer) RNA, which is in turn covalently attached to a small labeled DNA product. Upon ribonuclease or heat treatment, as illustrated in Fig. 2, this complex is converted to a small labeled DNA or covalent DNA–RNA hybrid molecule, thus registering as a positive "simultaneous detection" of reverse transcriptase and high molecular weight RNA from a reaction that contains neither component. Although such a complex, which has a size of 70 S, has not been reported for normal mammalian cells, in the absence of further data as described below positive results of this sort must be regarded as suggestive but not conclusive.

3. *Detection of Endogenous Reverse Transcriptase Activity*

Proof that an endogenous DNA polymerase activity is directed by RNA can be very difficult to obtain, especially with reaction complexes derived from cells. Sensitivity of the endogenous DNA polymerase activity to RNase, sometimes used as a sole criterion for reverse transcriptase activity, indicates that the reaction is dependent on RNA, but it does not prove that the reaction is directed by RNA. The problem is complicated by the presence of endogenous nucleases in subcellular fractions and in virus preparations; it is further complicated in at least one instance by an inhibitor of DNA synthesis, which is itself inhibited by

RNA (*264*). Destruction of endogenous RNA removes the constraint on this inhibitor, which then accordingly reduces DNA synthesis. This reaction is RNA-dependent only in the loosest sense of the term. Actinomycin D, which has been used to differentiate between DNA-directed and RNA-directed DNA synthesis (*82,123,227,232*), in our experience cannot be used to ascertain the template in an endogenous DNA polymerase reaction because its inhibition of mammalian tumor virus DNA polymerase is variable (*339;* Reitz and Gallo, unpublished observations) (50 µg/ml inhibits RLV DNA synthesis 0–90%, depending on the lot of actinomycin and the lot of the virus), and apparently DNA-directed DNA polymerase activity has a measurable, and also variable, resistance to the drug (*275*). Similarly, most other inhibitors, e.g., some derivatives of rifamycins, although initially believed to be relatively specific (*153*), really lack sufficient selectivity (*386*), especially in crude endogenous DNA polymerase systems. In our judgment, proof that such reaction is directed by RNA depends heavily on a careful and detailed analysis of the reaction product. The simultaneous detection test mentioned above indicates that the reaction product is associated with RNA, but in order to show a RNA-directed synthesis of DNA, it is necessary to show that the newly synthesized DNA is hydrogen bonded to RNA. This can be done by subjecting the reaction product to heat (100°) for 5–10 minutes and showing that the DNA product is melted off a RNA template, usually by demonstrating a shift in cesium sulfate gradients from the RNA to the DNA density regions after heat treatment. This approach has been combined with the simultaneous detection test mentioned above to strengthen the evidence for a reverse transcriptase activity only in the case of human leukemias (*19*).

Corroborating evidence has been provided more often by specific hybridization of the labeled DNA product to RNA from the analogous murine tumor viruses (i.e., Rauscher leukemia virus for leukemias, lymphomas, and sarcomas; mouse mammary tumor virus for breast cancer), indicating that the putative 70 S RNA template shared some nucleotide sequences with an appropriate and bona fide tumor virus RNA. Hybridization has usually been low. Unfortunately, no good animal virus models exist for the other tumors mentioned, so that it cannot be said whether these reverse transcriptase activities originate from an exogenous virus or from the cell itself, perhaps from an endogenous virus common to all cells of a species. The argument that they represent an infection from without is therefore only inferential and depends upon hybridization data. Typically, the hybridization evidence is a demonstration that the DNA transcript from a particular tumor will hybridize to RNA from the same tumor, but not to RNA from normal cells or other tumors. This is the sort of corroborating evidence reported for lymphomas (*206*), breast cancer (*9,309,310*), brain tumors (*59*), lung and gastrointestinal tract tumors (*58*), and malignant melanoma (*12*). Hybridization of synthesized DNA to RNA from the same cell is not surprising. If, for example, RNA and newly synthesized DNA were copied from opposite strands of a double-stranded DNA molecule, one would expect a positive hybridization result. Specific hybridization to RNA from a particular tumor does indicate that different messenger RNA is being transcribed in that tumor as compared to normal cells or other tumors, and the fact that this RNA is complementary to DNA synthesized by a cytoplasmic particulate fraction is of obvious interest and possible relevance to gene amplification processes or differentiation and proliferation. However, in the absence of evidence showing that a 70 S complex is predominantly composed of RNA and that the newly synthesized DNA is complementary to 70 S RNA from a bona fide RNA tumor virus, the relationship of the activity detected by the simultaneous detection assay to tumor viruses is somewhat speculative.

One difficulty of showing that nascent DNA is hydrogen bonded to RNA is that much of it from endogenous reactions of both viruses and subcellular fractions is small and/or covalently attached to an RNA primer molecule so that heat treatment leaves the DNA in the same density regions of Cs_2SO_4 gradients as untreated DNA, or simply causes it to lose its acid precipitability owing to its small size (see Fig. 3 for a schematic representation). The investigator cannot say what the template molecule is unless most of the radioactivity remains acid precipitable after heat treatment, which is a rare situation. An alternative approach is to digest the DNA product with a single strand-specific (S1) nuclease. Labeled DNA which disappears from the RNA density region of Cs_2SO_4 gradients is then attributable to a covalently linked DNA product—RNA primer molecule, and material in this region which is resistant to S1 nuclease is hydrogen bonded, almost certainly to RNA. This is also shown in Fig. 3. The test shows that the RNase-sensitive reaction from the high speed pellet fraction of normal phytohemagglutinin(PHA)-stimulated blood lymphocytes (36) is due at least in part to a DNA-directed RNA-primed DNA polymerase activity (275), while the same test reveals that a similar activity from at least some leukemic cells is directed by RNA (Fig. 4; Reitz and Gallo, unpublished observations).

Characterization of the endogenous reaction product depends in good part upon the quality and homogeneity of the product. This in turn depends on the relative purity and homogeneity of the endogenous DNA polymerase activity. Relative purity of such activities from cells is particularly important and can be difficult to attain. In human leukemic cells, a procedure involving repeated banding in isopycnic density gradients has resulted in a DNA polymerase activity whose presence persists at 1.16—1.18 gm/ml of the gradients but which is free of most of the ultraviolet-absorbing material initially banding at 1.16—1.18 gm/ml (109). [This may be true only for fresh, rather than frozen, cells (107).] This partially purified preparation synthesizes a DNA product which, by analysis on polyacrylamide gels after various treatments, is in part hydrogen bonded to a RNA molecule. This is essentially a gel electrophoresis analog of the simultaneous detection test. The DNA, in confirmation of the above reports, hybridizes to RNA from RLV, but not from AMV. In addition, higher hybridization (up to 50%) of the DNA from the acute and chronic myelogenous leukemia cell

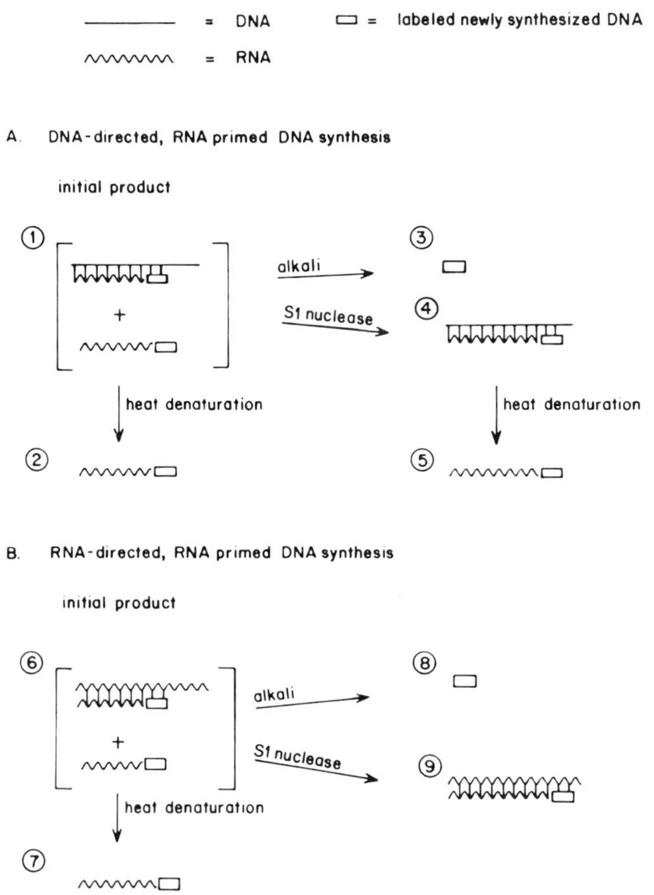

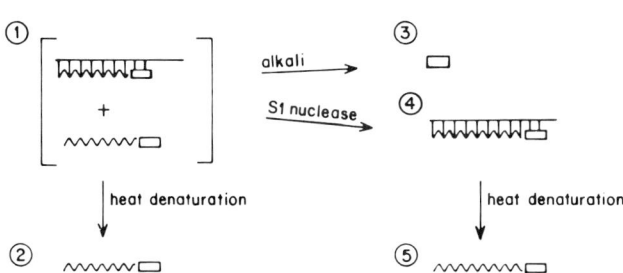

FIG. 3. Density analysis of newly synthesized DNA from an RNA-primed DNA polymerase reaction. Representation of the labeled complexes created by different treatments of DNA newly synthesized and attached to an RNA primer molecule. S1 nuclease treatment discriminates between complexes 1 and 6 when the labeled DNA and primer RNA are small, as complex 4 has a DNA-like density, while complex 9 has an RNA-like density. Hydrogen bonds are indicated by short vertical lines. (A) DNA is copied from DNA; (B) DNA is copied from RNA.

pellet DNA polymerase reactions is achieved to RNA from Kirsten murine sarcoma virus (KiSV), grown in normal rat kidney (NRK) cells (109) and/or SSV-1, grown in KiSV-infected nonproducer rat cells (KW23).[4] The particle of

---

[4] SSV-1 grown in KW23 cells, although containing rat cell nucleotide sequences (D. Gillespie, personal communication), contains 80% of the sequences represented in DNA synthesized by SSV-1 grown in marmoset cells (Reitz and Gallo, unpublished results). However, some uncertainty exists as to whether the detected hybridization is to SSV-1 or Kirsten-rat sequences.

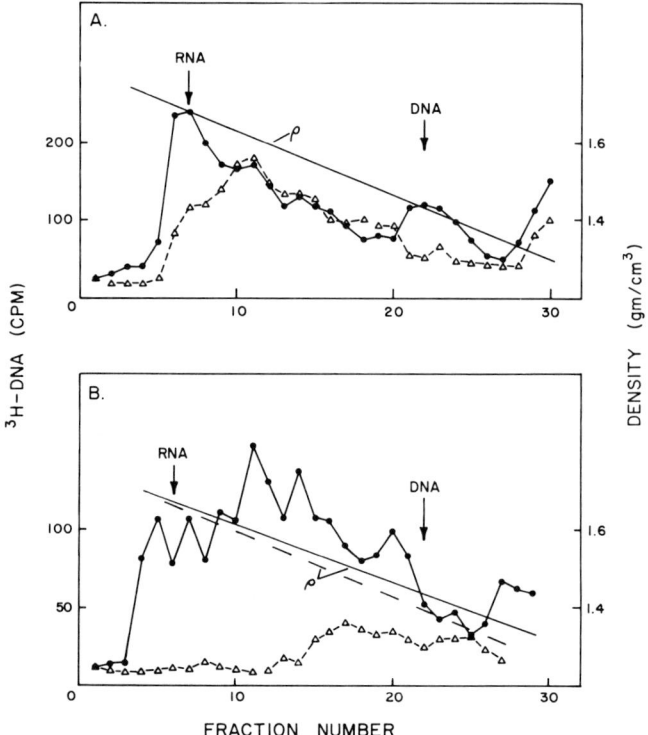

FIG. 4. Cs$_2$SO$_4$ density gradient analysis of endogenous human AML pellet DNA polymerase product. DNA product was prepared, purified, and analyzed by equilibrium density gradient centrifugation as described elsewhere (*300*). (1) DNA was analyzed without treatment (●——●) or after heat denaturation (△——△, 95°C, 10 minutes); (B) DNA was analyzed after S1 nuclease digestion (●——●) or alkali treatment (△——△, 0.3 N KOH, 95°C, 10 minutes).

myelogenous leukemic cells which synthesizes the virus-related DNA sequences is converted to a 1.23–1.25 gm/ml density when treated by low concentrations of nonionic detergent (*107*), a similar phenomenon to the conversion of type-C virions to cores (*334*). The size of the particle (about 1000 S) is reduced by detergent treatment, also similar to results with type-C virions. DNA synthesized from the detergent-generated 1.25 gm/ml particle of myelogenous leukemia cells also contains the virus-related sequences (*107*). The DNA thus shows a pattern of hybridization that one would expect from a human tumor virus, based on data using DNA synthesized by virions of various primate, murine, feline, and avian tumor viruses to various viral RNAs (*234*). In these studies, as in those above, a combination of physical characterization of the DNA product combined with corroborating hybridization data indicated that the endogenous reaction from myelogenous leukemic cells is probably directed by RNA.

In contrast, our results with other cellular endogenous DNA polymerase activities, including any activity from PHA-stimulated normal human lymphocytes, activities of large particles from any cells, and activities from low density (1.10–1.15 gm/ml) small particles from any cells, have not indicated a relatedness of the template to SSV/KW23 or KiSV 70 S RNA.

DNA synthesized by the comparable fraction from chronic lymphocytic leukemic cells or normal lymphocytes stimulated with PHA does hybridze to a lesser extent to 70 S from RLV or SSV-1 grown in NC37 cells, but SSV-1 grown in NC37 cells acquires information found in the DNA of normal human cells (see below) (*107*), and this may account for the hybridization of normal human pellet DNA product to this RNA. Hybridization to excess RLV RNA may reflect the detection of sequences from an endogenous human virus, similar to the baboon endogenous virus (BEV) and may not have any role in neoplasia. *In no case* has a biochemically characterized reverse transcriptase been obtained from the normal lymphocytes. The significance of the hybridization of the DNA from pellet DNA polymerase reactions of CLL and normal cells to RLV and SSV-1/NC37 RNA thus remains unknown. In no case have we detected hybridization of DNA synthesized by the lighter density small particles or the large particles to any viral RNA (*107*), and DNA synthesis by the large particles may be due in large part to mitochondrial DNA synthesis (*275*). Only with the small high density (1.16–1.18 gm/ml) particles from fresh human AML cells or CML blast phase cells is the endogenous activity maintained through repeated bandings. The less dense particles from these cells and all particles from other leukemias, normal lymphocytes, and frozen cells apparently degenerate and lose all endogenous DNA polymerase activity when repeatedly banded in sucrose. Whether this is an inherent property of the particles or is due to some other cellular factor(s) (proteases, lipases, nucleases) remains to be determined.

4. *Purified Reverse Transcriptase*

a. *Biochemical and Physical Properties of Reverse Transcriptase.* The DNA polymerase catalyzing the apparent reverse transcriptase activity of human leukemic cells can be purified by removal of endogenous nucleic acids by DEAE-cellulose chromatography and from most of the protein, including normal cellular DNA polymerases, by phosphocellulose chromatography. This purified preparation can then be more easily studied and its properties compared and contrasted with purified viral and normal cellular DNA polymerases. DNA polymerases purified from mammalian type-C viruses share certain unique properties, including: (1) marked preference for oligo (dT)·poly(rA) as a template over oligo(dT)·poly(dA) using Mg^{2+} or Mn^{2+} as the divalent cation (*14,280,111–113,139,210*); (2) efficient utilization of oligo (dG)·poly(rC) as template (*14, 111–113,139*); (3) the ability to transcribe heteropolymeric regions of natural

RNA, particularly viral 70 S RNA without oligo(dT) as a primer, and increased heteropolymer transcription in the presence of oligo(dT)[5] (*46,66,68,111–113, 186,240,274*, Abrell, Reitz, and Gallo, in preparation); and (4) a molecular weight of about 70,000 (*3,24,113,142,175,229,240,286,296,351,352,384*), except for the DNA polymerase from endogenous hamster virus (*365*). Normal cellular DNA polymerases, on the other hand, prefer oligo(dT)·poly(dA) over oligo(dT)·poly(rA), at least in the presence of Mg^{2+} as the divalent cation[6] (*95,107,111–113,139,217,218,280,323*), do not significantly use oligo(dG)·poly(rC) (*139,217,323*), and fail measurably to transcribe heteropolymeric regions of natural RNA (*36,323*). In addition, the molecular weights of the known cellular DNA polymerases (*17,37,48,49,50,88,107,113,218,322,323,376*), α = MW 150,000 (*48,49,218,323,376*) β = MW 40,000 (*48,49,218,323,376*), γ = ~MW 90,000 (*217*), distinguish them from type-C viral DNA polymerase.

A cautionary point regarding molecular weights is, however, worth making. A DNA polymerase from GaLV-infected cells, in contrast to the homologous enzyme from extracellular virions, apparently exists in two interconvertible molecular forms, one with the expected molecular weight of 70,000 and the other with a molecular weight of about 130,000 (*240*). High salt and nonionic detergent favor the presence of the low molecular weight form, while low salt and no detergent favor the larger form. Both forms are biochemically like reverse transcriptase in their template characteristics although the larger form is relatively more efficient in the transcription of 70 S RNA. Both forms are inhibited by antibody to GaLV virion DNA polymerase, but the inhibition of the smaller form is much greater. Whether the apparent aggregation is due to dimer formation or association with some cellular factor which is not found in the virion is not yet known, but the lack of this phenomenon with enzyme purified from virions favors the latter possibility. The same phenomenon is observed with the viruslike reverse transcriptase from human cells, including inhibition by anti-GaLV and SSV-1 DNA polymerase, and therefore this observation has some practical importance since antibody testing will give negative results if the enzyme is not in the low molecular weight form. Mizutani and Temin have reported similar findings for avian reticuloendotheliosis virus (*236*).

Using the approach of studying the biochemical characteristics of DNA polymerases purified from RNase-sensitive endogenous DNA polymerase activities of

---

[5] Although *E. coli* DNA polymerase I can copy heteropolymeric portions of 70 S RNA (*149, 221, 237, 297*), poly(dT) and poly(dA) are synthesized to a greater extent by one to two orders of magnitude than heteropolymeric transcripts, large excesses of enzyme are required and DNA templates are vastly preferred (*297*). None of the normal eukaryotic cell DNA polymerases, α, β, and γ, have been shown to transcribe heteropolymeric regions of natural RNA (*37, 280, 323*).

[6] DNA polymerase γ (*88*) greatly prefers oligo(dT)·poly(rA) over oligo(dT)·poly(dA) in the presence of Mn^{2+}, the preferred divalent cation, but with Mg^{2+} shows the opposite preference (*218*).

human cells, we have shown that the leukemic particle DNA polymerases from blood cells of ~50% of patients with AML (*112,113,32*) and some ALL patients (*112,113,300*) have all the expected properties of viral reverse transcriptase except molecular size. Although this was not appreciated at the time, the above-mentioned aggregation phenomenon was probably responsible for the apparent higher molecular weights in these reports. The apparent absence of this enzyme from some cases of AML and ALL may simply be due to technical failures. In our experience, DNA polymerases purified from the blood cells of patients with chronic meylogenous or chronic lymphocytic leukemia have not had all the characteristics expected for virus-related reverse transcriptase (*107*), for example, significant transcription of oligo(dG)·poly(rC) or heteropolymeric regions of viral 70 S RNA. They have shown some properties unlike cell DNA polymerases, however, and may represent some enzyme form intermediate between the viruslike and the cellular DNA polymerases. Biochemically characterized reverse transcriptase has, however, been obtained from cells of one CLL patient in our laboratory. Although all the biochemical criteria were satisfied (*107*) the enzyme was not inhibited by antisera to reverse transcriptase of GaLV, SSV-1, MPMV, or BEV. We regard such results as being inconclusive for virus-related reverse transcriptase.

The major DNA polymerase from a small particle fraction of PHA-stimulated human lymphocytes which possesses a RNase-sensitive endogenous activity has been shown to have biochemical characteristics identical to normal cellular DNA polymerases (*36*). To date, none of the normal eukaryotic cellular DNA polymerases have been shown to transcribe heteropolymeric regions of 70 S RNA or to transcribe oligo(dT)·poly(rA) better than oligo(dT)·poly(dA) in the presence of Mg^{2+}, and only slight transcription of oligo(dG)·poly(rC) has been noted for DNA polymerase γ (*107,112,113,218,280*). The only example of a biochemically and immunologically characterized viruslike reverse transcriptase from normal mammalian tissue is from a normal rhesus placenta-embryo (first trimester pregnancy) (*229*) which by electron microscopy was producing type-C particles. This polymerase activity was inhibited by antisera to RD114 reverse transcriptase. RD114 is closely related immunologically to BEV (*319,351*), and about 8% of the nucleotide sequences of BEV and RD114 are related as determined by molecular hybridization experiments (*23,24*). More significant to the data with the rhesus placenta-embryo enzyme is that the reverse transcriptases of RD114 and BEV are relatively closely related (*319*). In fact, Benveniste and Todaro have suggested that these two viruses are closely enough related as to suggest a common progenitor (*28*). Since BEV is believed to be similar to the rhesus placenta virus, it was concluded that the reverse transcriptase of rhesus placenta-embryo is derived from endogenous type-C virus.

  b. Immunological Characteristics of Viruslike Reverse Transcriptase from Human Cells. Further identification of a particular viruslike DNA polymerase from cells as a virus-related reverse transcriptase can be obtained by testing the purified DNA polymerase with antisera against DNA polymerases from known RNA tumor viruses and against normal cell DNA polymerases. Specific inhibition by antiviral DNA polymerase is perhaps the best single criterion for identifying a viruslike reverse transcriptase from cells because: (1) the DNA polymerase can be related to a particular group of type-C virus (1,266,312,313); (2) the degree of relatedness can be assessed by the kinetics of inhibition; (3) while synthetic template response and 70 S RNA transcription are functions of the purity of the enzyme and, thus, require a more purified enzyme preparation, antisera inhibition experiments can be performed with less purified enzyme preparations (assuming one has a monospecific antiserum); (4) conditions for remarkable specificity with these antibodies can be achieved, allowing fine distinctions even among reverse transcriptase from viruses derived from closely related species.

This approach has provided further evidence that human AML cells contain a DNA polymerase related to reverse transcriptase from GaLV and SSV-1. Reverse transcriptase-like activity with an apparent molecular weight of 70,000 can be detected in the high speed pellet fraction of from at least some patients AML cells which is inhibited 80–90% by antisera to DNA polymerase from GaLV or SSV-1 (94,107,240,349,350). These antisera do not inhibit cellular DNA polymerases α, β, or γ from normal or leukemic human leukocytes (94,107,349,350), and this reverse transcriptase is not significantly inhibited by antibodies to cell DNA polymerase α (322), or by antibodies to reverse transcriptase purified from FeLV, RSV, RD114, or MPMV (94,240,349,350). Slight inhibition has been observed using antibody to RLV DNA polymerase (349,350). This pattern of inhibition by antisera to DNA polymerases of different viruses is quite similar to that observed with GaLV and SSV-1 DNA polymerase (312). DNA polymerases from SSV-1 and GaLV are neutralized by low levels of antisera against either polymerase, but are not neutralized by antibody against MPMV (312) BEV (319), RD114 (319), FeLV (313), or RSV (312,313). Some cross neutralization (up to 50%) is observed with antisera against RLV DNA polymerase (312,313,319), and approximately equivalent inhibition is observed when the reciprocal experiment (anti SSV-1 polymerase versus RLV DNA polymerase) is performed (319). In general, the reverse transcriptases of oncogenic RNA viruses can be placed by immunologic criteria into four groups: birds, reptiles, lower mammals, and primates. The relatedness of the various virus-related DNA polymerases are summarized in Table II. The apparent close relatedness of the human leukemic DNA polymerase to SSV-1 and GaLV DNA polymerase places it immunologically within the group of reverse transciprtases of primate oncogenic RNA viruses and permits more confidence in identifying the human reverse transcriptase as a viral marker enzyme. This appears to be the first protein of an RNA tumor virus identified in any human neoplasia. It should be emphasized that, although immunological relatedness to a known RNA tumor virus DNA polymerase is the best single criterion for the identification of a cellular DNA

TABLE II
SEROLOGIC RELATIONSHIPS OF RNA TUMOR VIRUS DNA POLYMERASES[a]

DNA polymerase source[b]	Inhibition by antisera to DNA polymerase of						
	SSV-1	GaLV	BEV	MuLV	FeLV	RD114	RSV or AMV
Human leukemic cells	+++	+++	ND	+ to ++	−	+	−
HL23V-1	+++	+++	ND	+	−	+	−
SSV-1	+++	+++	−	+ to ++	−	−	−
GaLV	+++	+++	−	+ to ++	−	−	−
BEV	−	−	+++	−	−	++ to +++	−
MuLV	++	++	−	+++	++	−	−
FeLV	−	−	−	++	+++	−	−
RD114	−	−	++ to +++	−	−	+++	−
RSV or AMV	−	−	−	−	−	−	+++

[a] Summary of the cross-neutralization patterns seen with RNA tumor virus DNA polymerases, and antisera to these enzymes. +++, 75–100% inhibition at antisera dilutions which maximally inhibit the homologous enzyme; ++, 25–75% inhibition at comparable dilutions; +, 10–25%; −, less than 10%; ND, not done.
[b] HLV, human leukemia-associated virus; SSV-1, simian sarcoma virus; GaLV, gibbon ape lymphoma virus; BEV, baboon endogenous virus; MuLV, murine leukemia virus; FeLV, feline leukemia virus; RSV, Rous sarcoma virus; AMV, avian myeloblastosis virus.

polymerase as a viruslike reverse transcriptase, no single criterion is sufficient for establishing the presence of this marker.

5. *Viral Structural Protein Antigens*

A second set of antigenic markers for identifying virus-related proteins resides on the structural proteins of the virion. Some of the proteins that have been most studied are p30 *(42)* (a 30,000 MW protein making up the major structural protein of the viral core), p15 *(42)* (an envelope protein), p12 *(42)*, and GP69-71 (the major envelope glycoprotein, MW = 69,000–71,000). An earlier nomenclature, using GS-I and GS-III to denote, respectively, the major intraspecies and interspecies antigenic determinants, *(6,40,126,253,259–261,302)*, has been largely superceded by a nomenclature system proposed at a conference in 1973 *(11)*, and we refer the reader to this and to Ref. *(38)* for a summary of viral protein nomenclature. By this convention a lettered prefix p denotes a protein, and gp denotes a glycoprotein; a number follows denoting the MW × 10^3; and a suffix specifies the antigenic site being considered, such as interspec. Thus p30 interspec refers to a GS-III activity of a protein whose molecular weight is 30,000. This convention was necessary because (1) some viral proteins carry both intra- and interspecies determinants *(174,258,330,331)* and (2) not all viruses share a common GS-3 antigen *(303)*.

The experimental approach most often used in testing for viral antigens in human cells is to prepare a pure labeled viral antigen and a monospecific antiserum against the same viral antigen, construct a standard competition curve by adding increasing amounts of unlabeled viral antigen to the reaction of the labeled antigen with the antiserum, and then to measure any competition by the addition of increasing amounts of protein prepared from human cells. Since the protein preparations that are tested are a mixture of proteins, purity and specificity of the reagents are obviously crucial. In addition, one must include many careful controls to avoid artifacts, the commonest and most serious of which stem from the presence of proteases. Since the tests usually employ some form of protein precipitation, proteolytic degration of the labeled purified antigen, present in less than chemical amounts to begin with, can resemble inhibition of the antigen–antibody reaction.

Using this approach, two sets of results have been presented on the presence of viral antigens in human cells. The first set of results employed reagents prepared from what we call Class II viruses, and generally give positive results only with neoplastic tissues. Sherr and Todaro (*321*) used antisera prepared against the p30 of SSV-1 or GaLV in a radioimmune competition assay as described above to identify a protein related to these p30s from a number of cell samples of patients with acute leukemia. Using similar methods and an antiserum against MuLV gp69, Bolognesi and his colleagues (*39*) have detected a protein with a related antigenic determinant in human leukemia, but not in normal cells. A viral p30-related protein has also been reported in cells from several bone tumors, including osteosarcoma, chondrosarcoma, and a giant cell tumor, by Bentvelzen and his colleagues (*388*). Their approach was to incubate cells with either rat antiserum to RLV p30 or guinea pig antiserum to SSV-1 p30. The cells were then treated with fluorescent antiserum to rat IgG or guinea pig IgG to form a fluorescent "sandwich" at the site of any cell surface p30-like antigens. The cells were examined under a fluorescent microscope for the presence of antigen. Positive results were obtained with the tumor cells, but not with normal controls. Interestingly, only one of a number of antisera gave positive results, even though all had high interspecies (GS-3) reactivity, indicating a relatedness but nonidentity of the detected protein to the viral p30 used to prepare the antisera.

The second set of results has been obtained using either reagents from Class I viruses or a heterologous set of reagents, which include a Class I virus. Antiserum against the p30 of BEV has been used to detect by radioimmunoassay a related protein in some human tumors (*320*). However, the expression of this protein in humans, as in baboons (*318*), does not appear to be specific to tumors, but is rather expressed sporadically. Strand and August (*332*) have also detected a virus-related antigen in both normal and neoplastic cells by using a radioimmunoassay system. Unlike the above reports, which employed viral reagents of narrow specificity, these assays were performed with an RLV antigen and anti-RD114 antiserum. Since these two viruses are at most minimally related, this system would survey the broadest possible spectrum of antigenic determinants, perhaps one common to all mammalian oncornaviruses (including Class I, of which RD114 is a member).

In general, the above results suggest partial expression of a Class II-like virogene in human neoplasia, as well as a sporadic expression of possible Class I virogenes in both neoplastic and normal cells. These results therefore stand in good agreement with the detection of Class II viruslike reverse transcriptase only in neoplastic cells, as described above, as well as the detection of a Class I viruslike reverse transcriptase from normal rhesus placenta–embryo.

6. *RNA Tumor Virus-Related Nucleotide Sequences in Human Cellular RNA*

Numerous studies have been performed to determine whether or not virus-related RNA exists in human neoplastic cells which is absent from normal human cells. Detected differences would indicate either a lack of proviral information in the DNA of normal cells which is present in neoplastic cells or simply a differential expression of common virus-specific DNA into RNA between the two cell types. The former possibility would result from an infection from without, while the latter situation could arise, for example, by mutation or modification of cellular genes which control expression of endogenous viruses (*102*).

One method for measuring virus-specific RNA in cellular RNA preparations involves preparing labeled DNA transcripts of tumor virus RNA. Virus-specific DNA is often prepared in endogenous DNA polymerase reactions using partially permeabilized virions or using purified viral reverse transcriptase and added viral 70 S RNA. Precautions must be taken that the DNA does not contain a transcript of the poly(A) regions, as this will hybridize with any poly(A)-containing RNA. The formation of self-complementary DNA should also be avoided if possible, since its presence makes interpretation of hybridization results more difficult. Many investigators use actinomycin D to minimize the formation of double-stranded DNA, but it has been reported (*339*) and is also our experience that little double-stranded DNA is formed in endogenous DNA polymerase reactions of mammalian tumor viruses even in the absence of actinomycin.

The purified single-stranded DNA product is then annealed with the appropriate RNA preparations, and its hybridization is measured by any of a number of assay methods. Hybridization assay methods that have found wide application include digestion with a single strand-specific (S1) nuclease (*32,211*), hydroxyapatite chromatography (*211*), Cs_2SO_4 equilibrium density gradient centrifugation (*211,327*), or hybridization to RNA covalently attached to phosphocellulose paper discs (*301*). [These are schematically illustrated in Fig. 5. Each method has its advantages, and each measures slightly different parameters. The assay using S1 nuclease digestion employs a single-strand specific nuclease such as the enzyme from *Aspergillus oryzae* described by Ando (*5*) to digest unpaired DNA.

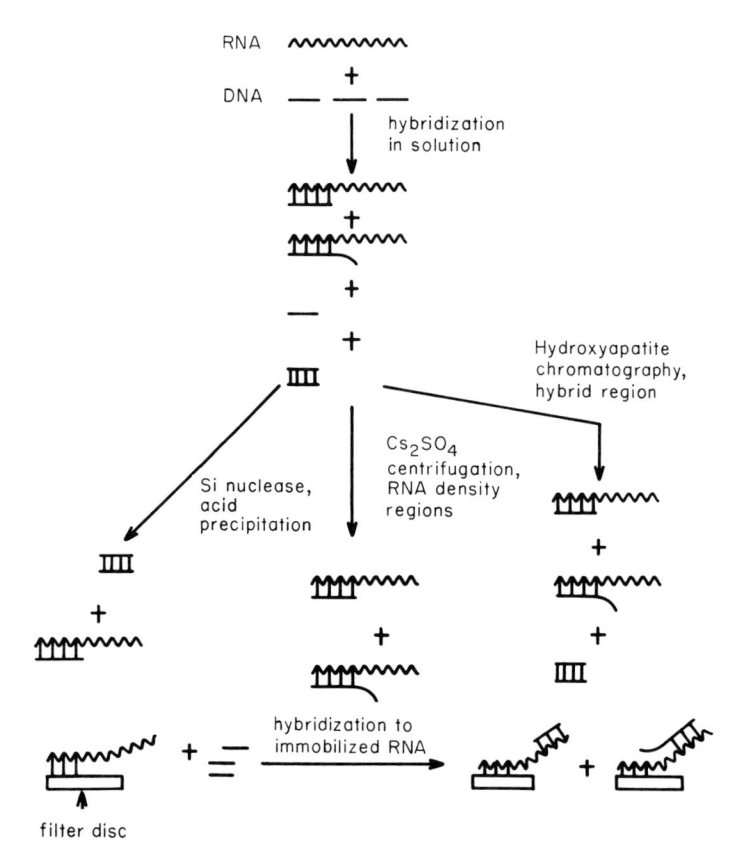

FIG. 5. Hybridization assay methods. Schematic representation of the most commonly used hybridization methods. Hydrogen bonds are indicated by short parallel lines.

Although the specificity has not been exactly determined (e.g., how extensively mismatched must hybridized DNA be before becoming susceptible to S1 nuclease), in general only DNA which is base-paired remains acid-precipitable after treatment with the nuclease. Unhybridized DNA covalently attached to hybridized DNA ("tails") is digested and not scored as hybrid. The method is fast and sensitive, but requires single-strand DNA and test RNA known to be free of DNA.

Hydroxyapatite chromatography, a second method of hybridization assay, relies on the unexplained ability of hydroxyapatite to bind double-stranded but not single-stranded nucleic acids at certain salt concentrations (e.g., 0.15 M PO_4). The exact length of double-stranded regions for binding to hydroxyapatite is not known, but in general with viral cDNA, both hybridized regions and unhybridized "tails" covalently attached to hybridized regions chromatograph as hybrids, making values from this assay somewhat higher than those with the S1 nuclease assay. Again, care must be taken to obtain a single-stranded cDNA and DNA-free test RNA. By passing buffer through the column at increasing temperatures, the degree of hybridization, as well as the quality of any hybrid formed can be ascertained. Hybridized DNA can be eluted by increasing the column temperature incrementally to melt the hydrogen bonds and regenerate single-stranded DNA. The thermal stability of the hybrid is determined by measuring the percentage of hybridized DNA which is eluted at each temperature. If the DNA is larger than a certain minimum size (~50 nucleotides), the thermal stability is determined by the precision of base-pairing between the RNA and DNA so that any mismatched bases would lower the thermal stability. Thermal stability is usually expressed as the temperature by which one half of the hybrid has been eluted. It is also affected by the base composition, since G-C bonds are stronger than A-T or A-U bonds. However, in most experiments with viral cDNA, the G-C content of the test RNA involved in the hybridization is tacitly assumed to be similar to that of the control RNA. This assay is somewhat more tedious than the S1 nuclease assay.

Another hybrid detection assay (Cs_2SO_4 density gradient centrifugation) takes advantage of the small size of the DNA and large size of the RNA, which gives hybrid complexes a density like that of RNA. Hybrid yield is estimated by the amount of radioactivity shifted from the DNA density regions of the gradient to the RNA regions. In general, this method is the most tedious and least quantitative of all the methods of hybrid detection. However, it can be used with denatured double-stranded DNA products, and the test RNA need not be free of DNA, since double-stranded DNA would not register as a hybrid. Like the hydroxyapatite assay, unhybridized DNA "tails" are scored as hybrid. A fourth system uses a method of hybrid formation with the RNA covalently attached to phosphocellulose discs. Hybrid formation is detected by washing unhybridized DNA from the discs. The immobilized RNA system, like the Cs_2SO_4 assay system, can also be used with denatured double-stranded cDNA, but the test RNA must be free of DNA. Although theoretically this method should also register unhybridized "tails" as hybrids, in practice the hybridization values are lower than the Cs_2SO_4 or S1 nuclease assays (*234, 274*). This is perhaps because the covalent attachment to a solid phase physically blocks some of the RNA from solution, making only short stretches of RNA available for hybridization. If the available region were short, formation of a stable hybrid might require a perfect base-pairing. Consistent with this notion is the apparent higher specificity of hybrid formation using this system (*274*).

One difficulty with these types of experiments is that the DNA is often an unrepresentative transcript of 70 S RNA, with 85% of the DNA sequences reportedly transcribed from only 15% of the genome, at least in the case of the avian viruses (*66,124,127,340,361*), although this is not necessarily true of the mammalian viruses. This imbalance in transcription is probably due to the fact that regions nearest the initiation sites are the most frequently transcribed. Since the polymerase reads away from the initiation site, the probability of termination of transcription by, for example, the inability of the polymerase to bridge a nick in the RNA, would be increased. [Virion 70 S molecules are known to be extensively nicked (*33*)]. DNA transcripts have been reported to be more related to nucleotide sequences from normal cells than the viral RNA itself and tend to hybridize preferentially to the more reiterated cell DNA sequences (*127,357, 362*). This may in turn mean that there are initiation sequences on 70 S RNA that are common to viruses and cells. However, recently it has been suggested that DNA transcripts of mammalian tumor virus DNA may be much more representative of the viral RNA as a whole than that of the avian system (*339*). Actinomycin D and Mn^{2+} as the divalent cation have been reported to help maximize and balance transcription. At any rate, hybridization results obtained with DNA transcripts must be interpreted with caution. The DNA product is usually prepared for hybridization by extraction with phenol, some form of chromatography (Sephadex, hydroxyapatite), precipitation with cetyltrimethyl ammonium bromide (*300*), or some combination of these methods, and removal of the RNA by alkaline hydrolysis.

Hybridization of cDNA to excess RNA has been used by Spiegelman and his colleagues to detect cellular RNA sequences related to RLV in leukocytes of human leukemia patients (*163*), lymphomas (*164*) including Burkitt's lymphoma (*205*) and Hodgkin's disease (*164*), sarcomas (*204*), and nasopharyngeal carcinoma (*205*). In all cases, hybridization was negative with equivalent amounts of RNA from normal lymphocytes. The detection of human RNA partly homologous to RNA from a murine virus is perhaps unexpected, but the assay system employed (centrifugation to equilibrium in Cs_2SO_4) would detect mismatched hybrids and would maximize positive results by including unhybridized viral DNA "tails." Also the use of a mouse virus may have been in part fortuitous, since DNA transcripts of RNA of the primate Class II viruses, GaLV and SSV-1, have been reported to hybridize to mouse cell DNA (*311*) and endogenous DNA from SSV-1 (grown and maintained in marmoset cells) hybridizes significantly to RNA from KiSV grown in rat cells (Reitz and Gallo, manuscript in preparation). Also, SSV-1 transcripts have been reported to hybridize to MuLV-AKR 70 S RNA (*27*), but it is not obvious from the manuscript whether the SSV-1 DNA transcript was prepared from SSV-1 grown in Kirsten virus-infected nonproducer normal rat kidney (NRK) cells or in human cells. SSV-1 grown in the rat cells might have picked up the Kirsten genome and register a false homology of SSV-1 RNA with MuLV-AKR RNA.

Thus far, in our experience RLV endogenous DNA transcripts, as well as those from FeLV, MuLV-AKR, and SSV-1 grown in KiSV-infected nonproducer NRK cells hybridize to RNA from leukemic lymphocytes (Reitz, Miller and Gallo unpublished results), as measured by resistance to S1 nuclease, Cs_2SO_4 density gradient centrifugation, or hybridization to immobilized RNA. However, hybridization is achieved to a nearly equal degree to RNA from PHA-stimulated normal human lymphocytes. This is partially consistent with the reciprocal hybridization experiments mentioned above, in which we find an equal degree of hybridization of normal and leukemic endogenous DNA transcripts to 70 S RNA from RLV and from SSV-1 grown in human (NC37) cells. The discrepancy between these and the above results may be due at least in part to the fact that PHA-stimulated lymphocytes are actively dividing, while many of the former studies used fresh unstimulated leukocytes as the normal control.

Other similar studies have shown that RNA from human breast tumors contains RNA homologous to that of mouse mammary tumor virus (*10*) and MPMV (*57*), and that these sequences are absent from normal human breast tissue. Human malignant melanoma, but not normal human tissue, has been reported to contain RNA sequences homologous to RNA from subcellular particles from hamster and mouse melanoma (*12*), the injection of which causes melanoma in recipient animals (*78*). Since these particles are strictly intracellular, the use of the term "virus" may be inappropriate. However, the RNA of these particles reportedly shares a slight homology to that of RLV (*162*).

The second experimental approach to detecting virus-related RNA in cells involves hybridizing excess labeled viral RNA to DNA from cells infected by and producing the same virus. To quantitate the RNA, a standard curve is constructed by adding unlabeled 70 S RNA from the same virus in increasing amounts to a hybridization mixture including labeled RNA from the same virus until hybridization of labeled RNA is down to nearly background levels. Similar experiments can then be done using unlabeled cell RNA instead of unlabeled 70 S RNA. The amount of viral specific RNA in the RNA preparation can then be quantitated by comparing the amount of cell RNA required to reduce the hybridization by a fixed amount to the amount of unlabeled viral 70 S RNA required for the same reduction. This technique has the advantage over those using labeled viral DNA transcripts of surveying the entire viral genome to an equal degree, thus eliminating uncertainties over the extent of trancription. Consequently, the percentage of the viral genome represented in the cell RNA in question can be more accurately ascertained. Difficulties are that the hybridization of RNA to infected cell DNA never proceeds to completion, owing in part to DNA—DNA reannealing, and in part to thermal degradation of the RNA during the course of the hybridization reaction. In addition, care must be taken to ensure than the RNA is in excess of the complementary sequences in the DNA; otherwise the added cold 70 S RNA will not effectively compete. Contamination with other RNAs in the labeled 70 S RNA can be a problem as well. For a more detailed description of the technical aspects of this system, we refer the reader to the review by Gillespie *et al.* (*135*). So far, this approach, although theoretically superior to those using DNA transcripts, has not been used in connection with human cells and tumor viruses. Success in either approach depends on selecting the relevant virus. Viral RNA sequences specific to RNA from BEV, for example, are found to a varying extent in different normal baboon tissues (23), but their distribution has no known relevance to neoplasia.

7. *RNA Tumor Virus-Related Nucleotide Sequences in Human Cellular DNA Related to Tumor Virus RNA*

Have neoplastic cells somehow acquired extra information from without? Experiments designed to detect viral information within the DNA of neoplastic, but not of normal, cells are the most direct and basic approach bearing on this question, since the results are independent of transcriptional and translational processes of the cell. Selection of a proper control cell type is thus somewhat less difficult. Since nuclear DNA contains complementary strands, either tumor virus RNA or transcripts of the RNA may be used for detection of viral sequences subject to the qualifications given in the preceding section. While detection of extra DNA sequences could mean that a virus has infected the cell in question from without, the extra sequences might alternatively be indicative of some kind of reshuffling of genetic information between cells or a loss of DNA from certain kinds of normal cells, such as occurs during the maturation of erythrocytes. The hybridization experiments can be performed in such a way as to determine whether any observed differences are due to a quantitative difference in the DNA preparations, that is, a difference in the number of copies of the same gene, or to a part or the whole of a given gene being completely absent from a given DNA preparation.

In practice this is done by incubating the hybridization mixture for a sufficiently long time period and adding a sufficient quantity of DNA to allow hybridization to proceed to completion even if the DNA sequences complementary to the test RNA were present in only one copy in only a fraction of the cells. The convention used in estimating what represents a sufficient time period and DNA concentration is the C_0t (43), which is the product of the time of hybridization in seconds multiplied by the concentration of DNA in moles per liter. A C_0t of 20,000 is required to hybridize nucleotide sequences which are not repeated within a cell genome, while higher values are required if not all cells have a copy of the sequence in question. If the final hybridization values are the same for two DNA preparations but occur at different C_0ts, then these DNAs differ in the number of copies of a particular sequence that each contain. On the other hand, if the final hybridization plateaus at a sufficiently high C_0t (>20,000) are different, then part of a given set of sequences must be absent from the DNA of at least some cells of one of the cell types. Alternatively, the possibility that a provirus might be carried as an episome, not integrated into cell RNA, should be considered, since with avian tumor viruses (*150,151,359,360*), the provirus is first formed in the cytoplasm, then later transported to the nucleus and integrated (*79,228*). DNA sequences thus might not be restricted to nuclear high molecular weight DNA.

It is possible that even where the degree of hybridization at a high C_0t is the same for different DNA preparations, nucleotide sequence differences may exist, since one given set of hybrid formation and detection conditions might detect hybrids which have a varying amount of mispaired bases. Obviously, care is required in selecting proper control cells to rule out the last-mentioned possibility. Detection of altered rather than additional DNA sequences in neoplastic DNA would result if an endogenous Class I virus had undergone mutation and acquired oncogenic potential (102) or if the genome of an exogenous infecting virus were partially homologous to that of an endogenous Class I virus. Therefore, measurement of the thermal stability of hybrids formed and experiments which measure hybrid under several sets of conditions allowing variable degrees of mismatching in hybrid formation and detection are also useful in comparing hybridization to different cellular DNAs. Varying the degree of mismatching allowed in hybrid formation is usually accomplished by varying the reaction conditions. Higher salt concentrations and lower temperatures require less precise base-pairing for the formation of hybrids. In general, hybrids that are less well base-paired can be better detected by physical methods, such as hydroxyapatite chromatography or binding to nitrocellulose, than by enzymic digestion with nucleases (see above for a discussion of hybridization assay methods), but increasing the salt concentration of the nuclease reaction mix also decreases the precision in base-pairing which is required for hybrid detection.

As an example of this type of experiment, the results obtained by hybridization of RNA from RLV to infected and uninfected cell DNA are worth mentioning. Using stringent hybrid formation and detection, RLV 70 S RNA anneals much more completely (~2-fold) to DNA from the infected cells, but, under conditions that allow and detect less well matched hybrids, the results are nearly comparable (383). This probably indicates that the endogenous mouse virogenes of normal mouse DNA are partially related but not identical to the Class II leukemia virus RLV. A similar situation exists with chickens, where an endogenous Class I virus, RAV-O, is carried in perhaps all chicken cells (15,285, 362,372,374), is nonpathogenic as far as is known, but shares a great deal of homology with exogenous Class II tumorigenic viruses, such as AMV and RSV (15,247,249). This in turn may indicate that the exogenous viruses in question arose from genes present in every normal cell by mutation and perhaps by recombination. These findings are also illustrative of the type of results one might obtain, as well as some of the difficulties one might experience, when using viral molecular probes and cellular DNA to investigate etiologic aspects of human neoplasia.

There also exist, however, precedents in animal systems for endogenous type-C viruses present in normal cells and apparently nonpathogenic for the host, which are totally unrelated to any known exogenous viruses tumorigenic for the same species. One example of such an unrelated pair of viruses is RD114 and FeLV in cats. The genetic information for RD114, the Class I feline virus, is apparently in the DNA (*16,134,248,290*) and RNA (*254*) of all normal cats. This virus will not productively infect cat cells (*84,220,299*) and is not known to cause any cat diseases. FeLV and FeSV (Class II feline viruses), on the other hand, cause leukemia as well as a variety of other diseases such as sarcoma, lymphoma, anemia, arthritis, and autoimmune disease (*125,180,181,278,324*) and are not highly related to sequences in the DNA of normal cats (*134*). A second similar situation is found among a pair of primate type-C RNA viruses. The information for BEV, the Class I primate virus which has been reported to be distantly related to RD114 (*23,24,165*), is found in the DNA of all normal Old World simians, as judged by hybridization of viral DNA transcripts to cell DNA (*23,24*). This virus also does not grow in homologous host cells (*165,351*), has not been shown to be pathogenic, and is expressed as extracellular virus in normal early term placenta (*189,333*). This class of virus is also found expressed in rhesus (*305*) and possibly in human (*188*) placenta. GaLV and SSV-1 related DNA, on the other hand, are apparently found only in the DNA of infected cells, as measured by hybridization of DNA transcripts to cell DNA (*311*). Related DNA sequences are detectable in normal mouse DNA, and this led to the suggestion of the possibility that this virus originated from mouse some time in the distant past (*23*) and was somehow transmitted at some point in evolution to primates. Consistent with this is a substantial (>50%) hybridization of cDNA from SSV-1, grown and maintained in marmoset cells and never exposed to nonprimate cells, to 70 S RNA from KiSV grown in NRK cells, and which had never been exposed to cells or viruses other than murine and rate (Reitz and Gallo, unpublished results). This points to the possibility that a virus endogenous to and nonpathogenic for one species may be exogenously infectious and pathogenic for another species. The above examples are included because they are helpful in evaluating data obtained with animal virus molecular probes and human normal and neoplastic cell DNA.

Hybridization experiments have been performed in our laboratory using ^{125}I-labeled 70 S RNA and cellular DNA to assess whether or not human leukemic cell genomic DNA contains virus-related sequences not found in normal cell DNA. Neither conditions permitting the formation and detection of mismatched hybrids nor more stringent conditions showed any differences between DNA of leukemic and normal cells (*137, 107*). This is true for 70 S RNA from RLV, SSV-1 grown in either human (NC37) cells or in KiSV-infected nonproducer NRK cells, or GaLV grown in NC37 cells. Prehybridizing RLV 70 S RNA with normal cell DNA to a $C_0 t\ 10^3$ to remove sequences related to normal cell DNA and then using the remaining RNA did not alter this pattern. These results are puzzling in view of the data on hybridization of endogenous leukemic DNA product to viral 70 S RNA, as well as the presence of reverse transcriptase (*349,350*), gp69 (*39*), and p30 (*321,388*) which are immunologically cross-reactive with the analogous proteins from SSV-1. One interpretation is that there are simply transcriptional and translational differences between normal and leukemic cells, and a mutation of cellular genes regulating endogenous virus expression or of the virogene itself has resulted in the observed phenotypic changes. Since SSV-1 and GaLV-related DNA sequences are found in infected, but not in normal, primates, this possibility seems unlikely. A second interpretation is that technical problems obscure a real difference in the content of nucleotide sequences related to SSV-1 or GaLV, or both, between the DNA of normal and leukemic cells. Favoring the second possibility is the fact that these data are at variance with other similar studies from Spiegelman's laboratory, described below, which indicate that differences do exist. Regarding the apparent conflict between two sets of data, the above experiments were performed with the entire viral genome in the form of 70 S RNA, while the experiments described below were performed with DNA transcripts of endogenous cell pellet DNA polymerase, subsets of which were selected where described by hybridization to the appropriate 70 S RNA. The information surveyed by this technique may be very narrow, yet relevant to neoplasia. A third possibility is that the provirus is carried in an unintegrated or episomal form. Although there are no animal model systems in which data have been obtained to support this possibility, findings in our laboratory indicate that SSV-1-related sequences are enriched in "cytoplasmic" DNA of human leukemic cells (107; Saxinger, Gillespie, and Gallo unpublished results).

The most complete set of data on extra virus-specific sequences in DNA of human neoplastic cells comes from studies using DNA synthesized by an endogenous high-speed pellet DNA polymerase of human cells from Burkitt's lymphoma, Hodgkin's disease, and lymphosarcoma (207) and especially the leukemias (18,20,21). The data here are more complete partly because these diseases have animal viral models. Therefore, the DNA originally synthesized in a cell fraction may be related to a known virus and the data obtained can be compared to those from the animal model using the same virus. In addition, viral RNA can be used to select subsets of nucleotide sequences which are virus-related from the DNA synthesized in the cell pellet fraction. In the leukemic studies, the DNA synthesized in the cell pellet was annealed to a high C_0t to nuclear DNA from normal cells, duplexes were removed by hydroxyapatite chromatography, and the remaining DNA was annealed to normal or leukemic DNA. This is illustrated in Fig. 6. These remaining sequences formed duplexes only with DNA from the leukemic cells and with RLV 70 S RNA (21). These extra sequences are found in nuclear DNA from leukocytes of patients in remission (20), but not the nonleukemic twins of leukemic patients (21), which argues for the addition of a stable genetic element added postnatally to the hematopoietic cells of the patient. The sensitivity of the technique from a consideration of the C_0t value obtained would allow detection of 1/400th of a viral gene equivalent or one full gene equivalent in one out of 400 cells. This argues that the difference observed is not due to gene amplification, but does not indicate whether the sequences might be present in leukocyte progenitor cells (e.g., stem cells, myeloblasts,

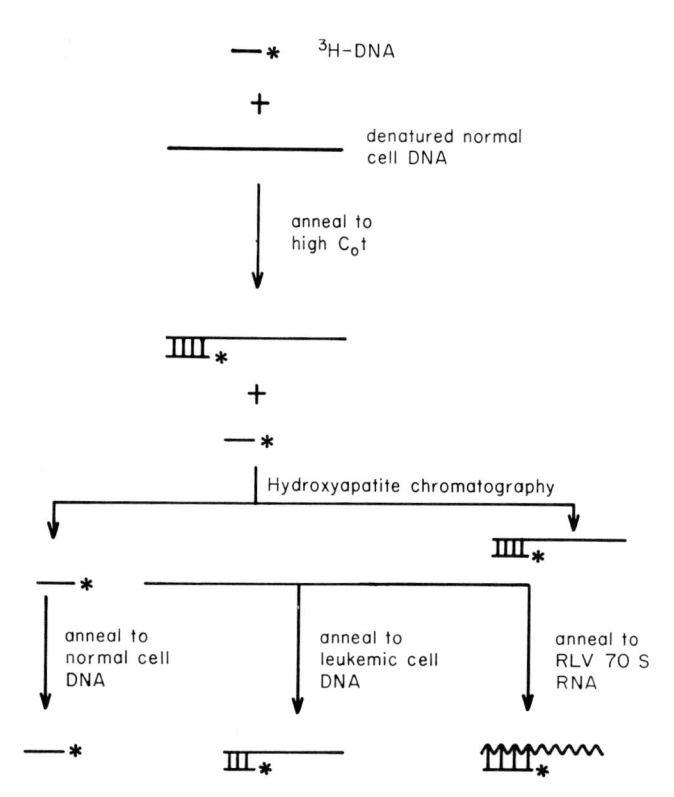

FIG. 6. Hybridization recycling. Schematic representation of a typical hybridization "recycling" experiment.

lymphoblasts) but lost during normal leukocyte differentiation. Extra sequences, are also detected in the DNA of patients with Hodgkin's disease, Burkitt's lymphoma, and lymphosarcoma (207) and (at least in the case of lymphosarcoma) are partially related to RLV 70 S RNA. The extra sequences of the Burkitt's and Hodgkin's cells are at least partially related to each other.

C. Isolation of Type-C Virus from Human Leukemic Cells

The value of these molecular approaches can be illustrated in the case of the recent isolation of a candidate human tumor virus from AML cells (91). First, without the great volume of data suggesting that a virus might be involved in AML (e.g., reverse transcriptase, hybridization data with model animal virus probes, and subsequently the p30 data) the time and effort of isolating this virus might well not have been taken. Second, some confidence can be taken that this virus is not a laboratory contaminant because studies on fresh myelogenous leukemia cells (where contamination is not a problem) with viral molecular probes have predicted the characteristics that a virus relevant to human leukemia may have (at least the myelogenous type) when isolated. These include p30 (*307,388*) and reverse transcriptase (*32,92–117,119–121,293–295*) immunologically closely related to SSV-1 and GaLV (*94,240,349,350*) and more distantly to RLV, and an endogenous high molecular weight RNA transcribed by reverse transcriptase into DNA (*19,234*) whose pattern of hybridization to 70 S RNA from various tumor viruses fits a pattern similar to that for SSV-1 (*102, 109, 234*). Since the candidate human virus fits these criteria, more confidence can be placed in the identity of this virus as truly derived from these cells. Additional evidence supporting the identity of this virus as one truly derived from human leukemic cells has been provided by Mak *et al.*, who report transient release of viruslike particles from shortterm marrow cultures of leukemic patients in relapse or remission (*225*). Although these particles are not continually released and did not have all features of a mature type-C virus, such as budding, and are not reported to be infectious, they do contain a functional reverse transcriptase and 70 S RNA which, like that from the human virus isolate and from fresh leukemic cells, are closely related to that of SSV-1 and GaLV and less closely related to KiSV and RLV (*224*).

The type-C human virus has now been isolated three times. The first two isolates, which we call HL23V-1, were obtained from cultural leukocytes of a single bleed of a leukemic (AML) patient. The third isolate was from marrow obtained 14 months later from the same patient, and we call this Hl23V-2. The two virus isolates appear to be identical, are classical type-C particles, and have reverse transcriptase (R.C. Gallo and R.C. Gallagher, in preparation), p30 (R. Gilden, personal communication), and p12 (S. Aaronson, peronsal communica-

TABLE III

TYPE-C VIRAL COMPONENTS COMMON TO HUMAN ACUTE MYELOGENOUS LEUKEMIC CELLS AND HUMAN TYPE-C VIRUS ISOLATE (HLV)

	Reverse transcriptase serologically related to SSV-1, GaLV[a]	RNA related to SSV-1, GaLV	p30 related to SSV-1, GaLV	p12 related to SSV-1
Fresh leukemic cells	Yes[b]	Yes[c]	Yes[d]	Not done
HL23V	Yes	Yes	Yes	Yes

[a] SSV-1, simian sarcoma virus; GaLV, gibbon ape lymphoma virus.

[b] Detected in about 25% of cases of acute myelogenous leukemia in our laboratory.

[c] Detected in our laboratory in about 50% of cases of acute myelogenous leukemia (see also Ref. 224).

[d] Detected in 5 of 5 cases of acute myelogenous leukemia (*321*), but many negatives were unreported.

tion) closely related to SSV-1 and GaLV. Although the host range has not yet been completely ascertained, the virus can productively infect WHE-2 (whole human embryo), A-204 (human rhabdomyosarcoma), K-NRK (KiSV-infected nonproducer rat kidney), and dog thymus cells (N. Teich, R. Weiss, R. Gallagher, D. Gillespie, and R.E. Gallo). Although only one patient has yielded the virus, its biochemical properties are like those observed with fresh leukemic *cells* from many patients with AML. These common properties are summarized in Table III.

It is hoped that the increasing use of techniques using molecular probes will lead to the isolation and identification of other similar viruses from other human neoplasias. Some immediate uses of this virus will be for the preparation of viral nucleic acids for hybridization experiments and for the preparation of antibodies specific for viral structural antigens in looking for related viral components in other related cancers. In any event, the availability of this and related viruses may allow a greater understanding of the pathogenesis of the disease, and they should provide the best available "molecular probes."

IV. Summary

Molecular probes from tumor viruses have found wide and increasing application to the study of human malignancies. Even in the absence of suitable animal models, inferential results can be drawn by preparing viruslike molecular probes, as in the detection of extra RNA sequences in certain malignancies, as noted above. As with any sensitive technique, care must be taken in the experimental approach and interpretation of results. However, these approaches have proved to be of value, as seen most recently in the isolation of a candidate human leukemia virus (*91*) and in the recent discovery of a DNA provirus in human leukemic cells (Reitz *et al., Proc. Nat. Acad. Sci. U.S.,* in press).

REFERENCES

1. Aaronson, S. Parks, W., Scolnick, E., and Todaro, G. (1971). Antibody to the RNA-dependent DNA polymerase of mammalian C-type RNA tumor viruses. *Proc. Nat. Acad. Sci. U.S.* **68**, 920.
2. Aaronson, S., Todaro, G., and Scolnick, E. (1971). Induction of murine C-type viruses from clonal lines of virus-free BALB/3T3 cells. *Science* **174**, 157.
3. Abrell, J.W., and Gallo, R.C. (1973). Purification, characterization, and comparison of the DNA polymerases from two primate RNA tumor viruses. *J. Virol.* **12**, 431.
4. Allison, A.C., and Burke, D. (1962). The nucleic acid content of viruses. *J. Gen. Microbiol.* **27**, 181.
5. Ando, T. (1966). A nuclease specific for heat-denatured DNA isolated from a product of *Aspergillus oryzae. Biochim. Biophys. Acta* **114**, 158.
6. Aoki, I., Boyse, E., and Old, L. (1968). Wild-type Gross leukemia virus. I. Soluble antigen (GSA) in the plasma and tissue of infected mice. *J. Nat. Cancer Inst.* **41**, 89.
   Aoki, T., Old, L., and Boyse, E. (1966). Serological analysis of the leukemia antigens of the mouse. *Nat. Cancer Inst. Monogr.* **22**, 449.

8. Aurelian, L., Royston, I., and Davis, H. (1970). Antibody to genital herpes simplex virus: Association with cervical atypia and carcinoma *in situ. J. Nat. Cancer Inst.* **45**, 455.
9. Axel, R., Gulati, S., and Spiegelman, S. (1972). Particles containing RNA-instructed DNA polymerase and virus-related RNA in human breast cancers. *Proc. Nat. Acad. Sci. U.S.* **69**, 3133.
10. Axel, R., Schlom, J., and Spiegelman, S. (1972). Presence in human breast cancer of RNA homologous to mouse mammary tumor virus RNA. *Nature (London)* **235**, 32.
11. August, J.T., Bolognesi, D., Fleissner, E., Gilden, R., and Nowinski, R. (1974). A proposed nomenclature for the virion proteins of oncogenic RNA viruses. *Virology* **60**, 595.
12. Balda, B., Hehlmann, R., and Spiegelman, S. (1975). Evidence for a reverse transcriptase and high molecular weight RNA in human melanoma related to particles from mouse melanoma. *Proc. Nat. Acad. Sci. U.S.* (in press).
13. Baltimore, D. (1970). Viral RNA-Dependent DNA polymerase. *Nature (London)* **226**:1209.
14. Baltimore, D., and Smoler, D. (1971). Primer requirement and template specificity of the DNA polymerase of RNA tumor viruses. *Proc. Nat. Acad. Sci. U.S.* **68**, 1507.
15. Baluda, M. (1972). Widespread presence in chickens of DNA complementary to the RNA genome of avian leukosis viruses. *Proc. Nat. Acad. Sci. U.S.* **69**, 576.
16. Baluda, M., and Roy-Burman, R. (1973). Partial characterization of RD114 virus by DNA-RNA hybridization studies. *Nature (London), New Biol.* **244**, 59.
17. Baril, E., Brown, O., Jenkins, M., and Laszlo, J. (1971). Deoxyribonucleic acid polymerase with rat liver ribosomes and smooth membranes. Purification and properties of the enzymes. *Biochemistry* **10**, 1981.
18. Baxt, W. (1974). Sequences present in both human cell nuclear DNA and Rauscher leukemia virus. *Proc. Nat. Acad. Sci. U.S.* **71**, 2853.
19. Baxt, W., Hehlmann, R., and Spiegelman, S. (1972). Human leukemic cells contain reverse transcriptase associated with a high molecular weight virus-related RNA. *Nature (London), New Biol.* **240**, 72.
20. Baxt, W., and Spiegelman, S. (1972). Nuclear DNA sequences present in human leukemic cells and absent in normal leukocytes. *Proc. Nat. Acad. Sci. U.S.* **69**, 3737.
21. Baxt, W., Yates, J., Wallace, H., Holland, J., and Spiegelman, S. (1973). Leukemia-specific DNA sequences in leukocytes of the leukemic member of identical twins. *Proc. Nat. Acad. Sci. U.S.* **70**, 2629.
22. Bellamy, A., Gillies, S., and Harvey, J. (1974). Molecular weight of two oncornavirus genomes: derivation from particle molecular weights and RNA content. *J. Virol.* **14**, 1388.
23. Benveniste, R., Heinemann, R., Wilson, R., Callahan, R., and Todaro, G. (1974). Detection of baboon type-C viral sequences in various tissues by molecular hybridization. *J. Virol.* **14**, 56.
24. Benveniste, R., Lieber, M., Livingston, D., Scherr, C., Todaro, G., and Kalter, S. (1974). Infectious type-C virus isolated from a baboon placenta. *Nature (London)* **248**, 17.
25. Benveniste, R., Lieber, M., and Todaro, G. (1974). A distinct class of inducible murine type-C viruses that replicate in the rabbit SIRC cell line. *Proc. Nat. Acad. Sci. U.S.* **71**, 602.
26. Benveniste, R., and Scolnick, R. (1973). RNA in mammalian sarcoma virus transformed nonproducer cells homologous to murine leukemia virus RNA. *Virology* **51**, 370.
27. Benveniste, R., and Todaro, G. (1973). Homology between type-C viruses of various species as determined by molecular hybridization. *Proc. Nat. Acad. Sci. U.S.* **70**, 3316.

28. Benveniste, R., and Todaro, G. (1974). Evolution of C-type viral genes: inheritance of exogenously acquired viral genes. *Nature (London)* **252**, 456.
29. Benveniste, R., and Todaro, G. (1974). Evolution of type-C viral genes: I. Nucleic acid from baboon type-C virus as a measure of divergence among primate species. *Proc. Nat. Acad. Sci. U.S.* **71**, 4513.
30. Benveniste, R., Todaro, G., Scolnick, E., and Parks, W. (1973). Partial transcription of murine type-C viral genomes in Balb/C cell lines. *J. Virol.* **12**, 711.
31. Bernhard, W. (1960). The detection and study of tumor viruses with the electron microscope. *Cancer Res.* **20**, 712.
32. Bhattacharyya, J., Xuma, M., Reitz, M., Sarin, P., and Gallo, R.C. (1973). Utilization of mammalian viral 70S RNA by a purified reverse transcriptase from human myelocytic leukemic cells. *Biochem. Biophys. Res. Commun.* **54**, 324.
33. Bishop, D.H.L., Ruprecht, R., Simpson, R., and Spiegelman, S. (1971). Deoxyribonucleic acid polymerase of Rous sarcoma virus: Reaction conditions and analysis of the product nucleic acids. *J. Virol.* **8**, 730.
34. Biswal, N., Grizzard, M., McCombs, R., and Benyesh-Melnick, M. (1968). Characterization of intracellular ribonucleic acid specific for the murine sarcoma leukemia complex. *J. Virol.* **2**, 1346.
35. Bittner, J. (1956). Some possible effects of nursing on the mammary gland tumor incidence in mice. *Science* **84**, 162.
36. Bobrow, S., Smith, R.G., Reitz, M., and Gallo, R.C. (1972). Stimulated normal human lymphocytes contain a ribonuclease-sensitive DNA polymerase which is distinct from viral RNA-directed DNA polymerase. *Proc. Nat. Acad. Sci. U.S.* **69**, 3228.
37. Bollum, F. (1960). Calf thymus polymerase. *J. Biol. Chem.* **235**, 2399.
38. Bolognesi, D. (1974). Oncogenic RNA tumor viruses and the host cell membrane. In "Cell Membranes and Viral Envelopes" (H.A. Blough and J.M. Tiffany, eds.), Academic Press, New York. (in press).
39. Bolognesi, D. (1975). Personal Communication.
40. Bolognesi, D.P., and Bauer, H. (1970). Polypeptides of avian RNA tumor viruses. I. Isolation and physical and chemical analysis. *Virology* **42**, 1097.
41. Bolognesi, D.P., and Graf, T. (1971). Size differences among the high molecular weight RNA's of avian tumor viruses. *Virology* **43**, 214.
42. Bolognesi, D., Luftig, R., and Shaper, J. (1973). Localization of RNA tumor virus polypeptides. *Virology* **56**, 549.
43. Britten, R., and Kohne, D. (1968). Repeated sequences in DNA. *Science* **161**, 529.
44. Brodey, R., McDonough, S., Frye, F., and Hardy, W. (1970). Epidemiology of feline leukemia (lymphosarcoma). In "Comparative Leukemia Research, 1969," (R.M. Dutcher, ed.), p. 333. Karger, Basel.
45. Brutlag, D., Schekman, R., and Kornberg, A. (1971). A possible role for RNA polymerase in the initiation of M13 DNA synthesis. *Proc. Nat. Acad. Sci. U.S.* **68**, 2826.
46. Canaani, E., and Duesberg, P. (1972). Role of subunits of 60 to 70S avian tumor virus ribonucleic acid in its template activity for the viral deoxyribonucleic acid polymerase. *J. Virol.* **10**, 23.
47. Canaani, E., Helm, K.V.D., and Duesberg, P. (1973). Evidence for 30–40S RNA as precursor of the 60–70S RNA of Rous sarcoma virus. *Proc. Nat. Acad. Sci. U.S.* **72**, 401.
48. Chang, L., and Bollum, F. (1971). Low molecular weight deoxyribonucleic acid polymerase in mammalian cells. *J. Biol. Chem.* **246**, 5835.
49. Chang, L., and Bollum, F. (1972). Low molecular weight deoxyribonucleic acid polymerase from rabbit bone marrow. *Biochemistry* **11**, 1264.

50. Chang, L., and Bollum, F. (1972). Antigenic relationships in mammalian DNA polymerase. *Science* **175**, 1116.
51. Chattopadhyay, S., Lowy, D., Teich, N., Levine, A., and Rowe, W. (1974). Evidence that the AKR murine-leukemia-virus genome is complete in DNA of the high virus DKR mouse and incomplete in the DNA of the "virus-negative" NIH mouse. *Proc. Nat. Acad. Sci. U.S.* **71**, 167.
52. Cheung, K.S., Smith, R.E., Stone, M., and Joklik, W. (1972). Comparison of immature (rapid harvest) and mature Rous virus particles. *Virology* **50**, 851.
53. Chopra, H., and Mason, M. (1970). A new virus in a spontaneous mammary tumor of a rhesus monkey. *Cancer Res.* **30**, 2081.
54. Churchill, A., and Biggs, P. (1967). Agent of Marek's disease in tissue culture. *Nature (London)* **215**, 528.
55. Churchill, A., and Biggs, P. (1968). Herpes-type virus isolated in cell culture from tumors of chickens with Marek's disease. II. Studies *in vivo*. *J. Nat. Cancer Inst.* **41**, 951.
56. Cotter, S., Essex, M., and Hardy, W. (1974). Serological studies of normal and leukemic cats in a multiple-case leukemia cluster. *Cancer Res.* **34**, 1061.
57. Colcher, D., Spiegelman, S., and Schlom, J. (1974). Sequence homology between the RNA of Mason-Pfizer monkey virus and the RNA of human malignant breast tumors. *Proc. Nat. Acad. Sci. U.S.* **71**, 4975.
58. Cuatico, W., Cho, J.R., and Spiegelman, S. (1974). Evidence of particle-associated RNA-directed DNA polymerase and high molecular weight RNA in human gastrointestinal and lung malignancies. *Proc. Nat. Acad. Sci. U.S.* **71**, 3304.
59. Cuatico, W., Cho, J.-R., and Spiegelman, S. (1973). Particles with RNA of high molecular weight and RNA-directed DNA polymerase in human brain tumors. *Proc. Nat. Acad. Sci. U.S.* **70**, 2789.
60. Darnell, J., Philipson, L., Wall, R., and Adesnik, M. (1971). Polyadenylic acid sequences: Role in conversion of nuclear RNA into messenger RNA. *Science* **174**, 507.
61. DeSchryver, A., Klein, G., Henle, G., Henle, W., Cameron, H., Santesson, L., and Clifford, P. (1972). Epstein-Barr virus-associated serology in malignant disease: antibody levels to viral capsid antigen (VCA) membrane antigens (MA) and early antigens (EA) in patients with various neoplastic conditions. *Int. J. Cancer* **9**, 353.
62. DiGiacoma, R. (1967). Burkitt's lymphoma in a white-handed gibbon (*Hylobates lar*). *Cancer Res.* **27**, 1178.
63. DiPaoli, A., and Garner, F. (1968). Acute lymphocytic leukemia in a white-cheeked gibbon (*Hylobates concolor*). *Cancer Res.* **28**, 2559.
64. Duesberg, P. (1968). Physical properties of Rous sarcoma virus RNA. *Proc. Nat. Acad. Sci. U.S.* **59**, 930.
65. Duesberg, P. (1970). On the structure of RNA tumor viruses. *Curr. Top. Microbiol. Immunol.* **51**, 79.
66. Duesberg, P., and Canaani, E. (1970). Complementarity between Rous sarcoma virus (RSV) RNA and the *in vitro*-synthesized DNA of the virus-associated DNA polymerase. *Virology* **42**, 783.
67. Duesberg, P., Canaani, E., van der Helm, K., Lai, M.M.C., and Vogt, P. (1973). News and views on avian tumor virus RNA. *In* "Possible Episomes in Eukaryotes" (L.G. Silvestri, ed.), p. 142. North-Holland Publ., Amsterdam.
68. Duesberg, P., Helm, K. V. D., and Canani, E. (1971). Comparative properties of RNA and DNA templates for the DNA polymerase of Rous sarcoma virus. *Proc. Nat. Acad. Sci. U.S.* **68**, 2505.
69. Duesberg, P., and Robinson, W. (1966). Nucleic acid and proteins isolated from the Rauscher mouse leukemia virus (MLV). *Proc. Nat. Acad. Sci. U.S.* **55**, 219.

70. Duesberg, P., and Vogt, P. (1970). Differences between the ribonucleic acids of transforming and nontransforming avian tumor viruses. *Proc. Nat. Acad. Sci. U.S.* **67**, 1673.
71. Duff, R., and Rapp, F. (1971). Properties of hamster embryo fibroblasts transformed *in vitro* after exposure to ultraviolet-irradiated herpes simplex virus type 2. *J. Virol.* **8**, 469.
72. East, J., Allen, P., Knesek, J., Chan, J., Bowen, J., and Dmochowski, L. (1973). Structural rearrangement and subunit composition of RNA from released Soehner-Dmochowski murine sarcoma virions. *J. Virol.* **11**, 709.
73. East, J., Knesek, J., Allen, P., and Dmochowski, L. (1973). Structural characteristics and nucleotide sequence analysis of genomic RNA from RD114 virus and feline RNA tumor viruses. *J. Virol.* **12**, 1085.
74. Edmonds, M., and Caramela, M. (1969). The isolation and characterization of adenosine monophosphate-rich polynucleotides synthesized by Ehrlich ascites cells. *J. Biol. Chem.* **244**, 1314.
75. Edmonds, M., Vaughn, M., and Nakazato, H. (1971). Polyadenylic acid sequences in the heterogenous nuclear RNA and rapidly-labeled polysomal RNA of HeLa cells: possible evidence for a precursor relationship. *Proc. Nat. Acad. Sci. U.S.* **68**, 1336.
76. Ellerman, V., and Bang, O. (1908). Experimentelle Leukämie bei Huhnern. *Centralbl. Bakteriol., Abt. 1 (Orig.)* **46**, 595.
77. Epstein, M.A., Achong, B., and Barr, Y. (1964). Virus particles in cultured lymphoblasts from Butkitt's lymphoma. *Lancet* **1**, 702.
78. Epstein, W.L., Fukuyama, K., Benn, M., Keston, A., and Brandt, R. (1968). Transmission of a pigmented melanoma in golden hamsters by a cell-free ultrafiltrate. *Nature (London)* **219**, 979.
79. Evans, R., Baluda, M., and Shoyab, M. (1974). Differences between the integration of avian myelobastosis virus DNA in leukemic cells and of endogenous viral DNA in normal chicken cells. *Proc. Nat. Acad. Sci. U.S.* **71**, 3152.
80. Fan, H., and Baltimore, D. (1973). RNA metabolism of murine leukemia virus: detection of virus-specific RNA sequences in infected and uninfected cells and identification of virus-specific messenger RNA. *J. Mol. Biol.* **89**, 93.
81. Fanshier, L., Garapin, A., McDonnell, J., Faras, A., Levinson, W., and Bishop, J. (1971). DNA polymerase associated with avian tumor viruses: Secondary structure of the deoxyribonucleic acid product. *J. Virol.* **7**, 77.
82. Faras, A., Fanshier, L., Garapin, A., Levinson, W., and Bishop, J. (1971). Deoxyribonucleic acid polymerase of Rous sarcoma virus: studies on the mechanism of double stranded deoxyribonucleic acid synthesis. *J. Virol.* **7**, 539.
83. Feldman, S., Schlom, J., and Spiegelman, S. (1973). Further evidence for oncornaviruses in human milk; the productio of cores. *Proc. Nat. Acad. Sci. U.S.* **70**, 1976.
84. Fischinger, P., Peebles, P., Nomura, S., and Haapala, D. (1973). Isolation of an Rd-114-like oncornavirus from a cat cell line. *J. Virol.* **11**, 978.
85. Flugel, R., and Wells, R.D. (1972). Nucleotides at the RNA-DNA covelent bonds formed in the endogenous reaction by the avian myelobastosis virus DNA polymerase. *Virology* **48**, 394.
86. Fox, R., Mendelsohn, J., Barbosa, E., and Goulian, M. (1973). RNA in nascent DNA from cultured human lymphocytes. *Nature (London) New Biol.* **245**, 234.
87. Frenkel, N., Roizman, B., Cassai, E., and Nahmias, A. (1972). A DNA fragment of Herpes simplex 2 and its transcription in human cervical cancer tissue. *Proc. Nat. Acad. Sci. U.S.* **69**, 3784.
88. Fridlender, B., Fry, M., Bolden, A., and Weissbach, A. (1972). A new synthetic RNA-dependent DNA polymerase from human tissue culture cells. *Proc. Nat. Acad. Sci. U.S.* **69**, 452.

89. Friend, C. (1957). Cell-free transmission in adult Swiss mice of a disease having the character of a leukemia. *J. Exp. Med.* **105**, 307.
90. Fujinaga, K., Parsons, T., Beard, J., Beard, D., and Green, M. (1970). Mechanism of carcinogenesis by RNA tumor viruses. III. Formation of RNA-DNA complex and duplex DNA molecules by the DNA polymerase(s) of avian myeloblastosis virus. *Proc. Nat. Acad. Sci. U.S.* **67**, 1432.
91. Gallagher, R.E., and Gallo, R.C. (1975). Type-C RNA tumor virus isolated from cultured human acute myelogenous leukemia cells. *Science* **187**, 350.
92. Gallagher, R.E., Mondal, H., Miller, D.P., Todaro, G.J., Gillespie, D.H., and Gallo, R.C. (1974). Relatedness of RNA and reverse transcriptase from human actue myelogenous leukemia cells and from RNA tumor viruses. *In* "Modern Trends in Human Leukemia" (R. Neth, R.C. Gallo, S. Spiegelman, and F. Stohlman, eds.), pp. 185–196. J.F. Lehmanns, Munich.
93. Gallagher, R.E., Smith, R.G., Gillespie, D.H., and Gallo, R.C. (1974). Primate type-C virus-related reverse transcriptase and RNA in human acute leukemia cells as potential diagnostic markers. *Ann. Clin. Lab. Sci.* **4**, 372.
94. Gallagher, R.E., Todaro, G.J., Smith, R.G., Livingston, D.M., and Gallo, R.C. (1974). Relationship between reverse transcriptase from human acute leukemic blood cells and primate type-C viruses. *Proc. Nat. Acad. Sci. U.S.* **71**, 1309.
95. Gallo, R.C. (1971). Reverse transcriptase, the DNA polymerase of oncogenic RNA viruses. *Nature (London)* **234**, 194.
96. Gallo, R.C. (1972). RNA-dependent DNA polymerase in viruses and cells: Views on the current state. *Blood* **39**, 117.
97. Gallo, R.C. (1973). Recent advances in molecular viral oncology and applications to human leukemia. *Proc. Congr. Ital. Cancer Soc.* **8**, 21.
98. Gallo, R.C. (1973). Reverse transcriptase and neoplasia. *Biomedicine* **18**, 446.
99. Gallo, R.C. (1973). On the etiology of human acute leukemia. *Med. Clin. No. Amer.* **57**, 343.
100. Gallo, R.C. (1973). Summary of recent observations on the molecular biology of RNA tumor viruses and attempts at application to human leukemia. *Amer. J. Clin. Pathol.* **60**, 80.
101. Gallo, R.C. (1973). Some recent observations on the molecular biology of RNA tumor viruses and attempts at application to human leukemia. *In* "Polyamines in Normal and Neoplastic Growth" (D.H. Russell, ed.), pp. 405–414. Raven Press, New York.
102. Gallo, R.C. (1974). On the origin of human acute myeloblastic leukemia: Virus "hot spot" hypothesis. *In* "Modern Trends in Human Leukemia" (R. Neth, R.C. Gallo, S. Spiegelman, and F. Stohlman, eds.), pp. 227–235. J.F. Lehmanns, Munich.
103. Gallo, R.C. (1975). New molecular biological findings on subviral components related to primate oncogenic RNA tumor viruses in human leukemia. *In* "Molecular Base of Malignancy, New Clinical and Therapeutic Evidences" (E. Deutsch, K. Moser, H. Rainer, and A. Stacher, eds.) Theime, Vienna (in press).
104. Gallo, R.C. (1975). New molecular biological findings on subviral (type-C) components in human leukemia. *Proc. Nat. Conf. Acute Leukemias* (in press).
105. Gallo, R.C. (1975). Viral oncogenesis, reverse transcriptase, and human malignancy. *In* "Textbook of Internal Medicine" (H.H. Fudenberg, ed.) Grune & Stratton, New York (in press).
106. Gallo, R.C., and Gallagher, R.E. (1974). Are viruses concerned in the etiology of human leukemia? *Ser. Haematol.* **7**, 224–273.
107. Gallo, R.C., Gallagher, R.E., Miller, N.R., Mondal, H., Saxinger, W.C., Mayer, R.J., Smith, R.G., and Gillespie, D.H. (1975). Relationships between components in primate RNA tumor viruses and in the cytoplasim of human leukemic cells: Implications to leukemogenesis. *Cold Spring Harbor Symp. Quant. Biol.* **39**, 933.

108. Gallo, R.C., Gallagher, R.E., Mondal, H., and Gillespie, D.H. (1974). Human acute leukemia: Increasing evidence for involvement of type-C RNA tumor viruses. *Proc. Tumor Virus-Host Interaction Symp.* pp. 337–352.
109. Gallo, R.C., Miller, N.R., Saxinger, W.C., and Gillespie, D. (1973). Primate RNA tumor virus-like DNA synthesized endogenously by RNA-dependent DNA polymerase in virus-like particles from fresh human acute leukemic blood cells. *Proc. Nat. Acad. Sci. U.S.* **70**, 3219.
110. Gallo, R.C., and Sarin, P.S. (1975). The DNA polymerase of oncornaviruses. *Advan. Mol. Biol.* (in press).
111. Gallo, R.C., Sarin, P.S., Sarngadharan, M.G., Reitz, M.S., Smith, R.G., and Bobrow, S.N. (1974). Viral 70S RNA directed DNA synthesis with a purified DNA polymerase from human acute leukemic cells. *In* "Molecular Studies in Viral Neoplasia," (University of Texas M.D. Anderson Hosp. and Tumor Inst. at Houston, 25th Annu. Symp. Fundman. Cancer Res. pp. 477–494. Williams & Wilkins, Baltimore, Maryland.
112. Gallo, R.C., Sarin, P.S., Sarngadharan, M.G., Smith, R.G., Bobrow, S.N., and Reitz, M.S. (1973). Biochemical properties of reverse transcriptase activities from human cells and RNA tumor viruses. *Proc. 6th Miles Int. Symp. Mol. Biol.* pp. 180–192.
113. Gallo, R.C., Sarin, P.S., Smith, R.G., Bobrow, S.N., Sarngadharan, M.G., Reitz, M.S., Jr., and Abrell, J.W. (1973). RNA directed and primed DNA polymerase activities in tumor viruses and human lymphocytes. *In* "DNA Synthesis in Vitro" Proc. 2nd Annu. Steenbock Symp., (R. Wells and R. Inman, eds.), pp. 251–286. Univ. Park Press, Baltimore, Maryland.
114. Gallo, R.C., Sarin, P.S., Wu, A.M., Sarngadharan, M.G., Reitz, M., Robert, M.S., Miller, N., Saxinger, W.C., and Gillespie, D. (1973). On the nature of the nucleic acids and RNA dependent DNA polymerase from RNA tumor viruses and human cells. *In* "Possible Episomes in Eukaryotes," Proc. IV Lepetit Colloq., (L. Silvestri, ed.), pp. 14–34. North-Holland Publ., Amsterdam.
115. Gallo, R.C., Saxinger, W.C., Gallagher, R.E., Miller, N. and Gillespie, D. (1975). Evolutionary nature of human reverse transcriptase and of viral-related DNA synthesized *in vitro* by human leukemic cells. *Proc. 6th Int. Symp. Comp. Leukemia Res.* pp. 569–576.
116. Gallo, R.C., Smith, R.G., Gillespie, D.H., and Gallagher, R.E. (1974). Evidence for components in human leukemic cells related to primate type-C RNA tumor viruses and potential prognostic and etiological relevance of these findings. *Advan. Biosci.* **14**, 547.
117. Gallo, R.C., Smith, R.G., Sarin, P.S., Sarngadharan, M.G., Reitz, M.S., and Bobrow, S.N. (1973). DNA replication in normal cells, in neoplastic cells, and in RNA tumor viruses. *Proc. 2nd Int. Symp. Metab. Membrane Permeability Erythrocytes, Thrombocytes, and Leucocytes* pp. 348–356.
118. Gallo, R.C. and Ting, R.C. (1972). Cancer viruses. *Crit. Rev. Clin. Lab. Sci.* **3**, 403–499.
119. Gallo, R.C., Yang, S.S., Smith, R.G., Herrera, F., Ting, R.C., Bobrow, S.N., Davis, C. and Fujioka, S. (1971). RNA- and DNA-dependent polymerases of human normal and leukemic cells. *In* "The Biology of Oncogenic Viruses" *Proc. 2nd Lepetit Colloq.* (L.G. Silvestri, ed.) pp. 210–220. North-Holland Publ., Amsterdam.
120. Gallo, R.C., Yang, S.S., Smith, R.G., Herrera, F., Ting, R.C., and Fujioka, S. (1971). Some observations on DNA polymerases of human normal and leukemic cells. *In* "Nucleic Acid-Protein Interactions and Nucleic Acid Synthesis in Viral Infection," Miami Winter Symp. 1971 (D.W. Ribbons, J.F. Woessner, and J. Schultz, eds.), pp. 353–376, North-Holland Publ., Amsterdam.
121. Gallo, R.C., Yang, S.S., and Ting, R.C. (1970). RNA dependent DNA polymerase of human acute leukaemic cells. *Nature (London)* **228**, 927.

122. Garapin, A.C., Leong, J., Fanshier, L., Levinson, W.E., and Bishop, J.M. (1971). Identification of virus-specific RNA in cells infected with Rous sarcoma virus. *Biochem. Biophys. Res. Commun.* **42**, 919.
123. Garapin, A., McDonnell, J., Levinson, W., Quintrell, N., Fanshier, L. and Bishop, J.M. (1970). Deoxyribonucleic acid polymerase associated with Rous sarcoma virus and avian myeloblastosis virus: Properties of the enzyme and its product. *J. Virol.* **6**, 589.
124. Garapin, A., Varmus, H., Faras, A., Levinson, W., and Bishop, J. M. (1973). RNA-directed DNA synthesis by virions of Rous sarcoma virus: Further characterization of the templates and the extent of their transcription. *Virology* **52**, 264.
125. Gardner, M., Rongey, R., Arnstein, P., Estecs, J., Sarma, P., Huebner, R., and Rickard, C. (1970). Experimental transmission of feline fibrosarcoma to cats and dogs. *Nature (London)* **226**, 807.
126. Geering, G., Aoki, T., and Old, L. (1970). Shared viral antigen of mammalian leukemia viruses. *Nature (London)* **226**, 265.
127. Gelb, L., Aaronson, S., and Martin, M. (1971). Heterogeneity of murine leukemia virus *in vitro* DNA; detection of viral DNA in mammalian cells. *Science* **172**, 1353.
128. Gianni, A., Smotkin, D., and Weinberg, R. (1975). Murine leukemia virus: Detection of unintegrated double-stranded DNA forms of the provirus. *Proc. Nat. Acad. Sci. U.S.* **71**, 1093.
129. Gielkens, A., Salden, M., and Bloemendal, H. (1974). Virus-specific messenger RNA on free and membrane-bound polyribosomes from cells infected with Rauscher leukemia virus. *Proc. Nat. Acad. Sci. U.S.* **71**, 1093.
130. Gilden, R., Frank, K., Hanson, M., Bladen, S., Toni, R., and Oroszlan, S. (1974). Similarity between gibbon ape and woolly monkey type-C virus internal antigens by quantitative micro-complement fixation. *Intervirology* **2**, 360.
131. Gilden, R., Toni, R., Hanson, M., Bova, D., Charman, H., and Oroszlan, S. (1974). Immunochemical studies of the major internal polypeptide of woolly monkey and gibbon ape type-C viruses. *J. Immunol.* **112**, 1250.
132. Gillespie, D., Gallagher, R.E., Smith, R.G., Saxinger, W.C., and Gallo, R.C. (1974). *Proc. Symp. Fundam. Aspects Neoplasia* (in press).
133. Gillespie, D., and Gallo, R.C. (1975). RNA processing and the origin and evolution of RNA tumor viruses. *Science* **188**, 802.
134. Gillespie, D., Gillespie, S., Gallo, R.C., East, J., and Dmochowski, L. (1973). Genetic origin of RD114 and other RNA tumor viruses assayed by molecular hybridization. *Nature (London), New Biol.* **244**, 51.
135. Gillespie, D., Gillespie, S., and Wong-Staal, F. (1975). RNA-DNA hybridization applied to cancer research; special references to RNA tumor viruses. *Methods Cancer Res.* (in press).
136. Gillespie, D., Marshall, S., and Gallo, R.C. (1972). RNA of RNA tumor viruses contains poly(A). *Nature (London) New Biol.* **236**, 227.
137. Gillespie, D., Saxinger, W.C., East, J.L., Wong-Staal, F., Dmochowski, L., and Gallo, R.C. (1974). Host effects on RNA tumor virus genetic information. *Proc. Nat. Acad. Sci. U.S.* (in press).
138. Gillespie, D., Saxinger, W.C., and Gallo, R.C. Information transfer in cells infected by RNA tumor viruses and extension to human neoplasia. *Progr. Nucleic Acid Res. Mol. Biol.* **15**, 1–108.
139. Goodman, N., and Spiegelman, S. (1971). Distinguishing reverse transcriptase of the RNA tumor viruses from other known DNA polymerases. *Proc. Nat. Acad. Sci. U.S.* **68**, 220.
140. Graffi, A., Bielka, H., Fey, F., Scharsach, F., and Weiss, R. (1955). Gehauffes Auftreten von Leukämien nach Injektion von Sarkom-Filtraten. *Wien. Klin. Wochschr.* **105**, 61.

141. Graham, F., van der Eb, A., and Heijneker, H. (1974). Size and location of the transforming region in human adenovirus DNA. *Nature (London)* **251**, 687.
142. Grandgenett, D., Gerard, G., and Green, M. (1972). Ribonuclease H: An ubiquitous activity in virions of ribonucleic acid tumor viruses. *J. Virol.* **10**, 1136.
143. Green, M., and Cartas, M. (1972). The genome of RNA tumor viruses contains polyadenylic acid sequences. *Proc. Nat. Acad. Sci. U.S.* **69**, 791.
144. Green, M., Rokutanda, M., Fujinaga, K., Ray, R., Rokutanda, H., and Gurgo, K. (1970). Mechanism of carcinogenesis by RNA tumor viruses. I. An RNA-dependent DNA polymerase in murine sarcoma viruses. *Proc. Nat. Acad. Sci. U.S.* **67**, 385.
145. Green, M., Rokutanda, H., and Rokutanda, M. (1971). Virus specific RNA in cells transformed by RNA tumor viruses. *Nature (London), New Biol.* **230**, 229.
146. Gross, L. (1951). "Spontaneous" leukemia developing in C3H mice following inoculation, in infancy, with AK-leukemic extracts, or AK-embryos. *Proc. Soc. Exp. Biol. Med.* **78**, 27.
147. Gross, L. (1970). "Oncogenic Viruses." Pergamon, Oxford.
148. Gulati, S.C., Axel, R., and Spiegelman, S. (1972). Detection of RNA-instructed DNA polymerase and high molecular weight RNA in malignant tissue. *Proc. Nat. Acad. Sci. U.S.* **69**, 2020.
149. Gulati, S., Kacian, D., and Spiegelman, S. (1972). Conditions for using the Kornberg enzyme I as an RNA-dependent DNA polymerase. *Proc. Nat. Acad. Sci. U.S.* **71**, 1035.
150. Guntaka, R., Bishop, J.M., and Varmus, H. (1975). *In* "Fundamental Aspects of Neoplasia" (A. Gottlieb, ed.) Springer-Verlag, Berlin and New York. in press.
151. Guntaka, R., Mahy, B., Bishop, J.M., and Varmus, H.E. (1975). Ethidium bromide inhibits appearance of closed circular viral DNA in duck cells infected by avian sarcoma virus. *Nature (London)* **253**, 507.
152. Gunven, P., Klein, G., Clifford, P., and Singh, S. (1974). Epstein-Barr virus-associated membrane-reactive antibodies during long term survival after Burkitt's lymphoma. *Proc. Nat. Acad. Sci. U.S.* **71**, 1422.
153. Gurgo, C., Ray, R., Thiry, L., and Green, M. (1971). Inhibitors of the RNA and DNA dependent polymerase activities of RNA tumor viruses. *Nature (London)* **229**, 111.
154. Hanafusa, H., and Hanafusa, T. (1971). Noninfectious RSV deficient in DNA polymerase. *Virology* **43**, 313.
155. Harewood, K., Vidrine, J., Carson, D., Wolff, J., Schidlovsky, G., and Mayassi, S. (1973). Biochemical and morphological studies of simian sarcoma virus, type 1. *Biochim. Biophys. Acta* **308**, 252.
156. Hartley, J., and Rowe, W. (1966). Production of altered cell foci in tissue culture by defective Moloney sarcoma virus particles. *Proc. Nat. Acad. Sci. U.S.* **55**, 780.
157. Hartley, J., Rowe, W., Capps, W., and Huebner, R. (1969). Isolation of naturally occurring viruses of the murine leukemia virus group in tissue culture. *J. Virol.* **5**, 221.
158. Harvey, J. (1964). An unidentified virus which causes the rapid production of tumours in mice. *Nature (London)* **204**, 1104.
159. Harvey, J., and East, J. (1969). Biological activity and separation of a leukaemogenic virus from murine sarcoma virus–Harvey (MSV-H). *Int. J. Cancer* **4**, 655.
160. Hatanaka, M., Kakefuda, T., Gilden, R.V., and Callan, E.A.O. (1971). Cytoplasmic DNA synthesis induced by RNA tumor viruses. *Proc. Nat. Acad. Sci. U.S.* **68**, 1844.
161. Hayward, W., and Hanafusa, H. (1971). Detection of avian tumor virus RNA in uninfected chicken embryo cells. *J. Virol.* **11**, 157.
162. Hehlmann, R., Balda, B., and Spiegelman, S. (1975). 70S RNA and reverse transcriptase activity from mouse melanoma. *Int. J. Cancer* (in press).
163. Hehlmann, R., Kufe, D., and Spiegelman, S. (1972). RNA in human leukemic cells related to the RNA of a mouse leukemia virus. *Proc. Nat. Acad. Sci. U.S.* **69**, 435.

164. Hehlmann, R., Kufe, D., and Spiegelman, S. (1972). Viral-related RNA in Hodgkin's disease and other human lymphomas. *Proc. Nat. Acad. Sci. U.S.* **69**, 1727.
165. Hellman, A., Peebles, P., Strickland, J., Fowler, A., Kalter, S., Oroszlan, S., and Gilden, R. (1974). Baboon virus isolate M7 with properties similar to feline virus RD114. *J. Virol.* **14**, 133.
166. Henle, G. and Henle, W. (1966). Immunofluorescence in cells derived from Burkitt's lymphoma. *J. Bacteriol.* **91**, 1248.
167. Henle, G., Henle, W., and Diehl, W. (1968). Relation of Burkitt's tumor associated herpes-type virus to infectious mononucleosis. *Proc. Nat. Acad. Sci. U.S.* **59**, 94.
168. Henle, W., Henle, G., Zajac, B., Pearson, G., Waubke, R. and Scriba, M. (1970). Differential reactivity of human sera with early antigens induced by Epstein-Barr virus. *Science* **169**, 188.
169. Hollinshead, A., Lee, O., McKelway, W., Melnick, J. and Rawls, W. (1972). Reactivity between herpes virus type 2-related soluble cervical tumor cell membrane antigens and matched cancer and control sera. *Proc. Soc. Exp. Biol. Med.* **141**, 688.
170. Hollinshead, A., and Tarro, G. (1973). Soluble membrane antigens of lip and cervical carcinomas: Reactivity with antibody for herpes virus nonvirion antigens. *Science* **179**, 699.
171. Houssaid, J., and Attardi, G. (1966). High molecular weight nonribosomal-type nuclear RNA and cytoplasmic messenger RNA in HeLa cells. *Proc. Nat. Acad. Sci. U.S.* **56**, 616.
172. Huebner, R. (1966). The murine leukemia-sarcoma virus complex. *Proc. Nat. Acad. Sci. U.S.* **58**, 835.
173. Huebner, R., Hartley, J., Rowe, W., Lane, W., and Capps, W. (1967). Rescue of the defective genome of Moloney sarcoma virus from a noninfectious hamster tumor and the production of pseudotype sarcoma viruses with various murine leukemia viruses. *Proc. Nat. Acad. Sci. U.S.* **56**, 1164.
174. Hunsmann, G., Moennig, V., Pister, L., Siefert, E., and Schafer, W. (1974). Properties of mouse leukemia viruses. *Virology* **62**, 307.
175. Hurwitz, S., and Leis, J. (1972). RNA-dependent DNA polymerase activity of RNA tumor viruses. I. Directing influence of DNA in the reaction. *J. Virol.* 9:116.
176. Jarrett, O., Pitts, J., Whalley, J., Clason, A., and Hay, J. (1971). Isolation of the nucleic acid of feline leukemia virus. *Virology* **43**, 317.
177. Jarrett, W. (1971). Feline leukemia. *Int. Rev. Exp. Pathol.* **10**, 243.
178. Jarrett, W., Crawford, E., Martin, W., and Davie, F. (1964). Leukemia in the cat. A virus-like particle associated with leukaemia (lymphosarcoma). *Nature (London)* **202**, 567.
179. Jarrett, W., Essex, M., Mackey, L., Jarrett, O., and Laird, H. (1973). Antibodies in normal and leukemic cats to feline oncornavirus-associated cell membrane antigens. *J. Nat. Cancer Inst.* **51**, 261.
180. Jarrett, W., Jarrett, O., Mackey, L., Laird, H., Hardy, W., and Essex, M. (1973). Horizontal transmission of leukemia virus and leukemia in the cat. *J. Nat. Cancer Inst.* **51**, 833.
181. Jarrett, W., Martin, B., Crighton, W., Dalton, R., and Stewart, M. (1964). Leukemia in the cat. Transmission experiments with leukemia (lymphosarcoma). *Nature (London)* 202:566.
182. Jelinek, W., Adesnik, M., Salditt, M., Sheiness, D., Wall, R., Molloy, G., Philipson, L., and Darnell, J. (1973). Further evidence on the nuclear origin and transfer to the cytoplasm of polyadenylic acid sequences in mammalian cell RNA. *J. Mol. Biol.* **75**, 515.
183. Jensen, E., Zelljadt, I., Chopra, H., and Mason, M. (1970). Isolation and propagation of

a new virus from a spontaneous mammary carcinoma of a rhesus monkey. *Cancer Res.* **30**, 2388.
184. Johnson, D., Wooding, W., Tonticharoenyos, P., and Bourgeois, C. (1971). Malignant lymphoma in the gibbon. *J. Amer. Vet. Med. Ass.* **159**, 563.
185. Josey, W., Nahmias, A., and Naib, Z. (1968). Genital infection with type 2 herpesvirus homines: present knowledge and possible relationship to cervical cancer. *Amer. J. Obstet. Gynecol.* **101**, 718.
186. Kacian, D., Watson, K., Burny, A., and Spiegelman, S. (1971). Purification of the DNA polymerase of avian myeloblastosis virus. *Biochim. Biophys. Acta* **246**, 365.
187. Kakefuda, T., and Bader, J. (1969). Electron microscopic observations on the ribonucleic acid of murine leukemia virus. *J. Virol.* **4**, 460.
188. Kalter, S., Helmke, R., Heberling, R., Panigel, M., Fowler, A., Strickland, J., and Hellman, A. (1973). C-type particles in normal human placentas. *J. Nat. Cancer Inst.* **50**, 1081.
189. Kalter, S., Helmke, R., Panigel, M., Heberling, R., Felsburg, P., and Axelrad, L. (1972). Observations of apparent C-type particles in baboon (*Papio cynocephalus*) placenta. *Science* **182**, 1151.
190. Kang, C., and Temin, H. (1972). Endogenous RNA-directed DNA polymerase activity in uninfected chicken embryos. *Proc. Nat. Acad. Sci. U.S.* **69**, 1550.
191. Kawai, Y., Nonoyama, M., and Pagano, J. (1973). Reassociation kinetics for Epstein-Barr virus DNA. Nonhomology to mammalian DNA and homology of viral DNA in various diseases. *J. Virol.* **12**, 1006.
192. Kawakami, T., Buckley, P., McDowell, Y., and DePaoli, A. (1973). Antibodies to simian C-type virus antigen in sera of gibbons (*Hylobates sp.*). *Nature (London) New Biol.* **246**, 105.
193. Kawakami, T., Huff, S., Buckely, P., Dungworth, D., Snyder, S., and Gilden, R. (1972). C-type virus associated with gibbon lymphosarcoma. *Nature (London), New Biol.* **235**, 170.
194. Kawakami, T., Theilen, G., Dungworth, D., Beall, S., and Munn, R. (1967). "C"-type viral particles in plasma of feline leukemia. *Science* **158**, 1049.
195. Kawakami, T. (1975). Personal communication.
196. Kirsten, W., Somers, K., and Mayer, L. (1968). Multiplicity of cell response to a murine erythroblastosis virus. *Proc. 3rd Int. Symp. Comp. Leukemia Res., 1967*, Bibl. Haematol. No. 30.
197. Kirsten, W., and Mayer, L. (1967). Morphologic responses to a murine erythroblastosis virus. *J. Nat. Cancer Inst.* **39**, 311.
198. Kirsten, W., Mayer, L., Wollman, R., and Pierce, M. (1967). Studies on a murine erythroblastosis virus. *J. Nat. Cancer Inst.* **38**, 117.
199. Klein, G., Clifford, P., Klein, E., Smith, R.T., Minowada, J., Kourilsky, K., and Burchenal, J. (1967). Membrane immunofluorescence reactions of Burkitt's lymphoma cells from biopsy specimens and tissue cultures. *J. Nat. Cancer Inst.* **39**, 1027.
200. Klein, G., Giovanella, B., Lindahl, T., Fialkow, P., Singh, S., and Stehlin, J. (1974). Direct evidence for the presence of Epstein-Barr virus DNA and nuclear antigen in malignant epithelial cells from patients with poorly differentiated carcinoma of the nasopharynx. *Proc. Nat. Acad. Sci. U.S.* **71**, 4737.
201. Klein, G., Pearson, G., Nadkarni, J.S., Nadkarni, J.J., Klein, E., Henle, G., Henle, W., and Clifford, P. (1968). Relation between Epstein-Barr viral and cell membrane immunofluorescence of Burkitt tumor cells. I. Dependence of cell membrane immunofluorescence on presence of EB virus. *J. Exp. Med.* **128**, 1011.
202. Kotler, M., Haspel, O., and Becker, Y. (1974). dsDNA made by RNase-sensitive DNA polymerase from RSV-transformed cells. *Nature (London)* **249**, 441.

203. Kramarsky, B. Sarkan, N., and Moore, D. (1971). Ultrastructural comparison of a virus from a rhesus-monkey mammary carcinoma with four oncogenic RNA viruses. *Proc. Nat. Acad. Sci. U.S.* **68**, 1603.
204. Kufe, D., Hehlmann, R., and Spiegelman, S. (1972). Human sarcomas contain RNA related to the RNA of a mouse leukemia virus. *Science* **175**, 182.
205. Kufe, D., Hehlmann, R., and Spiegelman, S. (1973). RNA related to that of a mouse leukemia virus in Burkitt's tumors and nasopharyngeal carcinomas. *Proc. Nat. Acad. Sci. U.S.* **70**, 5.
206. Kufe, D., Magrath, I., Ziegler, J., and Spiegelman, S. (1973). Burkitt's tumors contain particles encapsulating RNA-instructed DNA polymerase and high molecular weight virus-related RNA. *Proc. Nat. Acad. Sci. U.S.* **70**, 737.
207. Kufe, D., Peters, W., and Spiegelman, S. (1973). Unique nuclear DNA sequences in the involved tissues of Hodgkin's and Burkitt's lymphomas. *Proc. Nat. Acad. Sci. U.S.* **70**, 3810.
208. Lai, M.M.C., and Duesberg, P. (1972). Adenylic acid-rich sequence in RNA's of Rous sarcoma virus and Rauscher mouse leukemia virus. *Nature (London)* **235**, 383.
209. Laird, H., Jarrett, O., Crighton, G., and Jarrett, W. (1968). An electron microscopic study of virus particles in spontaneous leukemia in the cat. *J. Nat. Caccer Inst.* **41**, 867.
210. Leis, J., and Hurwitz, J. (1972). RNA dependent DNA polymerase activity of RNA tumor viruses. II. Directing influence of RNA in the reaction. *J. Virol.* **9**, 130.
211. Leong, J., Garapin, A., Jackson, N., Fanshier, L., Levinson, W., and Bishop, J.M. (1972). Virus-specific ribonucleic acid in cells producing Rous sarcoma virus. *J. Virol.* **9**, 891.
212. Levine, P., Ablashi, D., Bernard, G., Carbone, P., Wiggoner, D., and Malan, L. (1971). Elevated antibody titers to Epstein-Barr virus in Hodgkin's disease. *Cancer* **27**, 416.
213. Levine, P., O'Connor, G., and Bernard, C. (1972). Antibodies to Epstein-Barr virus (EBV) in American patients with Burkitt's lymphoma. *Cancer* **30**, 601.
214. Levy, J. (1973). Xenotropic viruses: murine leukemia virus associated with NIH Swiss, NZB, and other strains. *Science* **182**, 1151.
215. Levy, J. (1975). Host range of murine xenotropic virus: replication of avian cells. *Nature (London)* **253**, 140.
216. Levy, J., and Pincus, T. (1970). Demonstration of biological activity of a murine leukemia virus of New Zealand black mice. *Science* **170**, 326.
217. Lewis, B., Abrell, J., Smith, R.G., and Gallo, R.C. (1974). DNA polymerases in human lymphoblastoid cell lines infected with simian sarcoma virus. *Biochim. Biophys. Acta* **349**, 148.
218. Lewis, B., Abrell, J., Smith, R.G., and Gallo, R.C. (1974). Human DNA polymerase III (R-DNA polymerase): Distinction from DNA polymerase I and reverse transcriptase. *Science* **183**, 867.
219. Lindahl, T., Klein, G., Reedman, E., Johansson, B., and Singh, S. (1974). Relationship between Epstein-Barr virus (EBV) and the EBV-determined nuclear antigen (EBNA) in Burkitt's lymphoma biopsies and other lymphoproliferative malignancies *Int. J. Cancer* **13**, 764.
220. Livingston, D., and Todaro, G. (1973). Endogenous type-C virus from a cat cell clone with properties distinct from previously described feline type-C viruses. *Virology* **53**, 142.
221. Loeb. L. Tartof, K., and Travagline, E. (1973). Copying natural RNA's with *E. coli* DNA polymerase I. *Nature (London), New Biol.* **242**, 66.
222. Long, C., Sachs, R., Novell, J., Huebner, R., Hatanaka, M., and Gilden, R. (1973). Specificity of antibody to RD114 viral polymerase. *Nature (London), New Biol.* **241**, 147.

223. Maia, J., Rougeon, F., and Chapeville, F. (1971). Chick embryo poly (rA:dT)-dependent DNA polymerase. *FEBS Lett.* **18**, 130.
224. Mak, T., Kurtz, S., Manaster, J., and Housman, D. (1975). Viral-related information in oncornavirus-like particles isolated from cultures of marrow cells from leukemic patients in relapse and remission. *Proc. Nat. Acad. Sci. U.S.* **72**, 623.
225. Mak, T., Manaster, J., Howatson, A., McCulloch, E., and Till, J. (1974). Particles with characteristics of leukoviruses in cultures of marrow cells from leukemic patients in remission and relapse. *Proc. Nat. Acad. Sci. U.S.* **71**, 4336.
226. Mangel, W., Delius, H., and Duesberg, P. (1974). Structure and molecular weight of the 60–70S RNA and the 30–40S RNA of the Rous sarcoma virus. *Proc. Nat. Acad. Sci. U.S.* **71**, 4541.
227. Manly, K., Smoler, D., Bromfeld, E., and Baltimore, D. (1971). Forms of deoxyribonucleic acid produced by virions of the ribonucleic acid tumor viruses. *J. Virol.* **7**, 106.
228. Markham, P., and Baluda, M. (1973) The integrated state of oncornavirus DNA in normal chicken cells and in cells transformed by avian myeloblastosis virus. *J. Virol.* **12**, 721.
229. Mayer, R.J., Smith, R.G., and Gallo, R.C. (1974). Reverse transcriptase in normal rhesus monkey placenta. *Science* **185**, 864.
230. McAllister, R.O., Nicholson, M., Gardner, M., Rongey, R., Rasheed, S., Sarma, P., Huebner, R., Hatanaka, M., Oroszlan, S., Gilden, R., Kabigting, A., and Vernon, L. (1972). C-type virus released from cultured human rhabdomyosarcoma cells. *Nature (London) New Biol.* **235**, 3.
231. McCain, B., Biswal, N., and Benyesh-Melnick, M. (1973). The subunits of murine sarcoma-leukemia virus RNA. *J. Gen. Virol.* **18**, 69.
232. McDonnell, J., Garapin, A., Levinson, A., Quintrell, W., Fanshier, L., and Bishop, J.M. (1970). DNA polymerases of Rous sarcoma viruses: Delineation of two reactions with actinomycin. *Nature (London)* **228**, 433.
233. Mendecki, J., Lee, Y., and Brawerman, G. (1972). Characteristics of the polyadenylic acid segment associated with messenger ribonucleic acid in mouse sarcoma 180 ascites cells. *Biochemistry* **11**, 792.
234. Miller, N.R., Saxinger, W.C., Reitz, M.S., Gallagher, R.E., Wu, A.M., Gallo, R.C., and Gillespie, D. (1974). Systematics of RNA tumor viruses and virus-like particles of human origin. *Proc. Nat. Acad. Sci. U.S.* **71**, 3177.
235. Minowada, J., Nonoyama, M., Moore, G., Rauch, A., and Pagano, J. (1974). The presence of the Epstein-Barr viral genome in human lymphoblastoid B-cell lines and its absence in a myeloma cell line. *Cancer Res.* **34**, 1898.
236. Mizutani, S., and Temin, H. (1973). Specific serological relationships among partially purified DNA polymerases of avian leukosis-sarcoma viruses, reticuloendotheliosis virus, and avian cells. *J. Virol.* **13**, 1020.
237. Modak, M., Marcus, S., and Cavaliere, L. (1974). Synthesis of DNA complimentary to AMV RNA using *E. coli* polymerase I. *Biochem. Biophys. Res. Commun.* **56**, 247.
238. Moloney, J. (1960). Biological studies on a lymphoid leukemia virus extracted from sarcoma S. 37. I. Origin and introductory investigations. *J. Nat. Cancer Inst.* **24**, 933.
239. Moloney, J. (1966). A virus-induced rhabdomyosarcoma of mice. *Nat. Cancer Inst. Monogr.* **22**, 139–142.
240. Mondal, H., Gallagher, R.E., and Gallo, R.C. RNA-Directed DNA polymerase from human leukemic blood cells and from primate type-C virus-producing cells: High and low molecular weight forms with variant biochemical and immunological properties. *Proc. Nat. Acad. Sci. U.S.* **72**, 1194.
241. Nahmias, A., Josey, W., Naib, E., Luce, C., and Guest, B. (1970). Antibodies to herpesvirus hominis types 1 and 2 in humans: II. Women with cervical cancer. *Amer. J. Epidemiol.* **91**, 547.

242. Nahmias, A., Condon, W., Catalano, L., Fuccillo, D., Sever, J., and Graham, C. (1971). Genital herpesvirus hominis type 2 infection: an experimental model in Cebus monkeys. *Science* **171**, 297.
243. Nahmias, A., Naib, Z., and Josey, W. (1969). Herpesvirus hominis type 2 infection: Association with cervical cancer and perinatal disease. *Perspect. Virol.* **8**.
244. Naib, Z., Nahmias, A., Josey, W., and Kramer, J. (1969). Genital herpetic infection: Association with cervical dysplasia and carcinoma. *Cancer* **23**, 940.
245. Nathins, A., Mergenhagen, S., and Howard, R. (1970). Effect of virus infections on the function of the immune system. *Annu. Rev. Microbiol.* **24**, 525.
246. Nayak, D., Murray, P., and Goldblatt, D. (1974). Endogenous guinea pig virus: Equability of virus-specific DNA in normal, leukemic, and virus-producing cells. *Proc. Nat. Acad. Sci. U.S.* **71**, 1164.
247. Nieman, P. (1972). Rous sarcoma virus nucleotide sequences in cellular DNA. *Science* **178**, 750.
248. Nieman, P. (1973). Measurement of RD114 virus nucleotide sequences in feline cellular DNA. *Nature (London), New Biol.* **244**, 62.
249. Nieman, P., Wright, S., McMillin, S., and MacDonnell, P. (1974). Nucleotide sequence relationships of avian RNA tumor viruses. *J. Virol.* **13**, 837.
250. Neubort, S., and Bases, R. (1974). RNA-DNA covalent complexes in HeLa cells. *Biochim. Biophys. Acta* **340**, 31.
251. Nonoyama, M., Huang, C., Pagano, J., Klein, G., and Singh, S. (1973). DNA of Epstein-Barr virus detected in tissue of Burkitt's lymphoma and nasopharyngeal carcinoma. *Proc. Nat. Acad. Sci. U.S.* **70**, 3265.
252. Nonoyama, M., and Pagano, J. (1973). Homology between Epstein-Barr virus DNA and DNA from Burkitt's lymphoma and nasopharyngeal carcinoma determined by DNA-DNA reassociation kinetics. *Nature (London)* **242**, 44.
253. Nowinski, R., Old, L., Sarkar, N., and Moore, D. (1970). Common properties of the oncogenic RNA viruses (oncornaviruses). *Virology* **42**, 1152.
254. Okabe, H., Gilden, R., and Hatanaka, M. (1973). Extensive homology of RD114 virus DNA with RNA of feline cell origin. *Nature (London), New Biol.* **244**, 54.
255. Okabe, H., Loringer, G., Gilden, R., and Hatanaka, M. (1972). The nucleotides at the RNA-DNA joint formed by the DNA polymerase of Rauscher leukemia virus. *Virology* **50**, 935.
256. Old, L., Boyse, E., Oettgen, H., de Harven, E., Geering, G., Williamson, B., and Clifford, P. (1966). Precipitating antibody in human serum to an antigen present in cultured Burkitt's lymphoma cells. *Proc. Nat. Acad. Sci. U.S.* **56**, 1699.
257. Old, L., Boyse, E., and Stockert, E. (1964). Typing of mouse leukemias by serological methods. *Nature (London)* **201**, 777.
258. Oroszlan, S., Copeland, T., Summers, M., and Gilden, R. (1972). Amino terminal sequences of mammalian type-C RNA tumor virus group-specific antigens. *Biochem. Biophys. Res. Commun.* **48**, 1549.
259. Oroszlan, S., Fisher, C., Stanley, T., and Gilden, R. (1970). Proteins of the murine C-type RNA tumor viruses: Isolation of a group-specific antigen by isoelectric focusing. *J. Gen. Virol.* **8**, 1.
260. Oroszlan, S., Foreman, C., Kelloff, G., and Gilden, R. (1971). The group specific antigen and other structural proteins of hamster and mouse C-type viruses. *Virology* **43**, 655.
261. Oroszlan, S., Hatanaka, M., Gilden, R., and Huebner, R. (1971). Specific inhibition of mammalian ribonucleic acid C-type virus deoxyribonucleic acid polymerases by rat antisera. *J. Virol.* **8**, 816.
262. Pagano, J. Personal communication (1974); Zur Hausen, H., Schulte-Holthausen, H., Wolf, H., Dörries, K., and Egger, H. (1974). Attempts to detect virus-specific DNA in

human tumors. II. Nucleic acid hybrizations with complementary RNA of human herpes group viruses. *Int. J. Cancer* **13**, 657.
263. Pagano, J., Huang, C., and Levine, P. (1973). Absence of Epstein-Barr viral DNA in American Burkitt's lymphoma. *N. Engl. J. Med.* **289**, 1395.
264. Page, A. and Oman, D. (1974). Identification of a polypeptide DNA polymerase inhibitor responsible for ribonuclease inhibition of an endogenous DNA polymerase reaction. *Biochem. Biophys. Res. Commun.* **61**, 1213.
265. Parks, W., Scolnick, E., Noon, M., Watson, C., and Kawakami, T. (1973). Radioimmunoassay of mammalian type-C polypeptides. IV. Characterization of woolly monkey and gibbon viral antigens. *Int. J. Cancer* **12**, 129.
266. Parks, W., Scolnick, E., Ross, J., Todaro, G., and Aaronson, S. (1972). Immunological relationships of reverse transcriptase from ribonucleic acid tumor viruses *J. Virol.* **9**, 110.
267. Peters, W., Kufe, D., Schlom, J., Frankel, J., Groupe, V., and Spiegelman, S. (1973). Biological and biochemical evidence for an interaction between Marek's disease herpesvirus and avian leukosis virus *in vivo. Proc. Nat. Acad. Sci. U.S.* **70**, 3175.
268. Rangan, S. (1974). Antigenic relatedness of simian C-type viruses. *Int. J. Cancer* **13**, 64.
269. Rauscher, F. (1962). A virus-induced disease of mice characterized by erythrocytopoiesis and lymphoid leukemia. *J. Nat. Cancer Inst.* **29**, 515.
270. Rawls, W., Gardner, A., and Kaufman, R. (1970). Antibodies to genital herpesvirus in patients with carcinoma of the cervix. *Amer. J. Obstet. Gynecol.* **107**, 760.
271. Rawls, W., Tomkins, W., and Melnick, J. (1969). The association of herpesvirus type 2 and carcinoma of the cervix. *Amer. J. Epidemiol.* **89**, 547.
272. Reedman, B., and Klein, G. (1973). Cellular localization of an Epstein-Barr virus (EBV)-associated complement-fixing antigen in producer and non-producer cell lines. *Int. J. Cancer* **11**, 499.
273. Reedman, B., Klein, G., Pope, J., Walters, M., Hilgers, I., Singh, S., and Johansson, B. (1974). Epstein-Barr virus-associated complement fixing and nuclear antigens in Burkitt's lymphoma biopsies. *Int. J. Cancer* **13**, 755.
274. Reitz, M., Gillespie, D., Saxinger, W.C., Robert, M., and Gallo, R.C. (1974). Poly (rA) tracts of tumor virus 70S RNA are not transcribed in endogenous or reconstituted reactions of viral reverse transcriptase. *Biochem. Biophys. Res. Commun.* **49**, 1216.
275. Reitz, M.S., Smith, R.G., Roseberry, E.A., and Gallo, R.C. (1974). DNA-directed and RNA-primed DNA synthesis in microsomal and mitochondrial fractions of normal human lymphocytes. *Biochem. Biophys. Res. Commun.* **57**, 934.
276. Rho, H., and Green, M. (1974). The homopolyadenylate and adjacent nucleotides at the 3'-terminus of 30–40S RNA subunits of the genome of murine sarcoma-leukemia virus. *Proc. Nat. Acad. Sci. U.S.* **71**, 2386.
277. Rickard, C., Barr, L., Noronha, F., Dougherty, E., 3rd., and Post, J. (1967). C-type virus particles in spontaneous lymphocytic leukemia in a cat. *Cornell Vet.* **57**, 302.
278. Rickard, C., Gillespie, J., Lee, F., Noronha, F., Post, J., and Salvage, E. (1968). Transmission and electron microscopy of lymphocytic leukemia in the cat. *Proc. 3rd Int. Symp. Comp. Leukemia Res., 1967*, pp. 282–284.
279. Rickard, C.G., Post, J., Noronha, F., and Barr, L. (1969). A transmissable virus-induced lymphocytic leukemia in the cat. *J. Nat. Cancer Inst.* **42**, 987.
280. Robert, M.S., Smith, R.G., Gallo, R.C., Sarin, P.S., and Abrell, J.W. (1972). Viral and cellular DNA polymerase: Comparison of activities with synthetic and natural RNA templates. *Science* **176**, 798.
281. Robinson, W., and Baluda, M. (1965). The nucleic acid from avian myeloblastosis virus compared with RNA from the Bryan strain of Rous sarcoma virus. *Proc. Nat. Acad. Sci. U.S.* **54**, 1686.

282. Robinson, W., Pitkanen, A., and Rubin, H. (1965). The nucleic acid of the Bryan strain of Rous sarcoma virus: Purification of the virus and isolation of the nucleic acid. *Proc. Nat. Acad. Sci. U.S.* **54**, 137.
283. Robinson, W., Robinson, H., and Duesberg, P. (1967). Tumors virus RNA's. *Proc. Nat. Acad. Sci. U.S.* **58**, 825.
284. Rokutanda, M., Rokutanda, H., Green, M., Fujinaga, K., Ray, R., and Gurgo, C. (1970). Formation of viral RNA-DNA hybrid molecules by the DNA polymerase of sarcoma-leukemia viruses. *Nature (London)* **227**, 1026.
285. Rosenthal, P., Robinson, H., Robinson, W., Hanafusa, T., and Hanafusa, H. (1971). DNA in uninfected and virus-infected cells complementary to avian tumor virus RNA. *Proc. Nat. Acad. Sci. U.S.* **68**, 2336.
286. Ross, J., Scolnick, E., Todaro, G., and Aaronson, S. (1971). Separation of murine cellular and murine leukemia virus DNA polymerases. *Nature (London), New Biol.* **231**, 163.
287. Ross, J., Tronick, S., and Scolnick, E. (1972). Polyadenylate rich RNA in the 70S RNA of murine leukemia-sarcoma virus. *Virology* **49**, 230.
288. Rous, P. (1911). Transmission of a malignant new growth by means of a cell-free filtrate. *J. Amer. Med. Ass.* **56**, 198.
289. Royston, I., and Aurelian, L. (1970). Immunofluorescent detection of herpesvirus antigens in exfoliated cells from human cervical carcinoma. *Proc. Nat. Acad. Sci. U.S.* **67**, 204.
290. Ruprecht, R., Goodman, N., and Spiegelman, S. (1973). Determination of natural host taxonomy of RNA tumor viruses by molecular hybridization: application to RD-114, a candidate human virus. *Proc. Nat. Acad. Sci. U.S.* **70**, 1437.
291. Sabin, A. (1974). Herpes simplex-genitalis virus nonvirion antigens and their implication in certain human cancers: unconfirmed. *Proc. Nat. Acad. Sci. U.S.* **71**, 3284.
292. Sabin, A., and Tarro, G. (1973). Herpes simplex and herpes genitalis viruses in etiology of some human cancers. *Proc. Nat. Acad. Sci. U.S.* **70**, 3225.
293. Sarin, P.S., Abrell, J.W., and Gallo, R.C. (1974). Comparison of biochemical characterviruses. In "Control of Transcription" (B. Biswas, R. Mandal, A. Stevens, and W. Cohn, eds.), pp. 345–354. Plenum Press, New York.
294. Sarin, P.S., and Gallo, R.C. (1973). Characteristics of reverse transcriptase from human acute leukemic cells and RNA tumor viruses. *Int. Res. Commun. System* **1**, 52.
295. Sarin, P.S., and Gallo, R.C. (1974). RNA directed DNA polymerase. In "International Review of Science" (K. Burton, ed.), Vol. 6. Chapter 8, Butterworth, London, and Med. and Tech. Publ., Oxford.
296. Sarin, P.S., and Gallo, R.C. (1975). Purification and properties of gibbon ape (*Hylobates lar*) virus DNA polymerase (in preparation).
297. Sarin, P.S., Reitz, M.S., and Gallo, R.C. (1974). Transcription of heteropolymeric regions of avian myeloblastosis virus high molecular weight RNA with *E. coli* DNA polymerase I. *Biochem. Biophys. Res. Commun.* **59**, 202.
298. Sarma, P., Gilden, R., and Huebner, R. (1971). Complement fixation test for feline leukemia and sarcoma viruses (the COCAL test). *Virology* **44**, 137.
299. Sarma, P., Tieng, J., Lee, Y., and Gilden, R.V. (1973). Virus similar to RD114 virus in cat cells. *Nature (London), New Biol.* **244**, 56.
300. Sarngadharan, M.G., Sarin, P.S., Reitz, M.S., and Gallo, R.C. (1972). Reverse transcriptase activity of human acute leukemic cells: Purification of the enzyme, response to AMV 70S RNA, and characterization of the DNA product. *Nature (London), New Biol.* **240**, 67.
301. Saxinger, W.C., Ponnamperuma, C., and Gillespie, D. (1972). Nucleic acid hybridization with RNA immobilized on filter paper. *Proc. Nat. Acad. Sci. U.S.* **69**, 2975.
302. Schafer, W., Fischinger, P., Lange, J., and Pister, L. (1972). Properties of mouse

leukemia viruses: 1. Characterization of various antisera and serological identification of viral components. *Virology* **47**, 197.
303. Schafer, W., Pister, L., Hunsmann, G., and Moennig, V. (1973). Comparative serological studies on type C viruses of various mammals. *Nature (London), New Biol.* **245**, 75.
304. Scherrer, K., Marcaud, L., Zajdela, F., London, I., and Gros, F. (1966). Patterns of RNA metabolism in a differentiated cell: A rapidly labeled unstable 60S RNA with messenger properties in duck erythroblasts. *Proc. Nat. Acad. Sci. U.S.* **56**, 1571.
305. Schidlovsky, G., and Ahmed, M. (1973). C-type virus particles in placentas and fetal tissues of rhesus monkeys. *J. Nat. Cancer Inst.* **51**, 225.
306. Schlom, J. (1974). Personal communication.
307. Schlom, J., Colcher, D., Spiegelman, S., Gillespie, S., and Gillespie, D. (1973). Quantitation of RNA tumor viruses and virus-like particles in milk by hybridization to polyadenylic acid sequences. *Science* **179**, 696.
308. Schlom, J., and Spiegelman, S. (1971). Simultaneous detection of reverse transcriptase and high molecular weight RNA unique to oncogenic RNA viruses. *Science* **174**, 840.
309. Schlom, J., Spiegelman, S., and Moore, D. (1971). RNA-dependent DNA polymerase activity in virus-like particle isolated from human milk. *Nature (London)* **235**, 32. (231–91).
310. Schlom, J., Spiegelman, S., and Moore, D. (1972). Detection of high molecular weight RNA in particles from human milk. *Science* **175**, 542.
311. Scolnick, E., Parks, W., Kawakami, T., Kohne, D., Okabe, H., Gilden, R., and Hatanaka, M. (1974). Primate type-C viral nucleic acid association kinetics: Analysis of model systems and natural tissues. *J. Virol.* **13**, 363.
312. Scolnick, E., Parks, W., and Todaro, G. (1972). Reverse transcriptases of primate viruses as immunological markers. *Science* **177**, 1119.
313. Scolnick, E., Parks, W., Todaro, G., and Aaronson, S. (1972). Immunological characterization of primate C-type virus reverse transcriptase. *Nature (London), New Biol.* **235**, 35.
314. Scolnick, E., Rands, E., Williams, D., and Parks, W. (1973). Studies on the nucleic acid sequences of Kirsten sarcoma virus: A model for formation of a mammalian RNA-containing sarcoma virus. *J. Virol.* **12**, 458.
315. Shanmugan, G., Veccio, G., Ahardi, D., and Green, M. (1972). Immunological studies on viral polypeptide synthesis in cells replicating murine sarcoma leukemia virus. *J. Virol.* **13**, 447.
316. Sharp, D., and Beard, J. (1954). Virions of avian erythromyeloblastic virus IV. Sedimentation, density, and hydration. *Biochim. Biophys. Acta* **304**, 1.
317. Sharp, P., Pettersson, V., and Sambrook, J. (1974). Viral DNA in Transformed Cells. I. A study of the sequences of adenovirus 2 DNA in a line of transformed rat cells using specific fragments of the viral genome. *J. Mol. Biol.* **86**, 709.
318. Sherr, C., Benveniste, R., and Todaro, G. (1974). Type-C viral expression in primate tissues. *Proc. Nat. Acad. Sci. U.S.* **71**, 3721.
319. Sherr, C., Lieber, M., Benveniste, R., and Todaro, G. (1974). Endogenous baboon type C virus (M7): Biochemical and immunologic characterization. *Virology* **58**, 476.
320. Sherr, C., and Todaro, G. (1974). Type-C viral antigens in man. I. Antigens related to endogenous primate virus in human tumors. *Proc. Nat. Acad. Sci. U.S.* **71**, 4703.
321. Sherr, C., and Todaro, G. (1975). Primate type-C virus p 30 antigen in cells from humans with acute leukemia. *Science* **187**, 855.
322. Smith, R.G., Abrell, J.W., Lewis, B.J., and Gallo, R.C. (1975). Serologic analysis of human DNA polymerases. *J. Biol. Chem.* **250**, 1702.
323. Smith, R.G., and Gallo, R.C. (1972). DNA-dependent DNA polymerase I and II from normal human blood lymphocytes. *Proc. Nat. Acad. Sci. U.S.* **69**, 2879.

324. Snyder, S., and Theilen, G. (1969). Transmissable feline fibrosarcoma. *Nature (London)* **221**, 1074.
325. Soeiro, R., Birnboim, H., and Darnell, J. (1966). Rapidly labelled HeLa cell RNA. II. Base composition and cellular localization of a heterogeneous RNA fraction. *J. Mol. Biol.* **19**, 362.
326. Solomon, J., Witter, R., Nazerian, K., and Burmester, B. (1968). Studies on the etiology of Marek's disease. I. Propagation of the agent in cell culture. *Proc. Soc. Exp. Biol. Med.* **127**, 173.
327. Spiegelman, S., Burny, A., Das, M., Keydar, J., Schlom, J., Travnicek, N., and Watson, K. (1970). RNA directed DNA polymerase activity in oncogenic RNA viruses. *Nature (London)* **227**, 1029.
328. Springgate, C., Battula, N., and Loeb, L. (1973). Infidelity of DNA synthesis by reverse transcriptase. *Biochem. Biophys. Res. Commun.* **52**, 49.
329. Stephenson, M., Scott, J., and Zamecnik, P. (1973). Evidence that the polyadenylic acid segment of "35 S" RNA of avian myeloblastosis virus is located at the 3'-OH terminus. *Biochem. Biophys. Res. Commun.* **55**, 8.
330. Strand, M., and August, J.T. (1973). Structural proteins of oncogenic ribonucleic acid viruses. *J. Biol. Chem.* **248**, 5627.
331. Strand, M., and August, J.T. (1974). Structural proteins of mammalian oncogenic viruses: Multiple antigenic determinants of the major internal protein and envelope glycoproteins. *J. Virol.* **13**, 171.
332. Strand, M. and August, T. (1974). Type C-virus expression in human tissue. *J. Virol.* **14**, 1584.
333. Strickland, J., Fowler, A., Kind, P., Hellman, A., Kalter, S., Heberling, R., and Helmke, R. (1973). Group specific antigen and RNA-directed DNA polymerase activity in normal baboon placenta. *Proc. Soc. Exp. Biol. Med.* **144**, 256.
334. Stromberg, K. (1972). Surface-active agents for isolation of the core component of avian myeloblastosis virus. *J. Virol.* **9**, 684.
335. Sugino, A., Hirose, S., and Okazaki, R. (1972). RNA-linked nascent DNA fragments in *Escherichia coli*. *Proc. Nat. Acad. Sci. U.S.* **69**, 863.
336. Sugino, A., and Okazaki, R. (1973). RNA-linked DNA fragments *in vitro*. *Proc. Nat. Acad. Sci. U.S.* **70**, 88.
337. Sweet, R., Goodman, N., Cho, J.-R., Ruprecht, R., Redfield, R., and Spiegelman, S. (1974). The presence of unique DNA sequences after viral induction of leukemia in mice. *Proc. Nat. Acad. Sci. U.S.* **71**, 1705.
338. Tarro, G., and Sabin, A. (1973). Nonvirion antigens produced by herpes simplex viruses 1 and 2. *Proc. Nat. Acad. Sci. U.S.* **70**, 1032.
339. Tavitian, A., Hamelin, R., Tchen, P., Olafsson, B., and Boiron, M. (1974). Extent of transcription of mouse sarcoma-leukemia virus by RNA-directed DNA polymerase. *Proc. Nat. Acad. Sci. U.S.* **71**, 755.
340. Taylor, T., Faras, A., Varmus, H., Levinson, W., and Bishop, J. (1972). RNA-directed DNA synthesis by the purified DNA polymerase of Rous sarcoma virus: Characterization of the enzymatic product. *Biochemistry* **11**, 2343.
341. Temin, H. (1962). Separation of morphological conversion and virus production in Rous sarcoma virus infection. *Cold Spring Harbor Symp. Quant. Biol.* **27**, 407.
342. Temin, H. (1964). Homology between RNA from Rous sarcoma virus and DNA from Rous sarcoma virus-infected cells. *Proc. Nat. Acad. Sci. U.S.* **52**, 323.
343. Temin, H. (1971). The proto virus hypothesis: Speculations on the significance of RNA-directed DNA synthesis for normal development and for carcino-genesis. *J. Nat. Cancer Inst.* **46**, III–VII.

344. Temin, H. (1974). The cellular and molecular biology of RNA tumor viruses especially avian leukosis-sarcoma viruses, and their relatives. *Advan. Cancer Res.* **19**, 47–104.
345. Temin, H., and Mizutani, S. (1970). RNA-dependent DNA polymerase in virions of Rouse sarcoma virus. *Nature (London)* **226**, 1211.
346. Theilen, G., Gould, D., Fowler, M., and Dungworth, D. (1971). C-type virus in tumor tissue of a woolly monkey (*Lagothrix*) with fibrosarcoma. *J. Nat. Cancer Inst.* **47**, 881.
347. Ting, R.C., Yang, S.S., and Gallo, R.C. (1972). Reverse transcriptase, RNA tumor virus transformation and derivatives of rifamycin SV. *Nature (London), New Biol.* **236**, 163.
348. Todaro, G., Benveniste, R., Lieber, M., and Scherr, C. (1974). Characterization of a type-C virus released from the procine cell line PK (15). *Virology* **58**, 65.
349. Todaro, G., and Gallo, R.C. (1973). Human leukemic cell reverse transcriptase: Inhibition by antibody to primate C-type viruses. *In* "Episomes in Eukaryotes," Proc. 4th Lepetit Colloq. (L. Silvestri, ed.), pp. 117–122. North-Holland Publ., Amsterdam.
350. Todaro, G.J., and Gallo, R.C. (1973). Immunological relationship of DNA polymerase from human acute leukaemia cells and primate and mouse leukaemia virus reverse transcriptase. *Nature (London)* **244**, 206.
351. Todaro, G. Scherr, C., Benveniste, R., Lieber, M., and Melnick, J. (1974). Type-C viruses of baboons: isolation from normal cell cultures. *Cell* **2**, 55.
352. Tronick, S., Scolnick, E., and Parks, W. (1972). Reversible inactivation of the DNA polymerase of Rauscher leukemia virus. *J. Virol.* **10**, 885.
353. Tronick, S., Stephenson, J., and Aaronson, S. (1974). Immunological properties of two polypeptides of Mason-Pfizer monkey virus. *J. Virol.* **14**, 125.
354. Tronick, S., Stephenson, J., and Aaronson, A. (1974). Comparative immunological studies of RNA C-type viruses: Radioimmunoassay for a low molecular weight polypeptide of woolly monkey leukemia virus. *Virology* **57**, 347.
355. Tronick, S., Stephenson, J., Aaronson, S., and Kawakami, T. (1975). Antigenic characterization of type C RNA virus isolates of gibbon apes. *J. Virol.* **15**, 115.
356. Tsuchida, N., Robin, M.S., and Green, M. (1972). Viral RNA subunits in cells transformed by RNA tumor viruses. *Science* **176**, 1418.
357. Varmus, H.E., Bishop, J.M., Nowinski, R., and Sarkar, N. (1972). Mammary tumor virus specific nucleotide sequences in mouse DNA. *Nature (London), New Biol.* **238**, 189.
358. Varmus, H.E., Bishop, J.M., and Vogt, R. (1973). Appearance of virus specific DNA in mammalian cells following transformation by Rous sarcoma virus. *J. Mol. Biol.* **74**, 613.
359. Varmus, H.E., Guntaka, R., Deng, C., and Bishop, J.M. (1975). *Cold Spring Harbor Symp. Quant. Biol.* **39**, 987.
360. Varmus, H., Guntaka, R., Fan, W., Heasley, S., and Bishop, J.M. (1974). Synthesis of viral DNA in the cytoplasm of duck embryo fibroblasts and in enucleated cells after infection by avian sarcoma virus. *Proc. Nat. Acad. Sci. U.S.* **71**, 3874.
361. Varmus, H., Levinson, W., and Bishop, J.M. (1971). Extent of transcription by the RNA-dependent DNA polymerase of Rous sarcoma virus. *Nature (London) New Biol.* **233**, 19.
362. Varmus, H., Weiss, R., Friis, R., Levinson, W., and Bishop, J.M. (1972). Detection of avian tumor virus-specific nucleotide sequences in avian cell DNA. *Proc. Nat. Acad. Sci. U.S.* **69**, 20.
363. Verma, I., Meuth, N., and Baltimore, D. (1972). Covalent linkage between ribonucleic acid primer and deoxyribonucleic acid product of the avian myeloblastosis virus deoxyribonucleic acid polymerase. *J. Virol.* **10**, 622.
364. Verma, I., Meuth, N., Bromfeld, E., Manly, K., and Baltimore, D. (1971). A covalently linked RNA-DNA molecule as the initial product of the RNA tumor virus DNA polymerase. *Nature (London) New Biol.* **233**, 131.

365. Verma, I., Meuth, N., Fan, H., and Baltimore, D. (1974). Hamster leukemia virus: Lack of endogenous DNA synthesis and unique structure of its DNA polymerase. *J. Virol.* **13**, 1075.
366. Vernon, M., Lane, W., and Huebner, R. (1973). Prevalance of type-C particles in viscera tissues of embryonic and newborn mice. *J. Nat. Cancer Inst.* **510**, 1171.
367. Viola, M., and White, L. (1973). Differences in murine leukemia virus-specific DNA sequences in normal and malignant cells. *Nature (London) New Biol.* **246**, 485.
368. Vogt, P. (1967) A virus released by "non-producing" Rous sarcoma cells. *Proc. Nat. Acad. Sci. U.S.* **58**, 801.
369. Vogt, P., and Rubin, H. (1962). The cytology of Rous sarcoma virus infection. *Cold Spring Harbor Symp. Quant. Biol.* **27**, 395.
370. Wang, L.-H., and Duesberg, P. (1974). Properties and location of poly(A) in Rous sarcoma virus RNA. *J. Virol.* **14**, 1515.
371. Watson, J.D. (1971). The structure and assembly of murine leukemia virus: Intercellular viral RNA. *Virology* **45**, 586.
372. Weiss, R. (1967). Spontaneous virus production from "non-virus producing" Rouse sarcoma cells. *Virology* **32**, 719.
373. Weiss, R. (1969). The host range of Bryan strain Rous sarcoma virus synthesized in the absence of helper virus. *J. Gen. Virol.* **5**, 511.
374. Weiss, R.H., Friis, R., Katz, E., and Vogt, P. (1971). Induction of avian tumor viruses in normal cells by physical and chemical carcinogens. *Virology* **46**, 920 (1971).
375. Weisbach, A., Bolden, A., Muller, R., Hanafusa, H., and Hanafusa, T. (1972). Deoxyribonucleic acid polymerase activities in normal and leukovirus-infected chicken embryo cells. *J. Virol.* **10**, 321.
376. Weissbach, A., Schlabach, A., Fridlender, B., and Bolden, A. (1971). DNA polymerases from human cells. *Nature (London), New Biol.* **231**, 167.
377. Wickner, W., Brutlag, D., Schekman, R., and Kornberg, A. (1972). RNA synthesis initiates *in vitro* conversion of M13 DNA to its replicative form. *Proc. Nat. Acad. Sci. U.S.* **69**, 965.
378. Wolf, H., Zur Hausen, H., and Becker, V. (1973). EB viral genomes in epithelial nasopharyngeal carcinoma cells. *Nature (London), New Biol.* **244**, 245.
379. Wolfe, L., and Deinhardt, F. Personal communication (1974).
380. Wolfe, L., Smith, R., and Deinhardt, F. (1972). Simian sarcoma virus type 1 (Lagothrix): Focus assay and demonstration of nontransforming associated virus. *J. Nat. Cancer Inst.* **48**, 1905.
381. Wolfe, L., Deinhardt, F., Theilen, G., Kamakami, T., and Bustad, L. (1971). Induction of tumors in marmoset monkeys by simian sarcoma virus type 1 (*Lagothrix*): a preliminary report. *J. Nat. Cancer Inst.* **47**, 1115.
382. Wong, P., and McCarter, J. (1974). Studies of two temperature-sensitive mutants of Mononey murine leukemia virus. *Virology* **58**, 396.
383. Wong-Staal, F., Saxinger, W.C., Prensky, W., Gallo, R.C., and Gillespie, D. (1975). Cellular origin of Rauscher leukemia virus: Identification of sequences related to a major portion of the viral genome in DNA from uninfected mice. *Cell* (submitted).
384. Wu, A., and Gallo, R.C. (1974). Interaction between murine type-C virus RNA directed DNA polymerases and rifamycin derivatives. *Biochim. Biophys. Acta* **340**, 419.
385. Wu, A.M., Reitz, M.S., Paran, M., and Gallo, R.C. (1974). On the mechanism of stimulation of murine type-C RNA tumor virus production by glucocorticoids: Posttranscriptional effects. *J. Virol.* **14**, 802.
386. Yang, S.S., Herrera, F., Smith, R.G., Reitz, M., Lancini, G., Ting, R., and Gallo, R.C. (1972). Rifamycin antibiotics; Inhibitors of Rauscher (murine) leukemia virus reverse transcriptase and of purified DNA polymerases from human normal and leukemic lymphoblasts. *J. Nat. Cancer Inst.* **49**, 7.

387. Zhdanov, V., Soloview, V., Berktemiror, T., Ilyin, K., Bykovsky, A., Mazarenko, N., Irlin, I., and Yershov, F. (1973). Isolation of oncornavirus from continuous human cell cultures. *Intervirology* **1**, 19.
388. Zurcher, C., Bentvelzen, P., Brinkhof, J., and de Man, J. (1975). Detection of type-C oncornoviral antigens by immunofluorescence in cultured human bone marrow cells. *Nature* (in press).
389. Zur Hausen, H., Diehl, V., Wolf, H., Schulte-Holthausen, A., and Schneider, V. (1972). Occurrence of Epstein-Barr virus genomes in human lymphoblastoid cell lines. *Nature (London), New Biol.* **237**, 189.
390. Zur Hausen, H., and Schulte-Holthausen, H. (1970). Presence of Epstein-Barr virus nucleic acid homology in a "virus-free" line of Burkitt tumor cells. *Nature (London)* **227**, 245.
391. Zur Hausen, H., Schulte-Holthausen, H., Klein, G., Henle, W., Henle, G., Clifford, P., and Santesson, L. (1970). EBV DNA in biopsies of Burkitt tumors and anaplastic carcinomas of the nasopharynx. *Nature (London)* **228**, 1056.

NOTE ADDED IN PROOF

HL23V1 and V2 have been shown to contain a second viral entity, closely related to BEV. This unexpected finding prompted a search in our laboratory for BEV-related components in uncultured human cells. The endogenous pellet DNA polymerase product from uncultured cells of patient HL23 was found to contain nucleotide sequences complementary to BEV RNA. In addition, a partial provirus, amounting to 50–70% of the BEV viral genome, has been detected in 7 out of 8 leukemic cell DNA samples from different patients, including HL23 (F. Wong-Staal *et al.*, in preparation). The significance of these findings awaits further study.

Pathogenesis of Marek's Disease

L. N. PAYNE, J. A. FRAZIER and P. C. POWELL

Houghton Poultry Research Station, Houghton, Huntingdon, Cambs., England

I.	Introduction	59
II.	Historical Concepts and Nomenclature	61
III.	Virus–Cell Relationships	62
	A. Infection of the Cell	63
	B. Replication of Virions	63
	C. Different Expressions of MDV Infection	69
IV.	Pathology	70
	A. Natural Occurrence	70
	B. Experimental Transmission	71
	C. Gross Lesions	72
	D. Microscopic Lesions	76
V.	Immunity	126
	A. Passively Acquired Immunity	126
	B. Actively Acquired Immunity	129
	C. Vaccinal Immunity	133
	D. Immunosuppressive Effects of Marek's Disease	138
VI.	Factors Affecting Pathogenesis and Immunity	140
	A. Virus Strain	140
	B. Genetic Constitution of Host	141
	C. Age of Host	144
	D. Sex	144
	References	145

I. Introduction

Marek's disease (MD) is a lymphomatous and neuropathic disease of domestic chickens, and uncommonly of other birds, which is apparently without an exact counterpart in man and other mammals. Nevertheless many of its features are of comparative interest in relation to human and animal pathology. MD has come into eminence for several reasons.

1. Until it was brought under control by vaccination, it was the commonest naturally occurring neoplasm of any species, and the major cause of mortality, carcase condemnation and economic loss to the poultry industry in many countries. In the United States, for example, where the situation was best documented, annual losses by the late 1960s were about 200 million dollars, and 1.5% of all broiler carcases were condemned because of leukotic tumors. In laying and breeding flocks, 10–15% mortality was common, and losses of up to 80% of the flock could be encountered. These heavy losses were the consequence of the highly pathogenic acute form of MD which was first reported in Delaware in the 1950s (Benton and Cover, 1957) and subsequently spread throughout the United States and to other countries. Even before the acute form of MD became common, however, the more chronic, neuropathic, classical form of MD, first reported by Marek (1907), was one of the commonest diseases of chickens. This form was known popularly as fowl paralysis or range paralysis.

2. The serious economic consequences of MD stimulated increased efforts toward discovery of its etiology and into methods of control. In 1967 a herpesvirus was identified as the cause (Churchill and Biggs, 1967; Solomon *et al.*, 1968; Nazerian *et al.*, 1968), and the general principle was established that herpesviruses could be oncogenic. Subsequently other herpesviruses were shown to be responsible for lymphomas in primates, for renal adenocarcinoma in frogs, probably for Burkitt's lymphoma in African children, and possibly for cervical carcinoma in women (Kaplan, 1973).

3. Much emphasis was placed on finding ways to control or prevent MD. Only limited success was achieved by measures based on prevention of infection by isolation and by breeding genetically resistant stock, and these approaches were largely superseded by the development of live virus vaccines based on attenuated MD virus (MDV) (Churchill *et al.*, 1969a; Biggs *et al.*, 1970), an apathogenic herpesvirus of turkeys (Witter *et al.*, 1970; Okazaki *et al.*, 1970) or apathogenic strains of MDV (Rispens *et al.*, 1972a, b). Many millions of chickens are now vaccinated every year against MD, and another general principle has been recognized, namely, that large-scale commercial vaccination against a common virus-induced neoplasm is possible.

4. During the course of research into MD many host, viral, and environmental factors have been identified that influence the outcome of infection by MDV, and an understanding of these has helped in the study of other infectious diseases.

Thus MD is of importance not only in its own right, but also as an experimental model from which pathological principles may be elucidated (Klein, 1972a, b; Payne, 1973a). In the search for the etiology of MD and for control methods, the pathology and pathogenesis of the disease have been relatively neglected. There is now some evidence that after successful control this imbalance is being redressed. In this review we have attempted to draw together for the first time detailed information on the pathogenesis of MD. For more general accounts of the disease, including topics beyond the scope of this review, the reader is referred to Biggs (1968, 1971, 1973), Purchase *et al.* (1971a), Calnek and Witter (1972), Purchase (1972), and Nazerian (1973).

II. Historical Concepts and Nomenclature

MD has long been recognized to present a complex and variable pathological picture in which both neoplastic and inflammatory changes feature. Depending on the most conspicuous lesions seen in different circumstances, and on the supposed relationship between the various lesions, two main views have been expressed about the essential nature of MD. These views are that (1) the main lesions represent an inflammatory hyperplasia of lymphoid tissue, and (2) the lymphoid reaction is neoplastic. The inflammatory concept was proposed by Marek (1907), who observed only neuropathic changes, which he termed a "neuritis interstitialis" and a "polyneuritis." The term "neuromyelitis gallinarum" was used by van der Walle and Winkler-Junius (1924), "neuritis" by Doyle (1926), and "neurogranulomatosis infectiosa gallinarum (Marek)" by Lerche and Fritzsche (1934). Campbell (1956) recognized that nerve lesions might show a neoplastic tendency but regarded this as a rare sequel to a chronic inflammatory change. Similarly Wight (1962a) considered that some cases with tumors "originated by neoplastic change in long standing fowl paralysis lesions."

The opposing viewpoint, that the lymphoid proliferation is essentially neoplastic, was originated by Pappenheimer *et al.* (1926; 1929a, b), who proposed the name "neurolymphomatosis gallinarum," and this term was subsequently widely used. Pappenheimer and his associates also noted that visceral lymphomata, originating usually in the ovary, were associated with some cases and this was confirmed by others (Seagar, 1933a; Dalling and Warrack, 1936; Furth, 1935). Campbell (1956, 1961), however, did not regard these lesions as true neoplasms, but termed them "lymphogranulomas," although he later acknowledged that a proportion could become neoplastic, particularly in acute MD (Campbell, 1969).

For many years there was controversy about whether neurolymphomatosis and visceral lymphomatosis were etiologically related to the avian leukoses described by Ellerman (1921), and many attempts were made to prove or disprove the relationship (Patterson *et al.*, 1932; Furth, 1935; Jungherr, 1937). Although there were pathological grounds for dissociating the lymphoid tumors associated with neurolymphomatosis from those of Ellerman's lymphoid leukosis (Campbell, 1956, 1961), it was not until an etiological difference was shown in transmission experiments (Biggs and Payne, 1964) that the dissociation was accepted. Progress was perhaps hindered by the use of the term "avian leukosis complex" to describe the mesenchymal neoplasms of fowl, and by the classification of lymphomatosis into neural and visceral forms, the latter embracing two different lymphoid neoplasms as discussed above (Anonymous, 1941). Although etiological unity was not implied, this classification tended to divert attention from the need to establish the nature of fowl paralysis. Because of this, a new nomenclature was proposed (Campbell, 1961; Biggs, 1961) which discarded the term lymphomatosis, retained the term lymphoid leukosis for the neoplasm produced by avian RNA tumor (ART) virus, and introduced the name Marek's disease to replace fowl paralysis and neurolymphomatosis. Sevoian (1967) suggested the classification of avian lymphoid neoplasms into type I, type II, and type III, for the neoplasms induced by RIF-type virus (i.e., ART virus), JM-type virus (i.e., MDV), and T-type virus (i.e., reticuloendotheliosis virus, Purchase et al., 1973), respectively, but this terminology has not been widely used. We agree with Sevoian that these variously induced neoplasms are all forms of "lymphoid leukosis," but disagree with his view that "the cell types of lymphoid tumors . . . stimulated by each of these agents are indistinguishable," and that subclassification should be based on etiology. It is appropriate that pathological classifications of these neoplasms should be based on histogenesis and pathogenesis. Such a classification has yet to be devised; the division of the avian lymphoid system into bursal and thymic components, and characterization of the lymphoid neoplasms in terms of their derivations, offers a possible basis for a new classification. Popular or eponymous terms, such as fowl paralysis or Marek's disease, are of value for common use, but should not, we believe, be used for pathological classification.

With the ability to transmit MD experimentally it has become possible to study the pathogenesis and nature of the disease in great detail. The early stages of classical MD showed attributes of neoplasia (Payne and Biggs, 1967), and study of the acute form leaves no doubt that a neoplastic or closely similar process is involved (Sevoian and Chamberlain, 1964; Purchase and Biggs, 1967). It is clear, however, that inflammatory and degenerative processes are also involved, even early in the pathogenesis. Some of these appear to be related to the neoplastic lesions, and others to be essentially independent. MD thus has the attributes of both an inflammatory and neoplastic disease, the predominating lesions depending on factors such as strain of virus and genetic susceptibility of the fowl.

III. Virus–Cell Relationships

Structurally MDV is a typical herpesvirus. In tissue culture it was found to be avidly cell-associated; infectious virus was not released from the cells, and intact cells were required to transmit infectivity (Churchill, 1968; Churchill and Biggs, 1968). Because of these properties it was placed in the B group of herpesviruses

(Melnick et al., 1964). Cell-free virus can be recovered from feather follicle epithelium of infected chickens (Calnek et al., 1970a), but in other tissues, and in tissue culture, replication and expression of the herpesvirus is incomplete.

A. INFECTION OF THE CELL

The entry of cell-free, and presumably mainly enveloped, MDV into cells has been little studied. However, it is reasonable to suppose that the mechanism of entry is the same as for other members of the herpesvirus group, namely by adsorption of virus to the cell wall, digestion of the viral envelope and capsid, and release of the core (Morgan et al., 1968) or by viropexis (Dales and Silverberg, 1969; Abodeely et al., 1970). Recent studies by Hamdy et al. (1974) indicate that adsorption of one strain of cell-free MDV to duck embryo fibroblasts proceeds fairly rapidly, 60% of the virus being adsorbed in less than 1 hour.

With cell-associated infectivity it is probable that virus passes from cell to cell by cell fusion (Stoker, 1958; Ross and Orlans, 1958). There is evidence for this mode of spread with cell-associated MDV in that most strains of MDV cause polykaryocytosis in susceptible cultures (Churchill, 1968; Nazerian and Burmester, 1968; Sharma et al., 1969; Nazerian and Purchase, 1970), although the strain of virus, cell type, and other conditions affect the extent of polykaryocytosis. In addition, the presence of ultraviolet-irradiated Sendai virus (which produces cell fusion and formation of intercellular bridges between cells) increases the transfer of MDV from infected to uninfected cultured chick kidney cells (Hlozanek, 1970). Polykaryocytes are usually seen only in MDV-infected cell culture and rarely in vivo (Nazerian, 1971; Matsui, 1973; Omar et al., 1973). Cell-associated transfer of infectivity would account for the ability of some viruses, including MDV, to spread from cell to cell in the presence of antibody.

Once herpesvirus particles have gained entry to the cell, they are uncoated by cellular enzymes, and naked viral DNA, but not the coat protein, is transported into the nucleus (Hochberg and Becker, 1968). This process has not been studied for MDV.

B. REPLICATION OF VIRIONS

Ultrastructural studies in vitro with cell-free MDV and herpesviruses other than MDV have shown that one of the earliest signs (about 4–6 hours after infection) of cell infection is irregular condensation and margination of nuclear chromatin (Nii et al., 1968a; Hamdy et al., 1974). In MD infection (Hamdy et al., 1974), margination of chromatin is accompanied by the formation of binucleate cells and giant cells, and complement-fixing antigen is demonstrable at this stage. At 8 hours small hexagonal particles, 35 nm in diameter and resembling the central cores of capsids, are seen in cell nuclei. These small particles have been observed in the nuclei of other herpesvirus-infected cells, and it has been suggested that they are a precursor of the DNA-protein cores (Hamdy *et al.*, 1974). The presence of the 35 nm particles precedes the appearance of MDV nucleocapsids which appear at about 10 hours in the nucleus. Envelopment of nucleocapsids occurs at about 18 hours post infection. Nuclear changes result in the production of intranuclear inclusion bodies which, when seen with the light microscope, are characteristic of herpesviruses (Nazerian and Burmester, 1968).

Nucleocapsids of MDV vary considerably in appearance in thin section (Fig. 1) (Nazerian and Burmester, 1968; Epstein *et al.*, 1968; Ahmed and Schidlovsky,

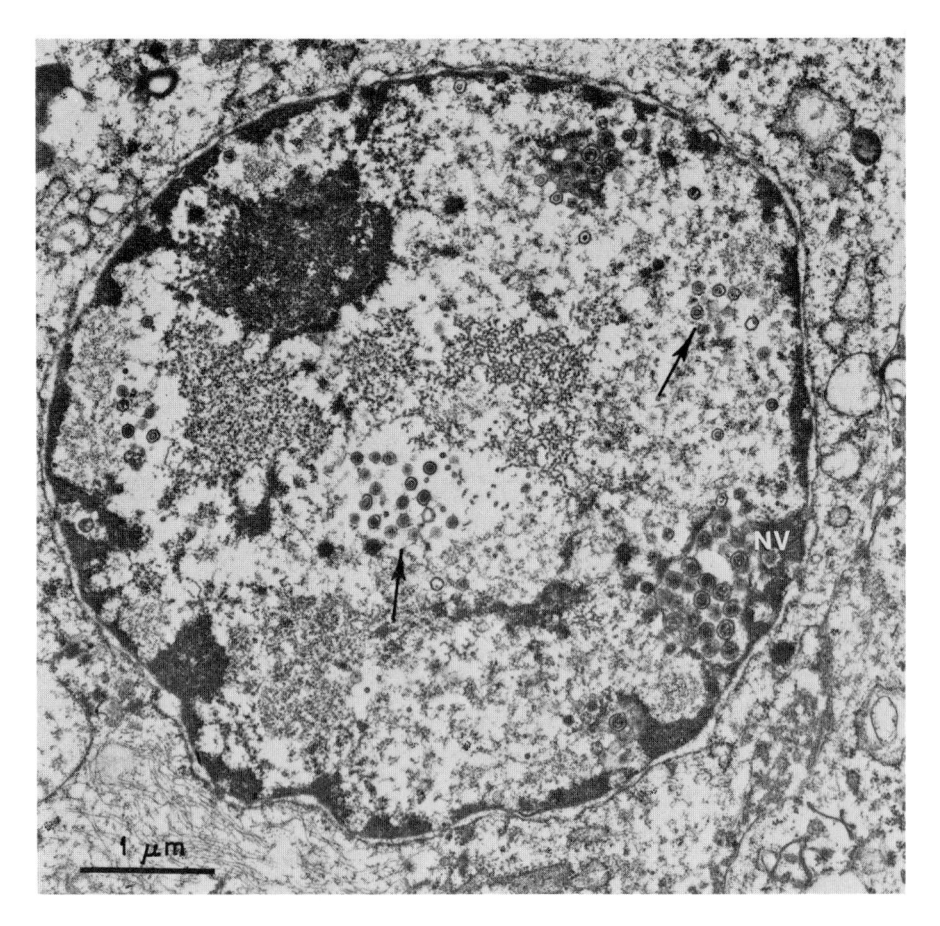

FIG. 1. Various morphological forms of unenveloped nucleocapsids of MDV (arrows) in the nucleus, and enveloped particles in nuclear vesicles (NV), of chick embryo fibroblast infected with HPRS-24 strain of MDV. × 17,800.

Unless stated otherwise, all figures of tissues of infected chickens come from the HPRS-RIR strain of chickens infected with Marek's disease virus (MDV) when 1 day old.

1968; Okada et al., 1972; Hamdy et al., 1974; Nazerian, 1974). Some capsids are empty whereas others have a round electron dense or electron lucent core. Other cores are bar shaped or horseshoe shaped. Occasionally, nucleocapsids containing from 1 to 6 small particles, often arranged in the form of an electron lucent cross (Fig. 2) are seen, particularly in cultures of a herpesvirus of turkeys, which is antigenically related to MDV (Nazerian et al., 1971; Okada et al., 1972). The pleomorphic character of the herpesvirus core is explained by the arrangement of DNA within the core (Furlong et al., 1972; Nazerian, 1974). Empty capsids are presumably devoid of DNA. Filamentous forms, which are probably aberrant forms of the virus, are also seen (Fig. 3). Other structures have been observed in MDV-infected cells (Epstein et al., 1968), and these include annulate lamellae (Fig. 4) in the cytoplasm and crystalline structures (Fig. 5, a and b).

Envelopment of MDV takes place at various sites. *In vitro*, the virus is most often enveloped at the nuclear membrane (Fig. 1) (Nazerian and Burmester, 1968; Epstein et al., 1968; Okada et al., 1972; Hamdy et al., 1974) and is usually seen in nuclear vesicles. This process of envelopment at the nuclear membrane has been described in detail by Darlington and Moss (1968) for other herpesviruses. When viral nucleocapsids come into contact with the inner nuclear membrane, this membrane becomes thicker at the point of contact. Immature nucleocapsids bud out from the nucleus into vesicles created by invagination of the nuclear membrane (Fig. 6). The enveloped particles measure about 120–170 nm in diameter. A similar process sometimes occurs at cytoplasmic membranes (Epstein et al., 1968). It seems likely that the nucleocapsid is enveloped by a portion of nuclear membrane modified by viral proteins inserted in it (Nii et al., 1968b; Nazerian and Chen, 1973).

Enveloped MDV particles are also seen in cytoplasmic inclusion bodies (Fig. 7), where they have a slightly different morphology from those enveloped at nuclear and cytoplasmic membranes (Nazerian and Witter, 1970). At this site the particles are often up to 200–250 nm in diameter. The envelope is swollen, and the nucleocapsid is often eccentrically located within the envelope. The space between the capsid and the envelope is filled with a material similar to that composing the cytoplasmic inclusion body. These inclusion bodies are seen infrequently in infected cell culture (Ahmed and Schidlovsky, 1968). They are, however, present in large numbers in the feather follicle epithelium of infected chickens (Nazerian and Witter, 1970; Calnek et al., 1970a), a site known to contain large amounts of cell-free virus. They are also seen in cultures of turkey herpesvirus, from which much more cell-free virus can be extracted than from most strains of MDV-infected cultures (von Bulow et al., 1975). It seems likely, therefore, that although MDV particles enveloped at sites other than cytoplasmic inclusion bodies may be infectious to some extent, the particles enveloped at cytoplasmic inclusion bodies could be far more stable than those enveloped elsewhere and are probably the major source of cell-free virus. It is known that

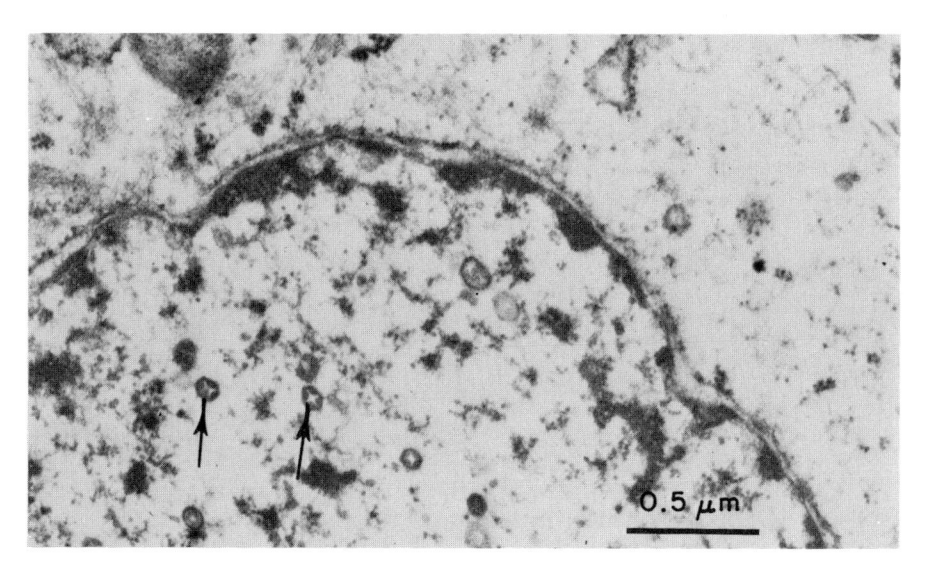

FIG. 2. Unenveloped virions in nucleus of chick embryo fibroblast infected with the herpesvirus of turkeys, showing characteristic electron lucent crosses (arrows). × 34,500.

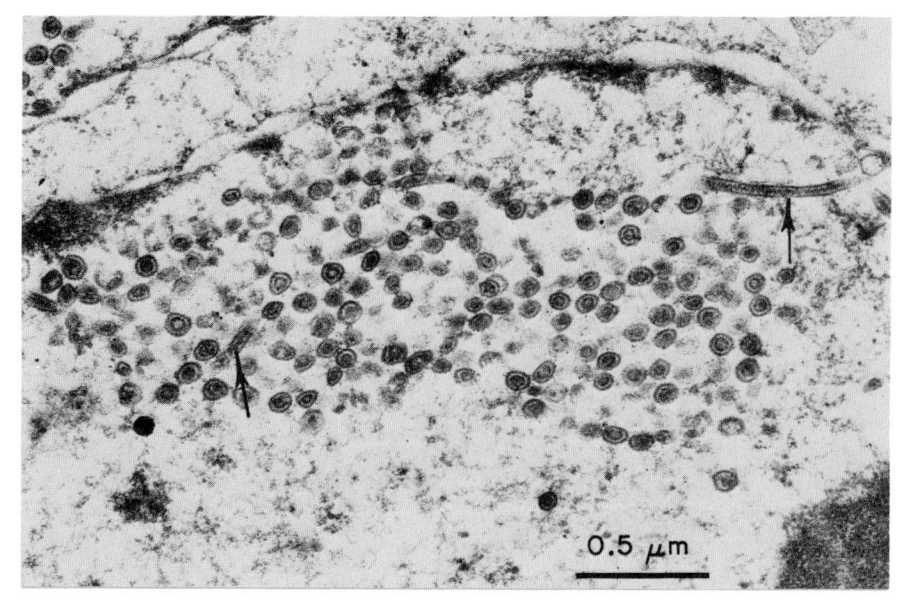

FIG. 3. Filamentous forms (arrows) of MDV in nucleus of chick embryo fibroblast infected with HPRS-24 strain of MDV. × 34,500

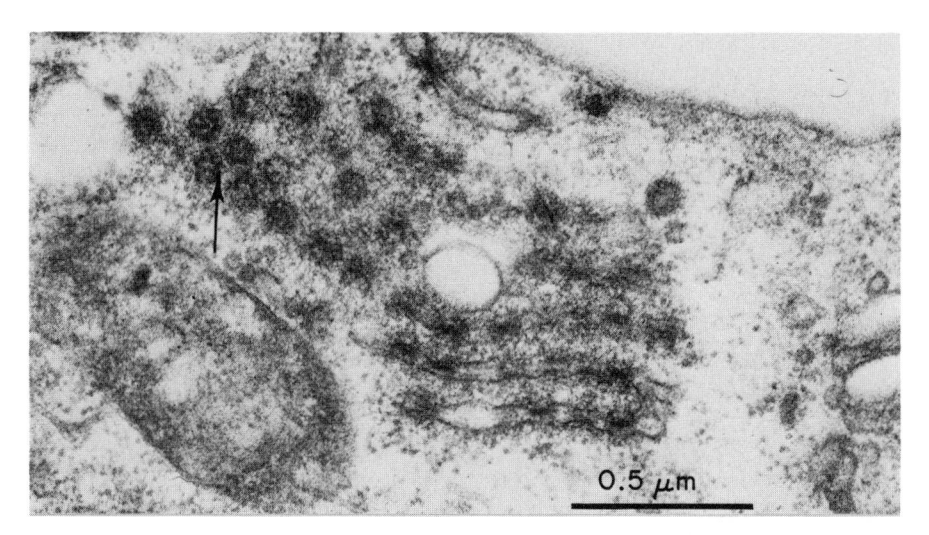

FIG. 4. Parallel arrays of annulate lamellae in the cytoplasm of HPRS line 1 of MD lymphoblastoid cells. Cross-sectional views (arrow) are also seen. × 46,900. From Frazier and Powell (1975).

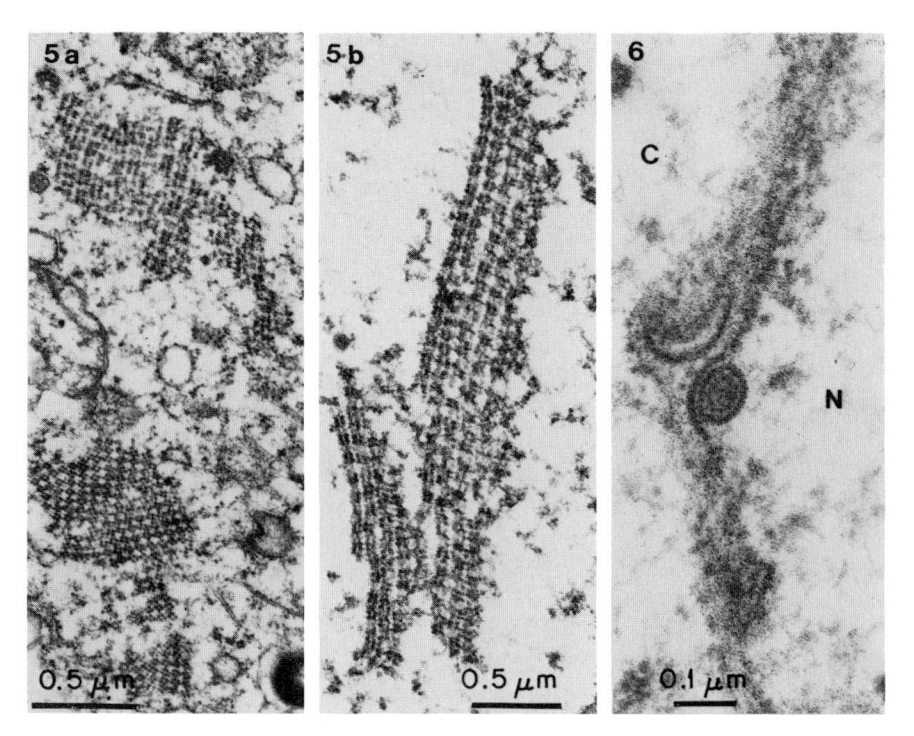

FIG. 5. Cytoplasmic cystalline structures in HPRS line 1 of MD lymphoblastoid cells. (a) × 23,200; (b) × 28,000. From Frazier and Powell (1975).

FIG. 6. Virion starting to bud through the nuclear membrane in thymic cell infected with HPRS-16 strain of MDV. C, cytoplasm; N, nucleus. × 82,600.

FIG. 7. Enveloped MD virions (arrows) in cytoplasmic inclusion bodies in feather follicle epithelium from chicken infected with HPRS-16 strain of MDV. × 20,300.

enveloped virus from feather follicle epithelium survives for long periods of time (over 16 weeks) at room temperature (Witter et al., 1968) and for 15 minutes at 56°C (Calnek and Adldinger, 1971).

It has been postulated that some herpesviruses are more cell-associated than others owing to inactivation of particles during their exit from the cell. Comparative ultrastructural studies of infectious laryngotracheitis virus (a group A herpesvirus) and MDV (Davis and Sharma, 1973) have revealed that the predominant site of envelopment is intracytoplasmic for laryngotracheitis virus and intranuclear for MDV. Enveloped infectious laryngotracheitis virus accumulated in cytoplasmic vacuoles and were released singly from the cell membrane, whereas MDV appeared to undergo cytoplasmic degradation. Davis and Sharma (1973) suggested that the perinuclear space and nucleus are the source of cell-free infectious MDV, which can be extracted from tissue culture cells by sonication (Calnek et al., 1970b) or by lysing cell cultures in demineralized water (Cook and Sears, 1970).

Thus, the presence of cell-free infectious virus in feather follicle epithelium is likely to be due to at least two factors. First, the specialized nature of the viral envelope elaborated at cytoplasmic inclusion bodies may protect the nucleocapsids more effectively than envelope elaborated at the nuclear membrane.

Second, the very nature and function of feather follicle epithelium, which results in gradual keratinization and death of the epithelial cells, may provide an environment more suited to the virus, with eventual release of cell-free enveloped particles along with sequestered portions of the stratum corneum. Exposure of the virus to active cytoplasm is thus probably minimal under these conditions.

Enveloped MDV has been observed *in vivo* in tissues (particularly the lymphoid organs) other than feather follicle epithelium (Calnek et al., 1970c; Ubertini and Calnek, 1970; Nazerian, 1971; Frazier and Biggs, 1972; Frazier, 1974a). However, such virus is usually enveloped at the nuclear membrane, although very rarely, enveloped particles in cytoplasmic inclusion bodies are seen (Frazier and Biggs, 1972). Cell-free virus has not, however, been extracted from tissues other than feather follicle epithelium (Adldinger and Calnek, 1973).

C. Different Expressions of MDV Infection

The reasons for the different behavior of MDV in different cells of the chicken can more readily be understood by considering the virus-cell relationships of other herpesvirus. Various herpesvirus–cell interactions have been defined (Roizman, 1972) as follows: (1) productive infection, in which death of the infected cell accompanies the release of infectious, cell-free virus; (2) restrictive or abortive infection, in which structural components and small amounts of usually intranuclear virus are produced; (3) nonproductive infection, in which no viral progeny are produced, no viral antigen can be detected, but viral genome is present. Since cell death is not a consequence of nonproductive infection, the cells survive and may express oncogenic functions.

Thus, in MDV-infected chickens, fully productive infection with release of much enveloped cell-free infectious virus occurs only in feather follicle epithelium (Calnek et al., 1970a; Nazerian and Witter, 1970). Restrictive infection, in which mainly nonenveloped intranuclear particles are produced, occurs in other tissues of infected chickens including lymphoid tissue, Schwann cells and lymphoid cells in peripheral nerve lesions, gonadal tumors, and renal epithelial cells (Schidlovsky et al., 1969; Calnek et al., 1970c; Ubertini and Calnek, 1970; Nazerian, 1971; Frazier and Biggs, 1972; Frazier, 1974a). Restrictive infections are particularly apparent in MDV-infected birds without maternal antibody.

Comparisons between cells abortively and productively infected with herpes simplex virus (Spring et al., 1968) have revealed that abortively infected cells contained 10-fold less virus-induced surface antigen than did productively infected cells. Thus, it seems likely that restrictively infected cells are defective and that the cell is unable to elaborate all the structural components necessary for the production of fully infectious virus. Small amounts of enveloped virus which may be produced are probably degenerated during passage out of the cell as discussed earlier. Two mechanisms for restrictive infection thus appear to operate. First, infections are restrictive owing to failure of the cell to produce some structural components of the virus. Second, any structurally mature virus which is produced is degenerated during egress from the cell. A balance between these two mechanisms presumably operates in the case of MDV, depending on the cell type. *In vivo*, only small numbers of intranuclear particles are seen in lymphoid cells, etc., whereas in tissue culture much larger numbers are common. Thus, a tissue culture cell is more able to produce at least some structural components of the virus than is a lymphocyte *in vivo*. A few enveloped particles are seen both *in vivo* and *in vitro*, but presumably the second mechanism operates and these particles are degraded during egress from the cell. Such particles can be rescued from infected tissue cultures by physical means (Calnek *et al.*, 1970b; Cook and Sears, 1970). In order to be fully productive a cell must therefore not only be able to produce infectious enveloped virus, but must have the ability to protect the virus during egress from the cell, e.g., by elaborating a special envelope or by providing a special compartment.

Fully and restrictively infected cells contain antigens that react with sera from MDV-infected birds in the immunoprecipitin (Churchill *et al.*, 1969b), immunofluorescence (Purchase, 1969; von Bulow and Payne, 1970; Spencer and Calnek, 1970), and immunoferritin tests (Nazerian *et al.*, 1972; quoted by Nazerian, 1973). Nazerian and Purchase (1970) found that immunofluorescent antigens were present only in cells that contained virus particles. Three structurally different antigens were detected: nuclear antigen, which often contained naked virions; diffuse cytoplasmic antigen, which only rarely contained virions; and granular cytoplasmic antigen, which never contained virions. In immunoferritin studies immune chicken and rabbit sera contained antibodies that reacted with viral capsid and envelope (Nazerian *et al.*, 1972; quoted by Nazerian, 1973). A membrane antigen has been reported in cells abortively infected with virulent virus by Chen and Purchase (1970), but its relation to other virus-associated antigens is as yet unclear.

The third or nonproductive type of virus infection is represented by the lymphoma cells in MD. These cells are able to infect chicks, and a small proportion of them (up to 1%) are infective in tissue culture; virus particles or viral antigens are rarely produced. Recent work suggests, however, that many if not all lymphoma cells harbor viral genome in a repressed form; this genome may cause changes in the cell, perhaps to the cell membrane, which lead to neoplastic transformation. This question is dealt with more fully in Section IV, D, 6, d.

IV. Pathology

A. Natural Occurrence

Three clinical manifestations of MD are recognized: the classical form, the acute form, and transient paralysis. The term "classical form" refers to the

TABLE I
EXPRESSION OF MAREK'S
DISEASE IN FLOCK AND
INDIVIDUAL

Flock incidence	Course	Individual lesion
High	Acute	Visceral
Low	Chronic	Neural

longer recognized and primarily neuropathic disease originally described by Marek (1907). "Acute form" refers to the more overtly leukotic manifestation described by Benton and Cover (1957) as "acute leukosis" but subsequently recognized as a form of MD (Biggs et al., 1965). Transient paralysis was first described by Zander (1959) and shown by Kenzy et al. (1973) to be an encephalitic manifestation of MDV infection. Although the terms classical (on the basis of current usage) and acute convey a general impression of the type of clinical disease, they cannot be used to describe precisely a disease outbreak in the flock or individual. For this purpose the incidence and course of an outbreak in the flock, and the predominating lesion seen in affected individual birds, must be stated. Terms that may be used are suggested in Table I. Thus the expression "a high, acute incidence of visceral MD" would convey the picture of heavy losses over a short period of time from the lymphomatous form of MD (i.e., typical "acute MD,") whereas "low, chronic incidence of neural MD" would indicate light losses over a long period of time from the neural form (i.e., typical "classical MD"). In the field and experimentally, various combinations of these flock and individual characteristics can be encountered, depending on host, viral, and environmental variables, which cannot be adequately described by the original two terms, but which can be defined by use of the proposed terminology.

B. Experimental Transmission

There are numerous publications describing early attempts to transmit Marek's disease experimentally (Biggs, 1968). Although success was claimed, and probably achieved, by some workers the experiments generally were not convincing, because of difficulty in regularly repeating results, of the occurrence of MD in control birds, and of diagnostic confusion between MD and the various forms of leukosis caused by the ART viruses.

The present era of MD research was ushered in by the successful transmission of acute MD by Sevoian et al. (1962) and of classical MD by Biggs and Payne (1963). Common features of these successful and repeatable transmissions were the use of young, highly susceptible chicks and the inoculation of viable blood or lymphoma cells from MD-affected birds. The JM isolate of Sevoian induced both neural and visceral lymphomatosis in 90–100% of inoculated chicks within 2–3 weeks; the HPRS-B14 isolate of Biggs and Payne induced neural lesions in 75% of chicks 4–10 weeks after inoculation, and 30% of affected female birds also developed ovarian lymphomas. Similar strains have been isolated by other workers: the best-known strains of acute MDV are JM, HPRS-16 (Biggs et al., 1965; Purchase and Biggs, 1967), GA (Eidson and Schmittle, 1968), Cal-1 (Bankowski et al., 1969), and Conn-B (Jakowski et al., 1969), and the best-known strains of classical MDV are HPRS-B14, Conn-A (Chomiak et al., 1967), and WSU-GF (Kenzy et al., 1964).

From the pathological standpoint the importance of these virus strains is that they allowed for the first time the production of cases of MD of known provenance for pathological study.

C. Gross Lesions

The gross changes seen in classical or acute MD are peripheral nerve enlargement, lymphoma formation in many organs and tissues, and degenerative changes in the bursa of Fabricius and thymus. Ocular changes have been commonly associated with classical MD in the field. There are no essential differences between the lesions seen in naturally occurring field cases and those in experimentally produced cases. No gross lesions are seen in transient paralysis.

1. Peripheral Nerves

Affected nerves are usually 2–3 times their normal thickness, and occasionally much more (Figs. 8 and 9). The enlargement is usually diffuse, but may be nodular. Affected nerves lose their cross striations, and show gray or yellow discoloration, and sometimes edema. Dorsal root ganglia may be enlarged. The distribution of macroscopic changes among different peripheral nerves in field cases was examined by Goodchild (1969) and Sugiyama et al. (1973). Goodchild observed that the autonomic nerves were frequently affected and that the celiac plexus was most often enlarged, in 78% of cases. The sciatic and brachial nerves and their plexi are often enlarged, and these nerves together with the celiac plexus, are recommended for routine examination.

2. Lymphoma Formation

Lymphoid tumors are typically seen in one or more organs or tissues in acute MD, and occasionally in classical MD, particularly in the ovary. In acute MD, ovarian (Fig. 10) and testicular lymphomas (Fig. 11) are commonly seen, but other tissues frequently involved are liver (Fig. 12), spleen, kidneys, lungs, heart, proventriculus, skeletal muscle, and skin (Table II). In the skin the lymphomas are usually associated with feather follicles. Tumorous involvement is usually diffuse, but occasionally nodular tumors occur. The organ distribution of lymphomas

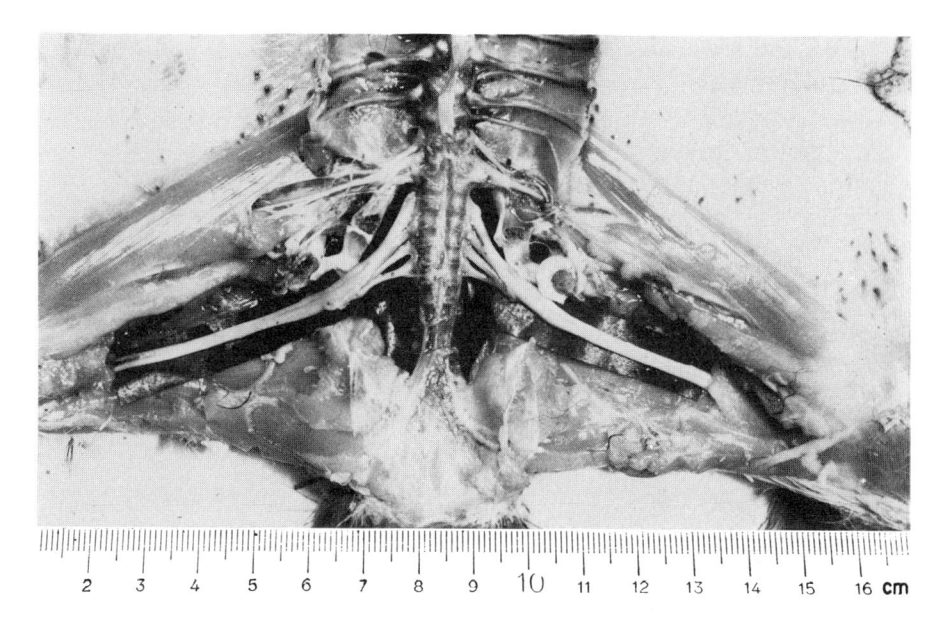

FIG. 8. Enlarged sciatic nerves of 63-day-old chicken infected at 2 days old with HPRS-B14 strain of MDV. From Payne and Biggs (1967).

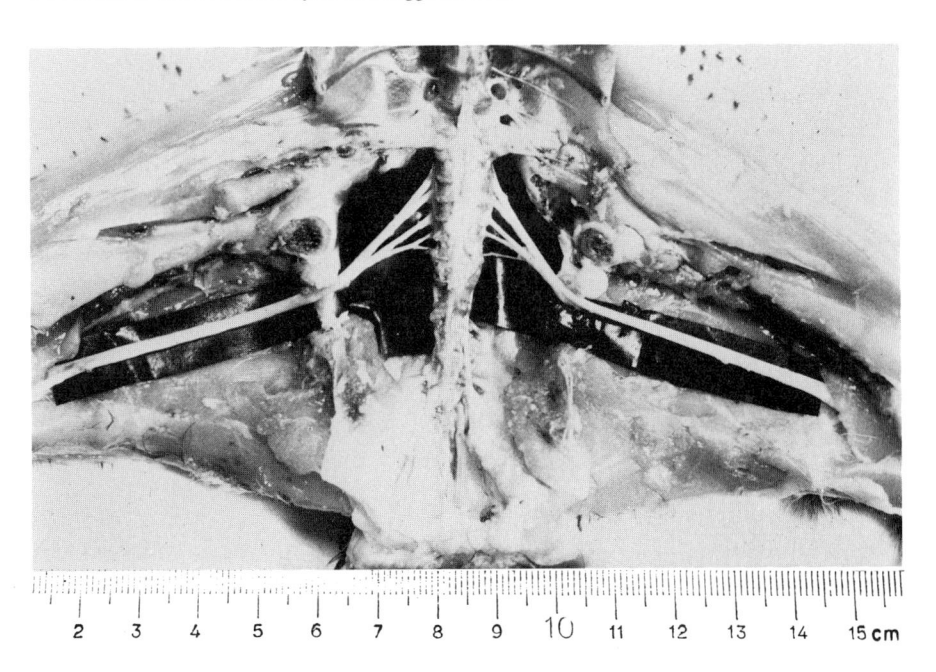

FIG. 9. Sciatic nerves of normal 63-day-old chicken, for comparison with Fig. 8. From Payne and Biggs (1967).

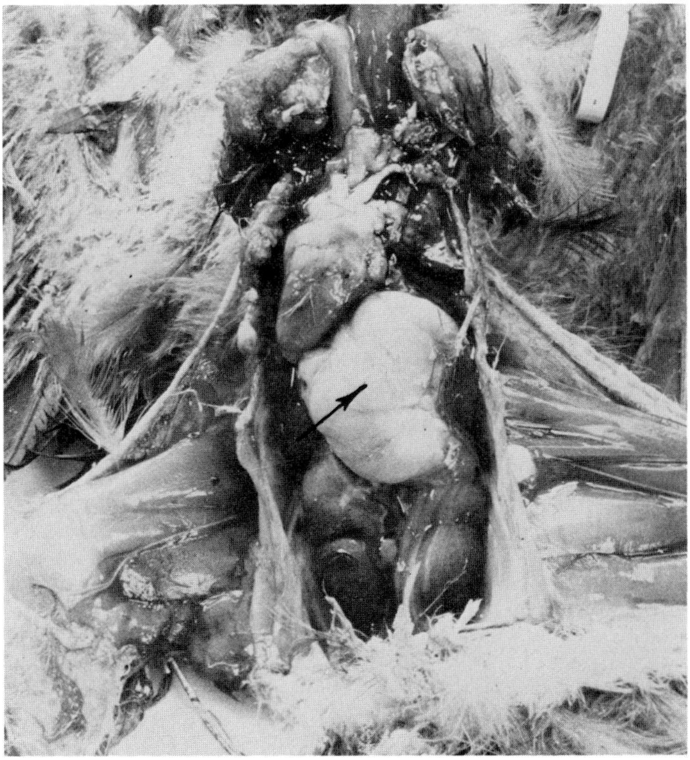

FIG. 10. Ovarian lymphoma (arrow) in 42-day-old chicken infected with HPRS-16 strain of MDV.

in field outbreaks of both classical and acute type have been detailed by Fujimoto et al. (1971) with findings similar to those in experimentally produced cases.

3. Eye

An iridocyclitis has frequently been observed in association with MD in the field (Pappenheimer et al., 1926, 1929a; McGaughey and Downie, 1930; Warrack and Dalling, 1932). Affected eyes show annular or patchy depigmentation of the iris, loss of ability of the iris to accommodate to light, and distortion of the pupil. In the past there has been some question of whether or not so-called "ocular lymphomatosis" is a manifestation of MD: Yamagiwa et al. (1967) were inclined to regard it as an independent disease, Simpson (1969a, b) found ultrastructural evidence for involvement of ART virus in the etiology, and Moriwaki and Horiuchi (1974) found no association between changes in the eye and lymphoproliferation in peripheral nerves or viscera. Usually ocular lesions

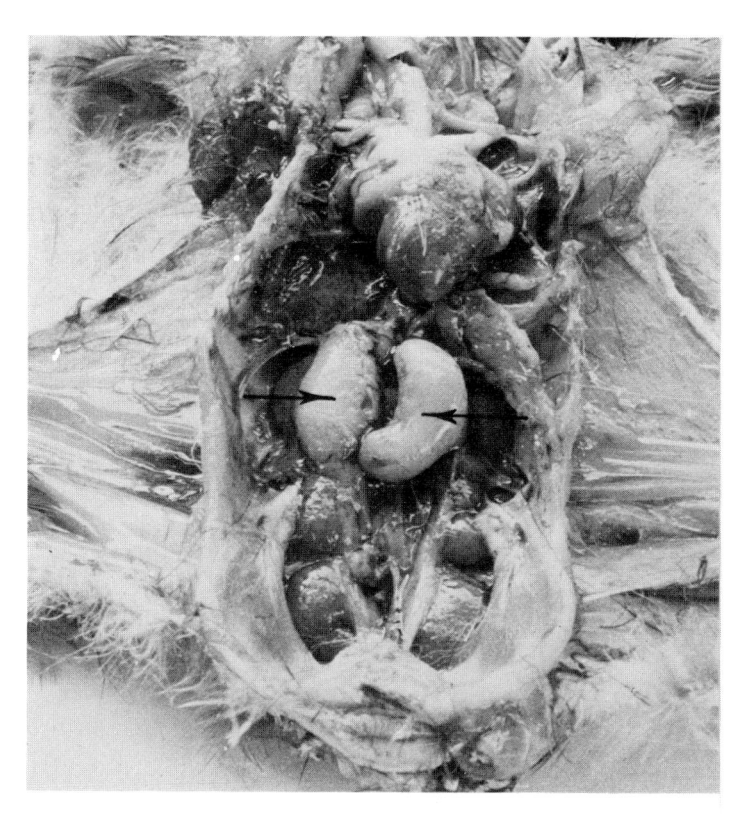

FIG. 11. Testicular lymphomas (arrows) in 42-day-old chicken infected with HPRS-16 strain of MDV.

have not been described as a feature of experimentally induced cases of MD. However, Sevoian and Chamberlain (1962, 1964) produced ocular changes in a high proportion of chicks inoculated with MD infective material into the anterior chamber of the eye, and perhaps more significantly in up to 5% of chicks inoculated intraperitoneally; more recently, Smith *et al.* (1974) produced ocular changes by intraocular and intra-abdominal inoculation of MDV in well controlled experiments. Cho (1974) has isolated MDV from the aqueous humor of a chicken with "the ocular form of Marek's disease." It now seems highly probable that MDV can cause iridocyclitis, but it is possible that there are other causes.

4. *Other Organs*

The bursa and thymus are often atrophic in acute MD. Muscular atrophy occurs in chronic cases (Wight, 1966).

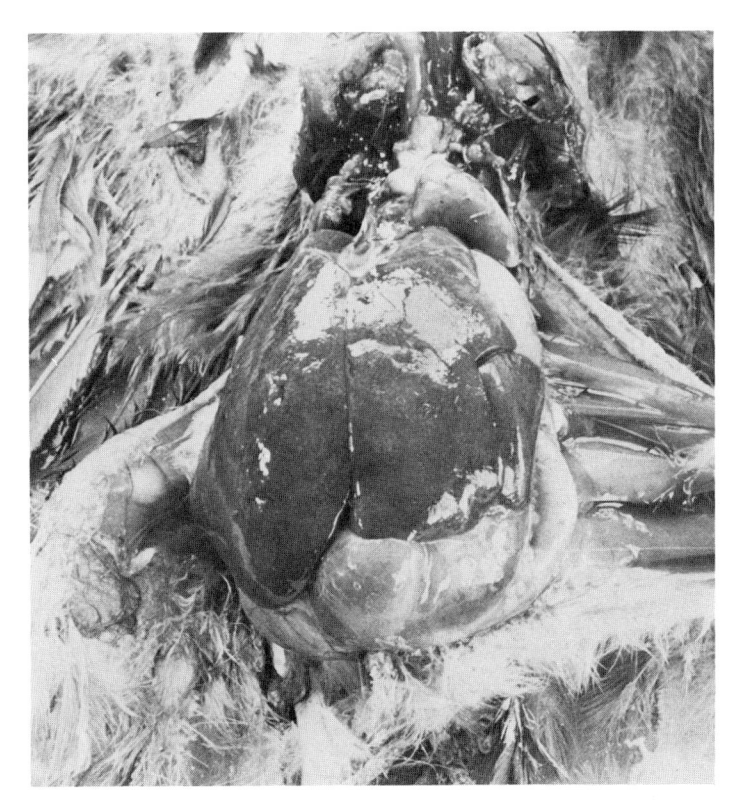

FIG. 12. Diffuse hepatic lymphomas in 42-day-old chicken infected with HPRS-16 strain of MDV.

D. Microscopic Lesions

The pathological changes in MD are more complex than was at one time realized. They include acute, subacute, and chronic inflammatory changes, degenerative and regressive changes, and lymphoproliferation, all in a variety of tissues. Knowledge of these changes has come from many investigations of both naturally occurring and experimentally induced cases. Recent studies allow the complex changes to be divided into several pathogenic processes: (1) initial infection of respiratory tract (following inhalation of MDV); (2) acute cytolytic infection of lymphoid tissues; (3) acute cytolytic infection of nonlymphoid tissues; (4) infection of feather follicle epithelium; (5) neuropathic changes; (6) lymphomagenesis; (7) hematological changes including leukemogenesis; (8) ocular changes. This order follows approximately the sequence of events

TABLE II
Distribution of Lymphomas in Chickens Inoculated with Isolates of Acute Marek's Disease Virus (HPRS-16, 18, 19, 20)[a]

Tissue	Percent with lymphomas (159 cases)
Gonad	97
Liver	59
Spleen	21
Lung	35
Muscle	27
Kidney	21
Heart	24
Proventriculus and intestine	9
Mesentary and serosa	6

[a] Data of Purchase and Biggs (1967).

after infection; some of the changes are interrelated whereas others appear to be essentially independent.

1. Initial Infection of Respiratory Tract

Under natural conditions MDV infection is believed to be acquired usually by inhalation of infective material derived from feathers, dander, and dust in poultry houses. After inhalation exposure of 4-week-old chicks to infectious feather material, Adldinger and Calnek (1973) detected viral antigen, by agar gel precipitin and immunofluorescent tests, in lungs at 24 hours post exposure. Infectious cell-associated virus was first detected at 5 days in lung tissue. In birds exposed when 1 week old, viral antigen was first detected in trachea and lung at 5 days by the precipitin test, and infectious virus was first detected in lung at 8 days. They concluded that the early presence of antigens in the respiratory tract probably indicated the presence of inhaled antigenic material, and that virus replication in the lungs was limited and perhaps not essential for virus dissemination. Possibly phagocytic alveolar cells take up the virus and carry it to other tissues. The presence of viral antigen in the lung several days after infection need not be indicative of a primary infection at this site, for Purchase (1970) found antigen by immunofluorescence tests in lung at 5 days after infection by the abdominal route. In the study of Adldinger and Calnek (1973) viral antigen was detected in buffy coat cells from peripheral blood and plasma by precipitin tests as early as 18 hours after infection, and the infection appeared at 3 days in the lymphoid organs. The early fate of virus inoculated intra-abdominally has not been determined, but uptake by phagocytic cells and blood-borne dissemination would seem likely.

2. *Acute Cytolytic Infection of Lymphoid Tissues*

In chicks lacking maternal antibody to MDV, striking changes occur in the lymphoid organs during the first week after infection. The first reports of this early response were by Jakowski *et al.* (1970). Essentially these changes consist of restrictively productive infection of cells in these organs, accompanied by an acute to subacute inflammatory response. The changes occur more or less simultaneously and equally in the bursa, thymus, and spleen and in other lymphoid tissue, suggesting that the target tissue is not specifically B or T cell-dependent. Mainly virological aspects of the acute infection are described by Phillips and Biggs (1972) and Adldinger and Calnek (1973), and mainly pathological aspects by Payne and Rennie (1973) and Frazier (1974a). Although these

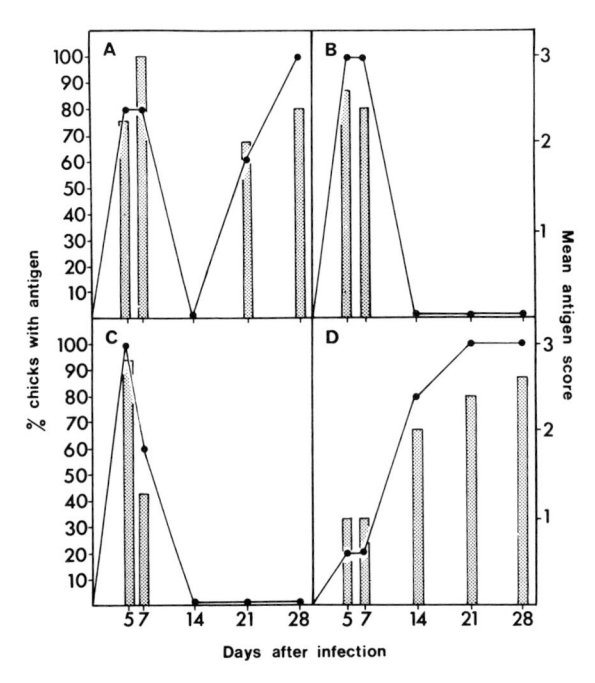

FIG. 13. MDV antigen in fluorescent antibody tests in (A) bursa, (B) thymus, (C) spleen, and (D) feather follicle epithelium and adjacent dermis of maternal antibody-free chicks at different times after infection with HPRS-16 strain of MDV. ●——●, Percentage of chicks with antigen; stippled area, mean antigen score of positive tissues. Scoring: 1 = a few single fluorescent cells; 2 = moderate numbers of fluorescent cells scattered singly or in groups; 3 = numerous fluorescent cells, usually in large groups. Note: At 5 and 7 days, fluorescent cells were only in dermal lymphoid foci near follicles. From Payne and Rennie (1973).

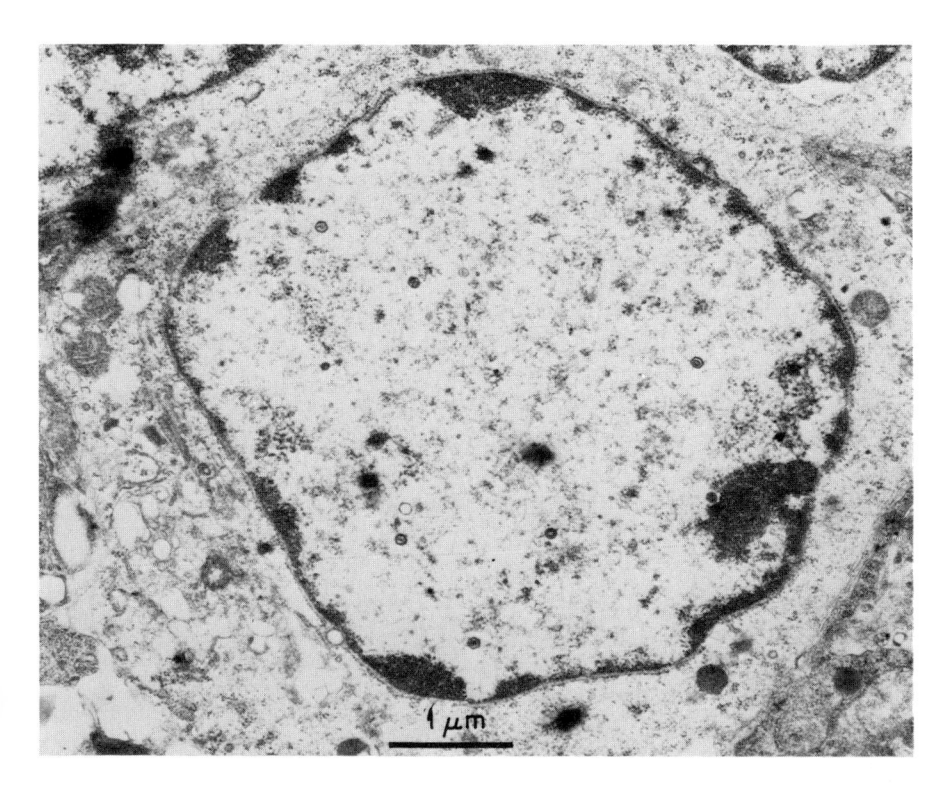

FIG. 14. Intranuclear unenveloped virions in lymphoid cell in spleen 4 days after infection of antibody-negative chick with HPRS-16 strain of MDV. × 16,000. From Frazier and Biggs (1972).

authors used different strains of birds, ages, and viruses, the results are remarkably consistent and allow a composite picture to be drawn.

Infection of the thymus, bursa, and spleen was first detected by the precipitin test at 3 days post exposure in birds infected when either 1 week old or 4 weeks old (Adldinger and Calnek, 1973). Infectivity of these organs reached a peak at about 5–7 days after infection, when measured for cell-associated infectivity, soluble antigens, and fluorescent antigens (Fig. 13). Infectivity levels tended to be higher in the thymus and spleen than in the bursa. The infection is of the restrictively productive type, since much viral antigen is produced, and cell-associated infectivity is high, but no cell-free virus can be extracted. Occasionally cytolysis is unaccompanied by viral antigen production. Naked herpesviruses are present in cell nuclei, but little or no coated virus is present (Fig. 14). The semiproductive infection causes marked degenerative and inflammatory changes in the affected organs. The earliest ultrastructural changes are seen at 3 days post infection, in the bursa, thymus, and spleen, and they precede obvious histopathological change. Electron dense, granular lymphocytes appear in the bursa and thymic cortex, of a type associated with cortisone-induced and physiological regression (Frazier, 1974a). Small dark reticular cells appear in the three lymphoid organs, and dense granular epithelial cells increase in the bursa and thymus. By 5–7 days after infection, lymphocytic regression is severe in the bursa and thymus, which show marked loss of weight (Payne and Rennie, 1973). Although cytolysis of lymphocytes occurs, this appears to be insufficient to account completely for lymphoid regression, and it seems likely that nonspecific factors released as a result of the stress of infection are involved. The value of this response to the bird is undetermined. The cortical cells of the thymus may almost completely disappear, and hyperplasia of reticulum cell elements in the medulla is present (Fig. 15). By conventional microscopy, primitive and activated reticulum cells are increased, and many cells contain intranuclear inclusion bodies (Fig. 16). Numerous cells that stain strongly for acid phosphatase, presumably macrophages, are present, as are metalophil cells (Figs. 17 and 18). Among these cells are scattered granulocytes (mainly heterophils and eosinophils from electron microscope studies), degenerating cells, lymphocytes, and blast cells. In immunofluorescence tests, abundant viral antigen is present (Fig. 19).

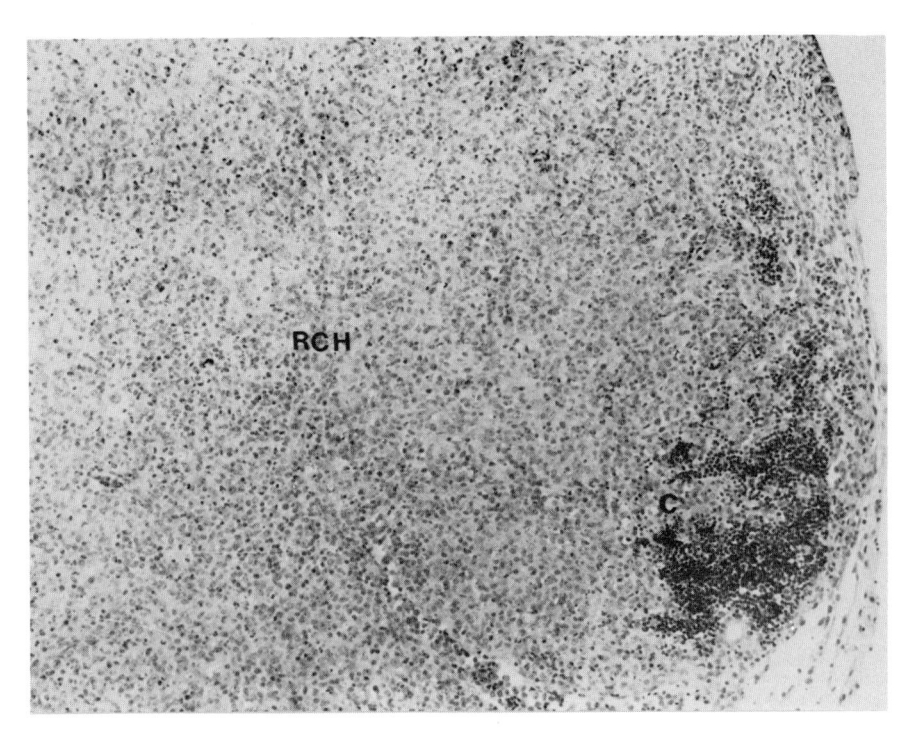

FIG. 15. Severe cortical regression (C) and medullary reticulum cell hyperplasia (RCH) in thymus of 8-day-old chick infected with HPRS-16 strain of MDV. × 160. From Payne and Rennie (1973).

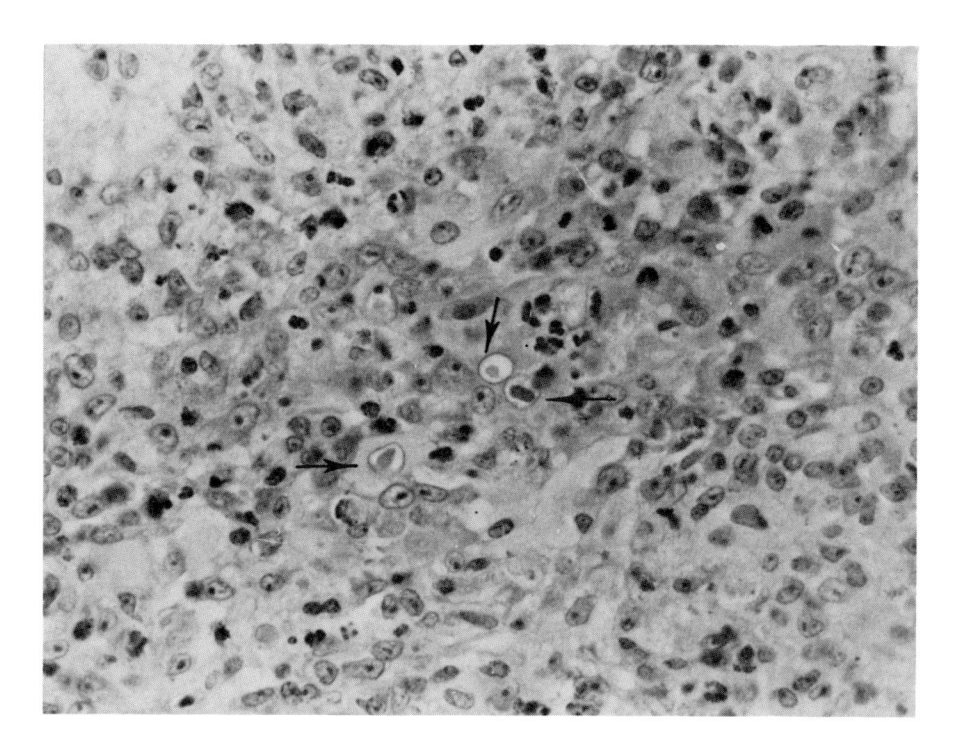

FIG. 16. Reticulum cell hyperplasia, with cells containing intranuclear inclusion bodies (arrows), in medulla of thymus of an 8-day-old chick infected with HPRS-16 strain of MDV. × 640. From Payne and Rennie (1973).

The reticulum cells appear to correspond to large pale cells seen under the electron microscope (Fig. 20) (Frazier, 1974a). These cells contain few ribosomes, and sparse to moderate quantities of mitochondria and endoplasmic reticulum. They are rarely seen in lymphoid organs of normal birds (Frazier, 1973, 1974b). Frequently they contain immature, intranuclear herpesvirus particles, and they may be the target cells for the virus, since they are the most common cell type to contain virus (Fig. 21). Also markedly increased are phagocytic mesenchymal reticulum cells or macrophages; these show many ultrastructural similarities to the large pale reticulum cells, which may therefore be their precursors (Fig. 22). Virus particles are rarely present in the nuclei of macrophages, and they are occasionally seen within phagocytosed cells. Among the lymphocytes at 5 days and subsequently are cells with nuclear projections, which have been associated with neoplastic change (see Section IV, D, 6, a). Syncytia, usually composed of cells resembling reticulum cells and often containing intranuclear herpesvirus particles, are sometimes present in the lymphoid organs 6–9 days after infection (Fig. 23). They presumably arise by cell fusion of infected and uninfected cells such as is seen in tissue culture (see Section III,

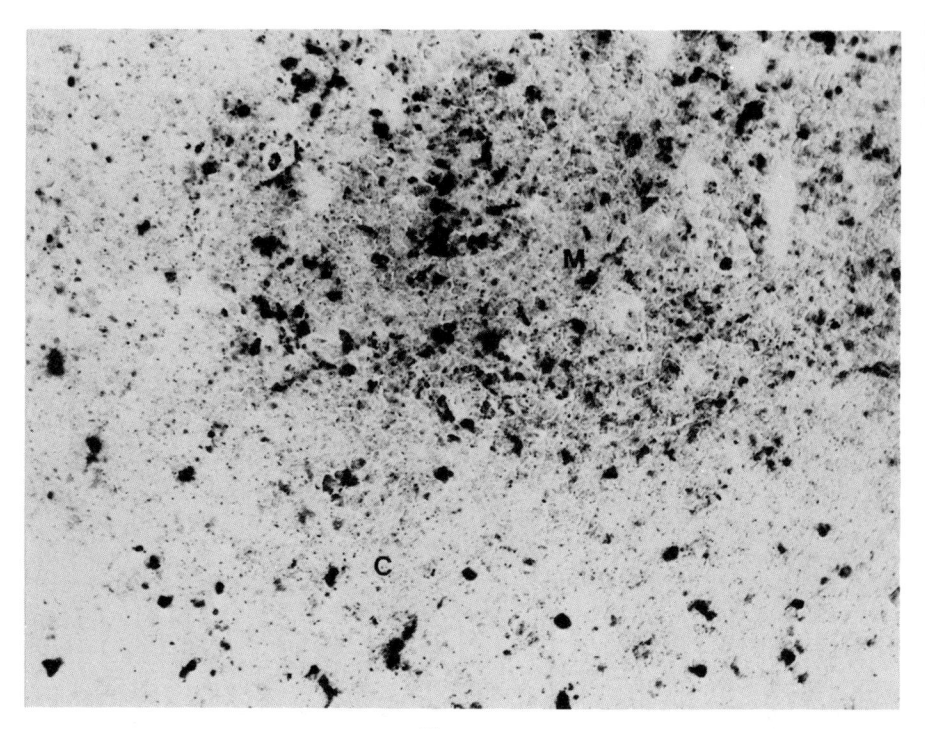

FIG. 17.

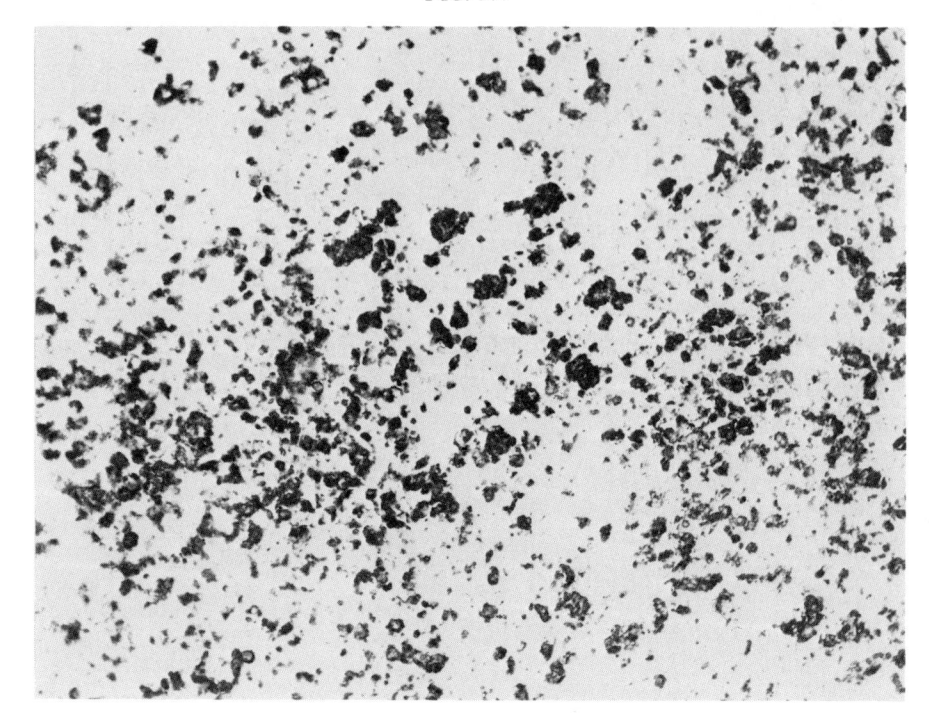

FIG. 18.

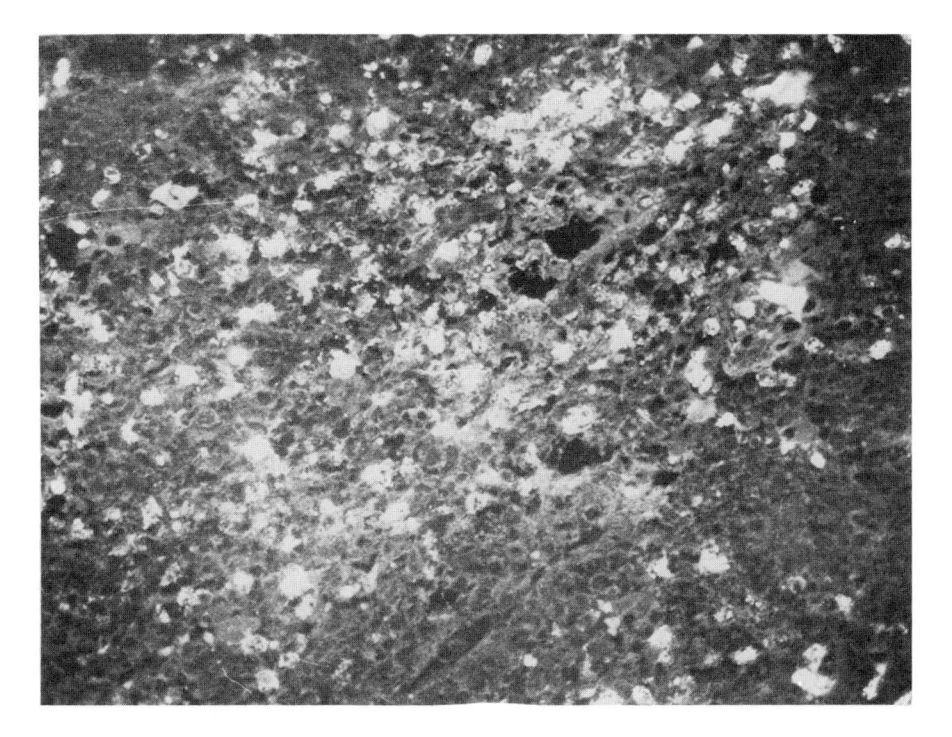

FIG. 19. Fluorescent MDV antigen-containing cells in thymus of a 6-day-old chick infected with HPRS-16 strain of MDV. The antigen is mainly in medullary cells. × 640. From Payne and Rennie (1973).

A) and provide a means of spread of the virus. Mainly intranuclear unenveloped herpesviruses are also present in lymphocytes and epithelial cells, although less often than in the reticulum cells.

The reticulum cell hyperplasia seen in the thymus occurs also in the bursa (Fig. 24), where the normal follicular architecture may be destroyed, in focal areas in the spleen, and in submucosal lymphoid tissue in the gut. In all these locations the reticulum cell response is associated with the presence of inclusion bodies, viral antigen, and unenveloped virions. In the spleen, where lymphoid regression is not a factor, the response results in weight increase. In addition, the cells of the sheathed capillaries show marked phagocytic activity, suggesting removal of

---

FIG. 17 (*top*). Acid phosphatase-positive cells, presumably macrophages, in medulla (M) and cortex (C) of normal thymus of 6-day-old uninfected chick. Gomori's method. × 256. From Payne and Rennie (1973).

FIG. 18 (*bottom*). Increased numbers of acid phosphatase-positive cells, presumably macrophages, in area of reticulum cell hyperplasia in thymic medulla of 6-day-old chick infected with HPRS-16 strain of MDV. Compare with Fig. 17. Gomori's method. × 256. From Payne and Rennie (1973).

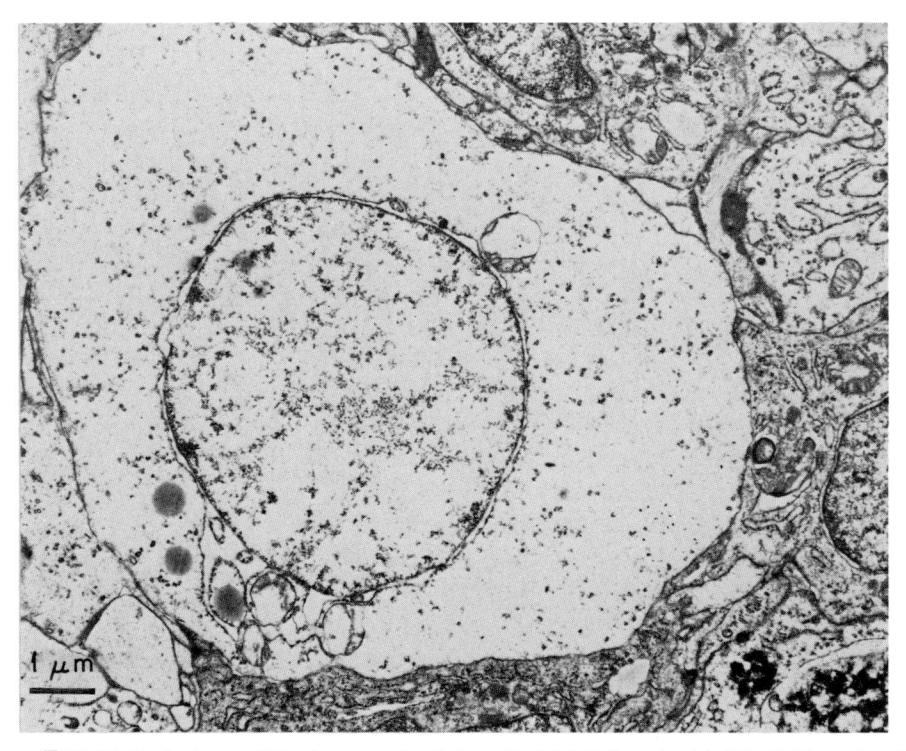

FIG. 20. Reticulum cell in thymus of a 6-day-old chick infected with HPRS-16 strain of MDV. × 8500. From Frazier (1974a).

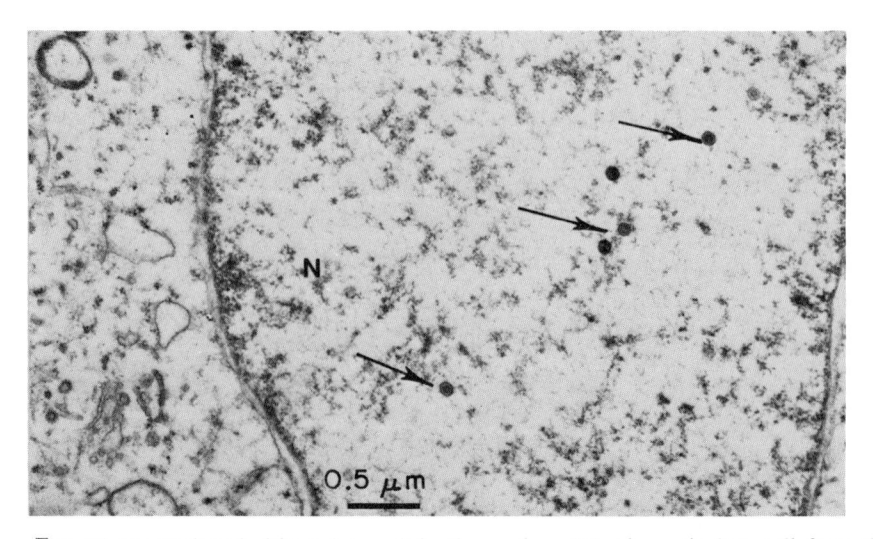

FIG. 21. Unenveloped virions (arrows) in the nucleus (N) of a reticulum cell from the thymus of an 8-day-old chick infected with HPRS-16 strain of MDV. × 18,400.

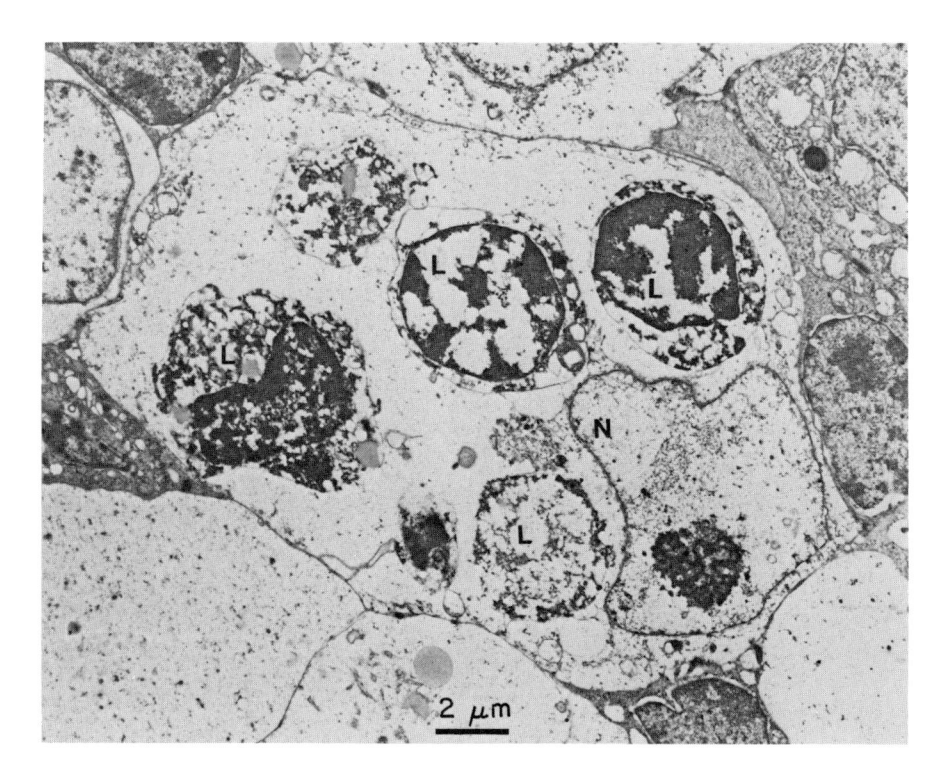

FIG. 22. Macrophage with virions in the nucleus (N) and containing several phagocytosed lymphocytes (L), in thymus of a 9-day-old chick infected with HPRS-16 strain of MDV. × 9400.

debris from the circulation, and the sheaths undergo hyperplasia. Occasionally intranuclear inclusion bodies are seen in the sheath cells. These changes stimulate an increase in acid phosphate-positive macrophages at the periphery of the sheaths.

The acute inflammatory changes in the various lymphoid organs, which might be termed an acute lymphoreticulitis, resolve after 7 days (Fig. 25). Inclusion bodies, viral antigen, and virions disappear, as do the reticulum cells and macrophages, and by 14 days the architecture of these organs is considerably restored. Although the inflammatory changes have disappeared by 14 days, lymphoid tissues in the thymic cortex and bursa are not fully restored, and these organs still weigh less than normal organs. After 14 days there is evidence of a resurgence of infection and of degenerative changes in the bursa. In the spleen, the areas of reticulum cell hyperplasia become progressively infiltrated by lymphocytes, converting them into areas of lymphoid hyperplasia, which maintains the increased weight of the infected spleens over uninfected spleens.

Infectivity and antigenicity of bone marrow, buffy coat cells, and blood plasma were studied by Adldinger and Calnek (1973). The results gave evidence

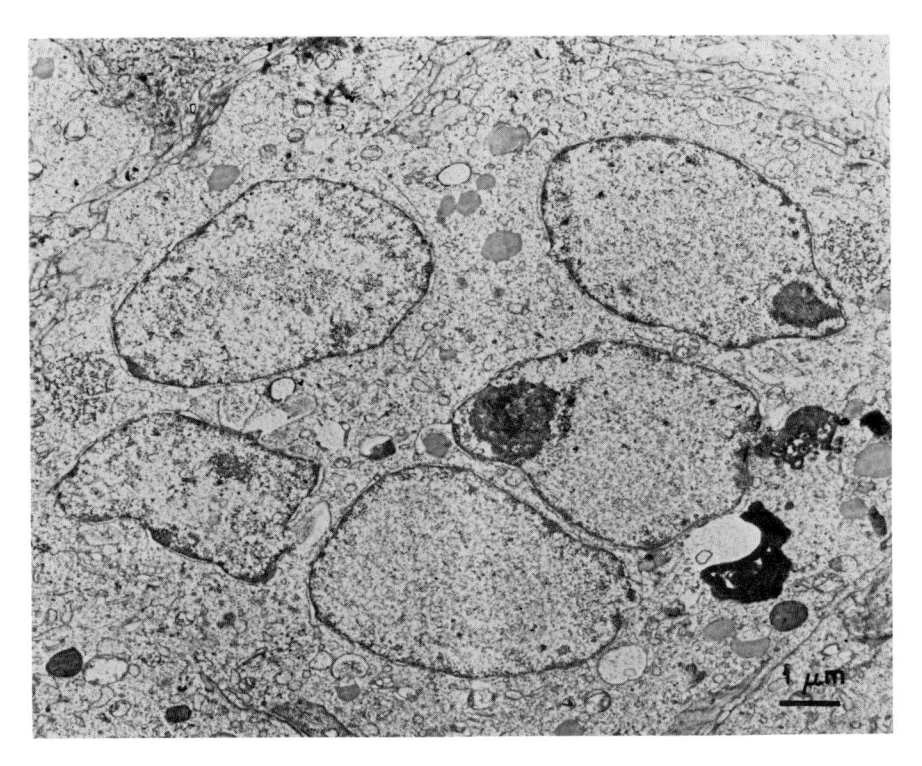

FIG. 23. Reticulum cell syncytia in bursa of 9-day-old chick infected with HPRS-16 strain of MDV. × 7700.

of a peak in bone marrow infectivity and cell-associated viremia at about 7 days after infection, suggesting that blood-borne dissemination of virus is marked at this time. Infection of the bone marrow may lead to aplasia and anemia (Jakowski et al., 1970). In our own studies, immature erythrocytes and granulocytes were present in the blood 7 days after infection of day-old chicks (Payne and Rennie, unpublished observations).

3. Acute Cytolytic Infection of Nonlymphoid Tissues

During the acute infection of lymphoid tissues other nonlymphoid tissues may show evidence of, usually, low grade MDV infection. Seven to 41 days after exposure of susceptible 4-week-old chicks, Adldinger and Calnek (1973) isolated cell-associated virus from proventriculus, kidney, liver, and gonad; earlier times were not studied, but in another strain infected at 1 week old no evidence of infectivity (in immunofluorescence tests) was found between 18 hours and 7 days. In our own study (Payne and Rennie, 1973) MDV antigen was observed between 3 and 10 days in the proventriculus (but in lymphoid foci) and lung, but not in kidney, liver, or gonad. In general the nonlymphoid tissues do not

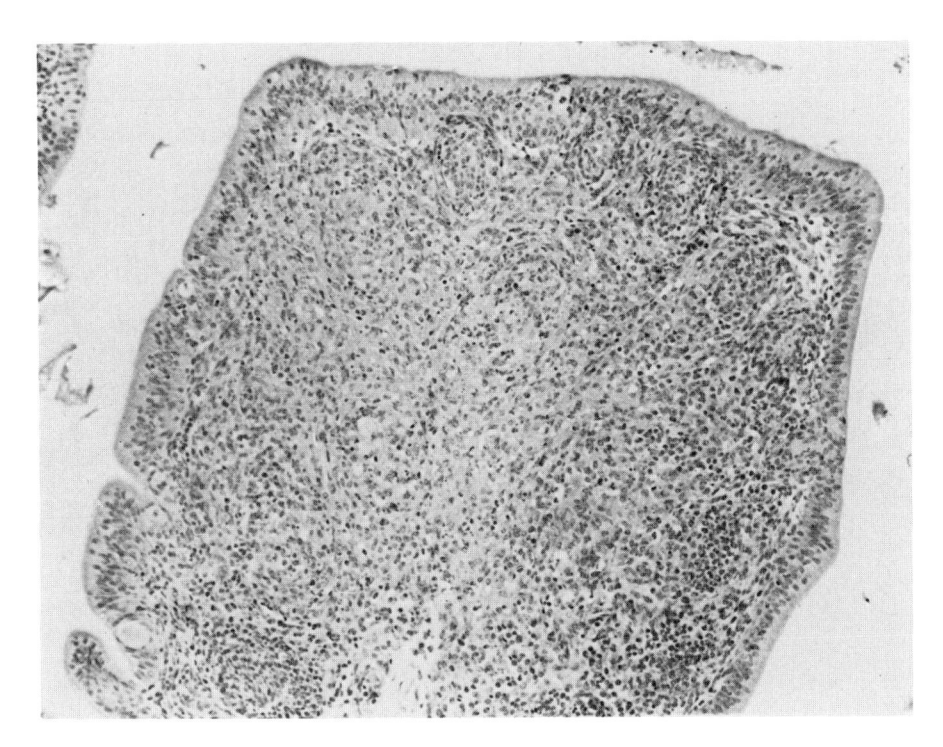

FIG. 24. Area of reticulum cell hyperplasia with loss of lymphoid follicles in bursa of 8-day-old chick infected with HPRS-16 strain of MDV. × 160. From Payne and Rennie (1973).

appear to be particularly susceptible to MDV infection. However, Calnek (1972a) observed focal necrosis of renal tubular epithelium with intranuclear inclusion bodies, glomerulitis or glomerular necrosis, and focal or generalized necrosis of pancreas, proventriculus, liver, and heart, and nuclear degeneration of proventriculus (with inclusion bodies), heart, and liver was reported by Ratz et al. (1972). Virions were observed in the nuclei of proventricular epithelial cells by Solisch (1972). We observed intranuclear inclusions in adrenal cortical cells. In Calnek's (1972a) report, some chicks died with degenerative lesions 10–17 days after infection, apparently from overwhelming MDV infection.

4. *Infection of Feather Follicle Epithelium*

In 1969 Calnek and Hitchner reported the presence in a high proportion of MDV-infected chickens of abundant viral antigen in feather follicle epithelium. It was subsequently shown that cellular and extracellular enveloped herpesvirus was present and that cell-free infectious virus could be removed from this site (Calnek et al., 1970a; Nazerian and Witter, 1970). Shed feathers, feather debris, and dander have been shown to be vehicles for MDV, and they clearly represent

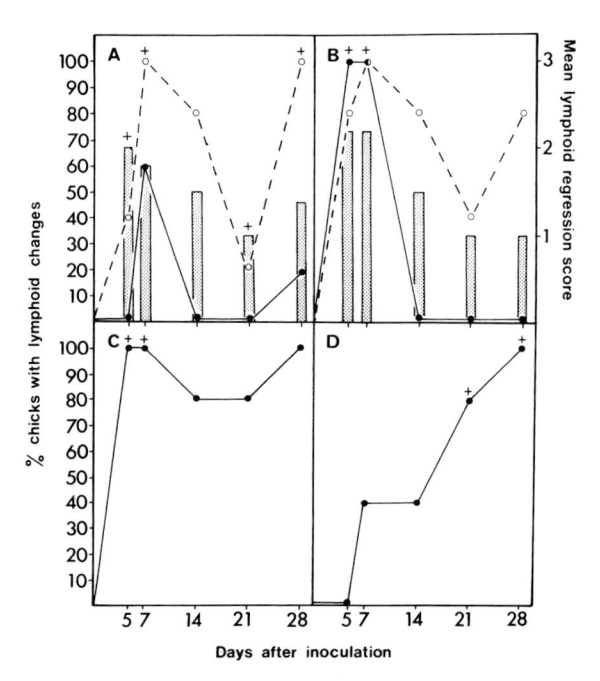

FIG. 25. Lymphoid regression and reticulum cell hyperplasia in (A) bursa and (B) thymus, and reticulum cell hyperplasia and lymphoid proliferation in (C) spleen and (D) feather follicle region of dermis in maternal antibody-free chicks at different times after infection with MDV. A, B: ●——●, percentage of chicks with reticulum cell hyperplasia; ○– – –○, percentage of chicks with lymphoid regression: stippled area, mean lymphoid regression score of positive tissues. Scoring: 1 = slight regression; 2 = moderate regression; 3 = severe regression. C,D: ●——●, percentage of chicks with reticulum cell hyperplasia (spleen), or lymphoid proliferation (spleen and feather follicle region). + = intranuclear inclusion bodies present. From Payne and Rennie (1973).

a major source of environmental contamination (Calnek et al., 1970a; Beasley et al., 1970). These findings were an important step in the understanding of the epidemiology of MDV, since they showed for the first time where virus replication takes place in the bird, and how infection spreads from bird to bird. The productive replication of MDV in the unique feather follicle site is an event necessary for the spread of MD, but one that seems to be essentially unrelated to the other pathogenic effects of MDV.

Infection of the feather follicle epithelium usually occurs later than the initial restrictively productive infection of lymphoid tissues (Fig. 13). Although antigen may be detected in feather follicle epithelium as early as 5 days after infection (Purchase, 1970), the majority of chicks do not show follicular antigen until 13–14 days post infection (Lapen et al., 1971; Payne and Rennie, 1973; Adldinger and Calnek, 1973). In our own study, viral antigen was seen at 5 days in lymphoid cell aggregates adjacent to feather follicles, before its presence in the follicle cells, suggesting that lymphocytes might carry the virus to the feather follicles. Subsequently, viral antigen can be found in the feather follicles of a high proportion of infected birds, for at least 6 weeks after infection. Viral antigen may also be detected on feather shafts by a radial diffusion technique in agar containing MDV antiserum (Haider *et al.*, 1970). Diffuse and granular viral antigen is seen intranuclearly and intracytoplasmically in the stratum corneum of the feather follicle epithelium. Intranuclear inclusion bodies are present in the corneous and transitional layers (Fig. 26), and affected cells undergo cloudy swelling and hydropic degeneration (Purchase, 1970; Lapen *et al.*, 1970). The viral antigen does not extend beyond the feather follicle epithelium into the epidermis of the skin. Occasionally viral antigen is present in the sheath and barb cells of the feather.

In thin sections (Calnek *et al.*, 1970c; Nazerian and Witter, 1970) virus-specific cytopathological changes are restricted to cells in the stratum transivativum. Basal cells and 3 or 4 adjacent inner layers of epithelial cells appear normal whereas degenerative changes are seen in the 3 or 4 rows of the outermost layer

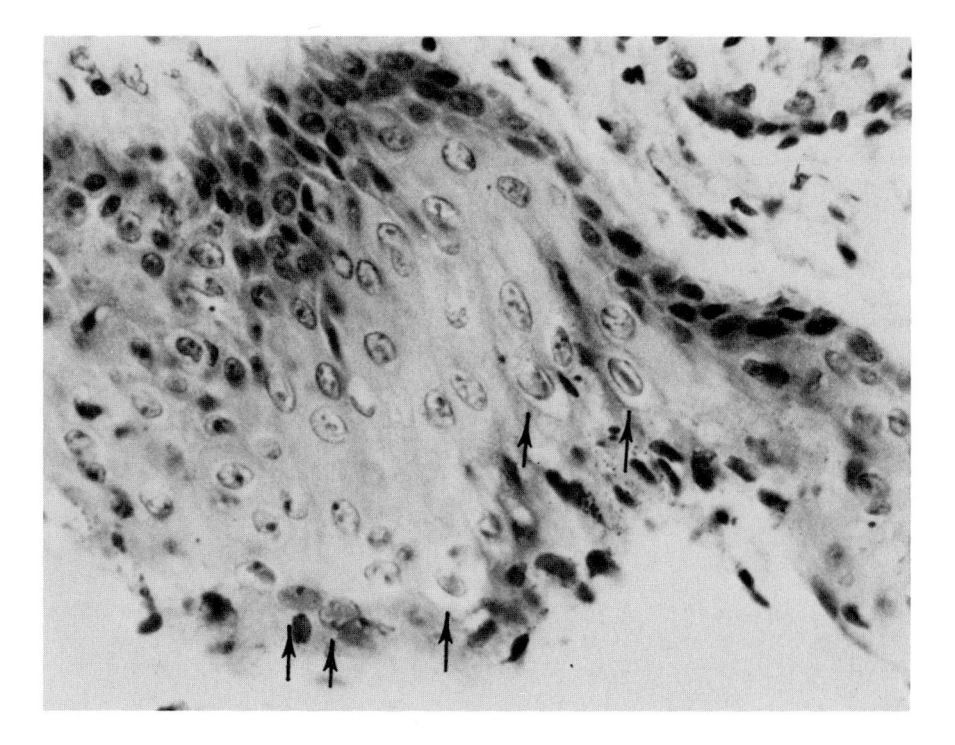

FIG. 26. Intranuclear inclusion bodies (arrows) in epidermis of feather follicle in 22-day-old chick infected with MDV. × 640. From Payne (1972).

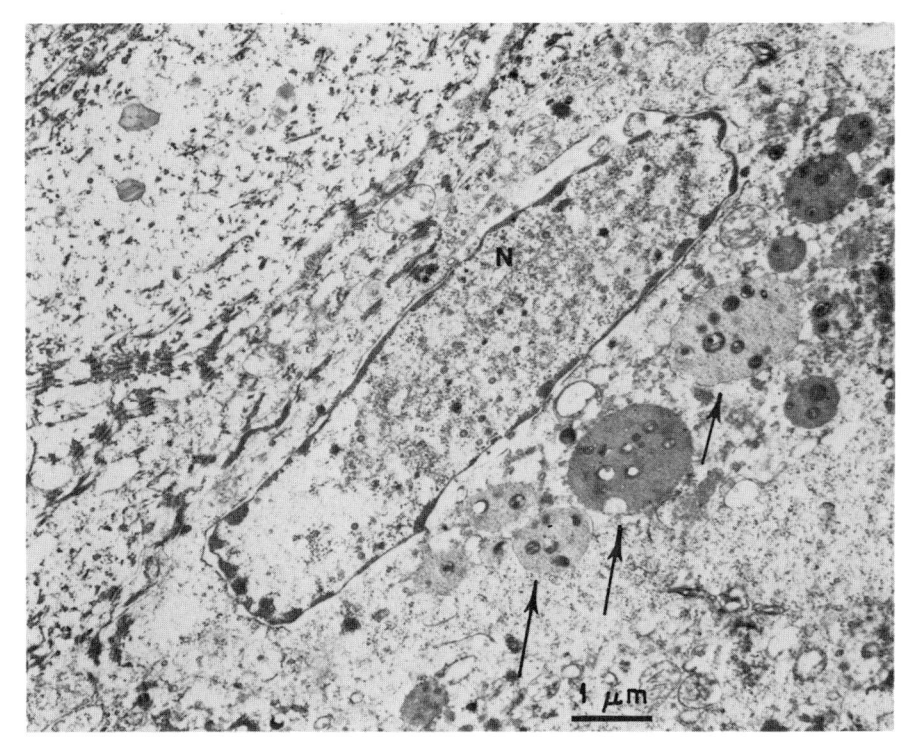

FIG. 27. Feather follicle epidermal cell with unenveloped nuclear virions in the nucleus (N), and enveloped virions (arrows) in intracytoplasmic inclusion bodies. × 10,300.

of the follicular epidermis, these changes originating in the inner cells and becoming more extensive in the outermost cells. Early changes are first seen in the nucleus and include margination of chromatin and appearance of intranuclear inclusion bodies. Naked and occasionally enveloped particles are present either at the periphery of the nucleus or in the nuclear inclusion bodies. Many cytoplasmic inclusion bodies are seen in later stages of infection, and the nuclear membrane often becomes ruptured. The cytoplasmic inclusions often occupy a major part of the cytoplasm and appear homogeneous, except for the presence of the virus particles (Figs. 7 and 27).

In the nucleus, the immature particles vary in structure from empty capsids to capsids that are almost entirely filled with nucleoid. Some particles acquire an envelope at the nuclear membrane and measure 150–170 nm in diameter, although the majority of the enveloped particles are found in the cytoplasmic inclusion bodies, where they measure up to 250 nm in diameter (see Section III, B). Occasionally, one envelope may contain two nucleocapsids. Envelopment of virus in cytoplasmic inclusion bodies seems to be a feature of feather follicle epithelium related to production of infectious cell-free virus.

Cells in the outermost layer of the feather follicle epithelium are often completely degenerate, and portions of these cells are found in the space between the epithelium and the feather shaft. Lack of exposure of virus to active cytoplasm may help to explain maintenance of virus infectivity. Cell debris found in this area includes intact nuclei with intranuclear inclusions, and inclusion bound and free-enveloped virus (Nazerian, 1971). These cells lining the inner surface of the feather follicle are degenerate even in uninfected birds, and it is clear that such a site provides a natural way in which the particles can be released into the air.

The appearance of viral antigen in the feather follicle is associated with perifollicular accumulation and proliferation of lymphoid cells (Fig. 28). These arise as perivascular lymphoid accumulations in the dermis, and are first seen at 7 days post infection (Payne and Rennie, 1973) (Fig. 25). They progressively increase in size and coalesce, and they may infiltrate into adjacent adipose tissue, smooth muscle (of pilomoter muscle), and subcutaneous nerves, giving rise in some birds to lymphomalike masses (Lapen et al., 1971). Occasionally the lymphoid cells may infiltrate the feather follicle epithelium and also the epidermis of the skin, causing an eczema. In some instances proliferating lymphoid

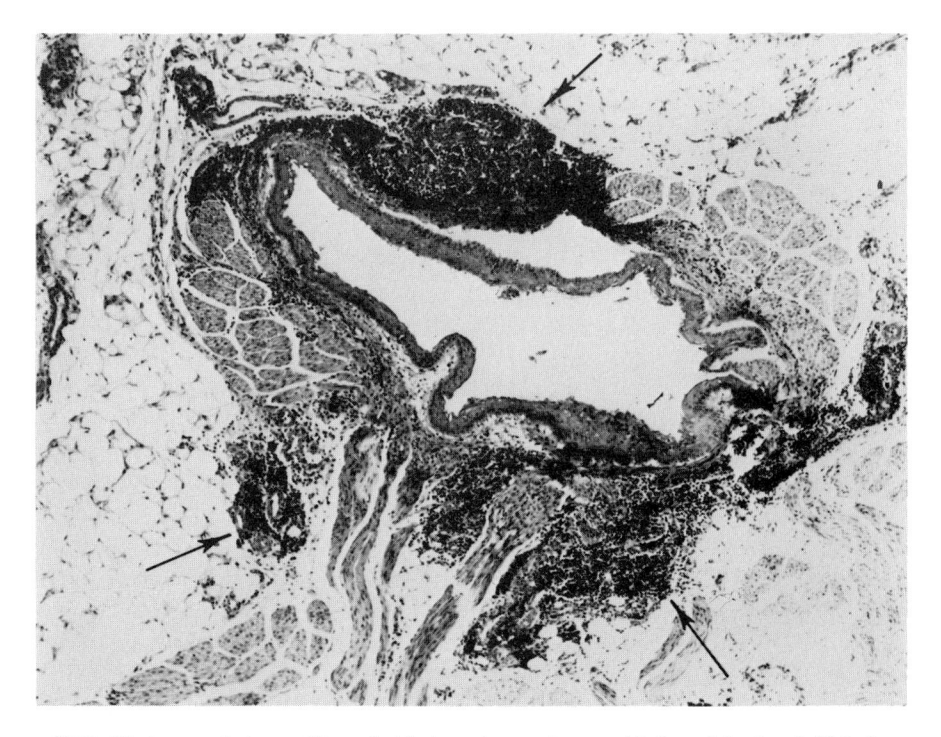

FIG. 28. Accumulations of lymphoid tissue (arrows) around infected feather follicle from 22-day-old chick infected with MDV. × 80. From Payne (1972).

cells are found in the pulp of the feather. In limited electron microscopical studies mainly medium to large lymphocytes, including some with nuclear projections, were observed in the dermis. They have not been seen to contain virus particles (Frazier, unpublished observations).

There is a correlation between the presence of lymphoid proliferation and viral antigen in the feather follicle. Lapen *et al.* (1971) suggested that MDV in the epithelium provides an antigenic stimulation for a perivascular lymphoid response. They discussed the question of whether the reactive lymphoid cells are (1) normal cells that respond to the antigenic stimulus, (2) cells that become neoplastically transformed at the site, or (3) cells that are transformed elsewhere but retain the ability to respond to antigen. At present the question cannot be answered. One possibility is that the cells that accumulate in response to follicular antigen are already sensitized during the preceding acute infection of lymphoid tissue. After their accumulation in the dermis, some of them undergo neoplastic transformation that may or may not lead to lymphoma formation, depending on host immune responses directed against tumor-specific antigens on the transformed cells.

5. *Neuropathic Changes*

MDV infection induces changes in both the peripheral and central nervous system; those in the peripheral nerves are the more severe and will be discussed first.

a. *Peripheral Nervous System.* The main features of the peripheral neuropathy of MD have been described by many workers, the more important early accounts being those of Marek (1907), Pappenheimer *et al.* (1926, 1929a), Lerche and Fritzsche (1934), and Potel (1939). Peripheral nerves of affected fowl were found to be variably infiltrated by lymphocytes, often with accompanying plasma cells and macrophages. Interneuritic edema was sometimes observed, and degeneration of the nerve fibers occurred particularly in heavily infiltrated nerves. Opinion differed on whether these changes were essentially inflammatory (Marek, 1907; Lerche and Fritzsche, 1934) or neoplastic (Pappenheimer *et al.*, 1926, 1929a; Furth, 1935). Present knowledge suggests that lesions of either type occur, depending on the stage or type of disease process. Another disputed question is whether changes in the neurites precede or follow lymphocytic infiltration, as discussed below.

The characteristics of the lymphoid cell infiltration in affected nerves have been used by several groups of workers to classify the lesions into pathological types and to suggest how the types might be related (Wight, 1962a; 1969; Payne and Biggs, 1967; Fujimoto *et al.*, 1971; Okada and Fujimoto, 1971). These schemes are summarized in Tables III and IV. The classifications of Wight and Fujimoto were derived from studies of 100 and 181 field cases, respectively, and might be expected therefore to embrace at least the commoner variations that occur; however, opinions expressed on the relationships between the different

TABLE III
CLASSIFICATIONS OF MAREK'S DISEASE NEUROPATHY

Predominant lesion	Wight (1962)	Payne and Biggs (1967)	Fujimoto et al. (1971)
Infiltration by small lymphocytes	Type I	—	T_I-type
Infiltration by mixed lymphocytes	Type I	A-type	T_{II}-type
Infiltration by lymphoblasts	Type III	—	—
Infiltration by reticular or undifferentiated mesenchymal cells	—	—	T_{III}-type
Sparse infiltration by small lymphocytes and plasma cells	—	C-type	—
Interneuritic edema, with infiltration by small lymphocytes and plasma cells	Type II	B-type	R-type

types of lesions must inevitably be rather speculative. The temporal relationships between the experimentally induced cases of Payne and Biggs (1967) are known, but this material has the disadvantage that the full spectrum of pathological responses may not have been encountered.

There is agreement between the classifications that the lesion characterized by interneuritic edema and sparsely scattered lymphocytes and plasma cells is inflammatory (i.e., a neuritis or polyneuritis). It has been designated variously as type II (Wight, 1962a), B-type (Payne and Biggs, 1967), and R-type (for "nontumorous response") (Fujimoto et al., 1971). There is less agreement about the more heavily infiltrative lesions. Mixed lymphoid cell proliferations were regarded as neoplastic by Payne and Biggs (1967) (A-type) and Fujimoto et al. (1971) (type T_{II}, a subdivision of "tumorous proliferation") but inflammatory by Wight (1962a) (type I). Infiltrations by small lymphocytes were classified as

TABLE IV
SUGGESTED NATURE OF MAREK'S DISEASE NEUROPATHY

Suggested nature of lesions and their relationship	Wight (1962)	Payne and Biggs (1967)	Fujimoto et al. (1971)
Inflammatory	Types I, II	B- and C-types	R-type
Neoplastic	Type III	A-type	T_I-, T_{II}-, T_{III}-type
Relationship	Type II→type I→type III	A-type↔B-type or C-type	T-types→R-type

inflammatory by Wight (1962a) (type I) but neoplastic by Fujimoto et al. (1971) (type T_I); they would be included in the A-type of Payne and Biggs (1967) and regarded as neoplastic. Proliferations of lymphoblastic cells were agreed to be neoplastic by Wight (type III) and Payne and Biggs (included in the A-type), and this class may be comparable to type T_{III} of Fujimoto et al. (1971), which was composed of "reticular or undifferentiated mesenchymal cells." The C-type lesion described by Payne and Biggs (1967) does not appear to have a counterpart in the other two classifications. We regard it as a mild inflammatory lesion.

In addition to lymphoid cell infiltration, nerves in MD also show a variety of changes in the neural tissue, including Schwann cell activation, demyelination and remyelination, and axon degeneration and regeneration. In our present state of knowledge these changes cannot be specifically related to particular types of infiltrative process, and they will be considered separately after discussion of the lymphoid changes.

In the sections that follow the nerve lesions of MD are discussed on the basis of our own experience and classification, and the results of others are discussed in this context. Our observations with the light microscope are derived from studies with the HPRS-B14 strain of classical MDV (Biggs and Payne, 1967; Payne and Biggs, 1967) and with the HPRS-16 strain of acute MDV (Purchase and Biggs, 1967; Payne and Rennie, 1973). Ultrastructural observations are derived from studies with HPRS-16- and HPRS-B14-infected chicks (Frazier, unpublished data). In these studies, 1-day-old MD antibody-free RIR chicks were inoculated with 10^3 PFU of HPRS-16 strain MDV. Sciatic plexus, celiac nerve, and dorsal root ganglia were removed from 2 control and 5 infected birds on each of the following days after infection: 7, 14, 21, 28, and 35 days. Other chicks were inoculated as above with 10^3 PFU of HPRS-B14 strain MDV, and brachial and sciatic plexi from 4 birds were examined at 41 days after infection. Material from HPRS-16-infected birds yielded A-type nerve lesions; that from HPRS-B14-infected birds, both A-type and B-type lesions.

i. *A-type lesion.* The mixed population of infiltrative and proliferative lymphoid and reticulum cells that typically constitutes the A-type lesion is the first change seen after infection under the light microscope (Fig. 29). The lymphorproliferation appears similar by light microscopy whether induced by classical or acute strains of MDV (Payne and Biggs, 1967; Purchase and Biggs, 1967; Payne and Rennie, 1973), but Frazier (see later) observed lymphocyte differences under the electron microscope. With HPRS-16 the earliest infiltrations were seen at 10 days post infection but were not present at 7 days. They consisted at first of small focal collections of blast cells, medium and small lymphocytes, activated reticulum cells, and so-called Marek's disease (MD) cells (Figs. 30 and 31). These last-named cells were about the same size as a blast cell and had a very basophilic, pyroninophilic, vacuolated cytoplasm. The nucleus was reddish when stained with hematoxylin and eosin, and the nuclear detail was not clearly

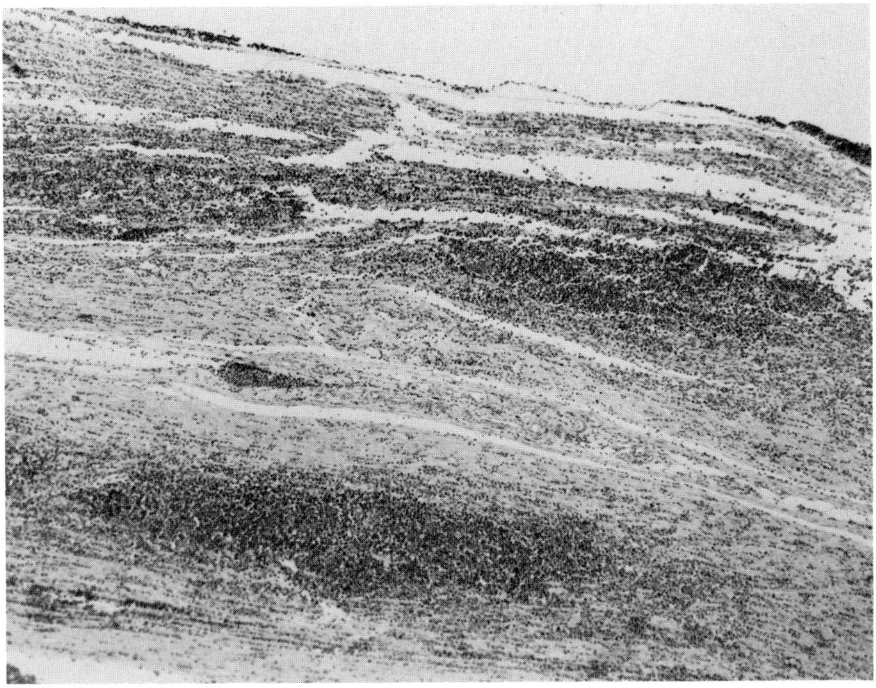

FIG. 29. A-type nerve lesion, showing lymphoid cell infiltration between neurites, in peripheral nerve of 28-day-old chick infected with HPRS-B14 strain of MDV. × 64. From Payne (1972).

visible. MD cells occur scattered among the other lymphoid cells and appear to represent a degenerative process occurring in a blast cell. Ubertini and Calnek (1970) identified MD cells under the electron microscope as degenerating lymphoblastoid cells that contained immature herpesvirions in the nucleus and, more rarely, coated virions at the nuclear border.

The lymphoid cell collections subsequently increase in size, and by 21 days and later nerves may be almost solidly infiltrated. In our experience the infiltrates appear to originate adjacent to capillaries and to increase in size by accumulation of blood-borne cells and by local proliferation. However, Sevoian and Chamberlain (1964) considered that the mononuclear cells in the nerve originated by hyperplasia of primitive mesenchymal cells of the tunica adventitia of the arterioles and of neurilemmal cells. Further work is needed to determine the origin of the proliferative and infiltrative cells.

In ultrastructural studies on the developing A-type lesion induced by HPRS-16 strain of MD, small numbers of medium to large lymphoid cells, some with nuclear projections, were observed at 14 days post infection. Mast cells were sometimes present, confirming the observations of Wight (1967). The nuclei of

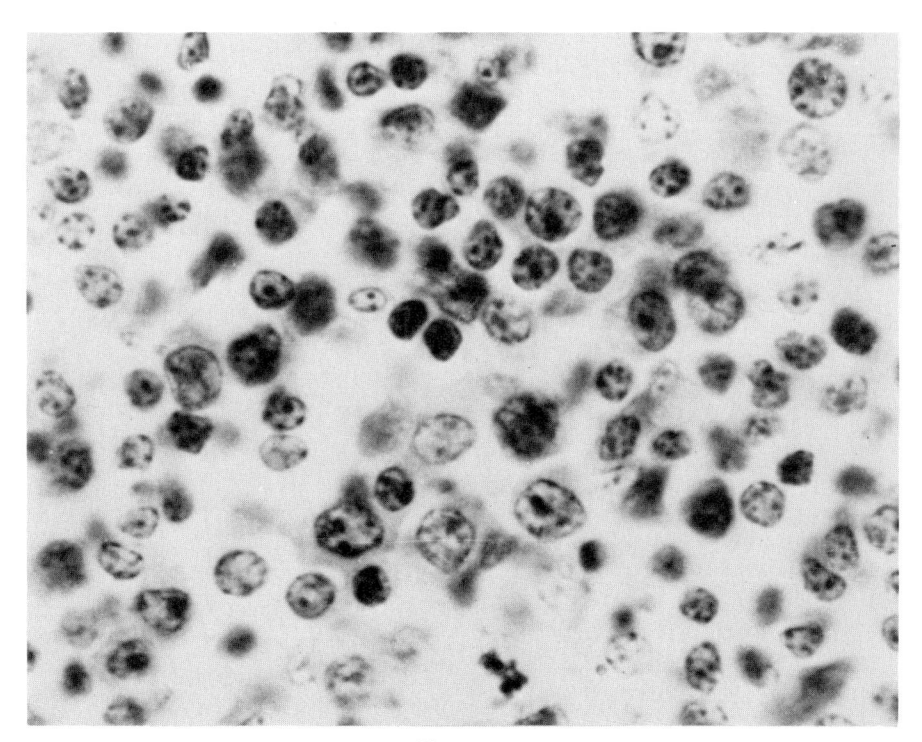

FIG. 30.

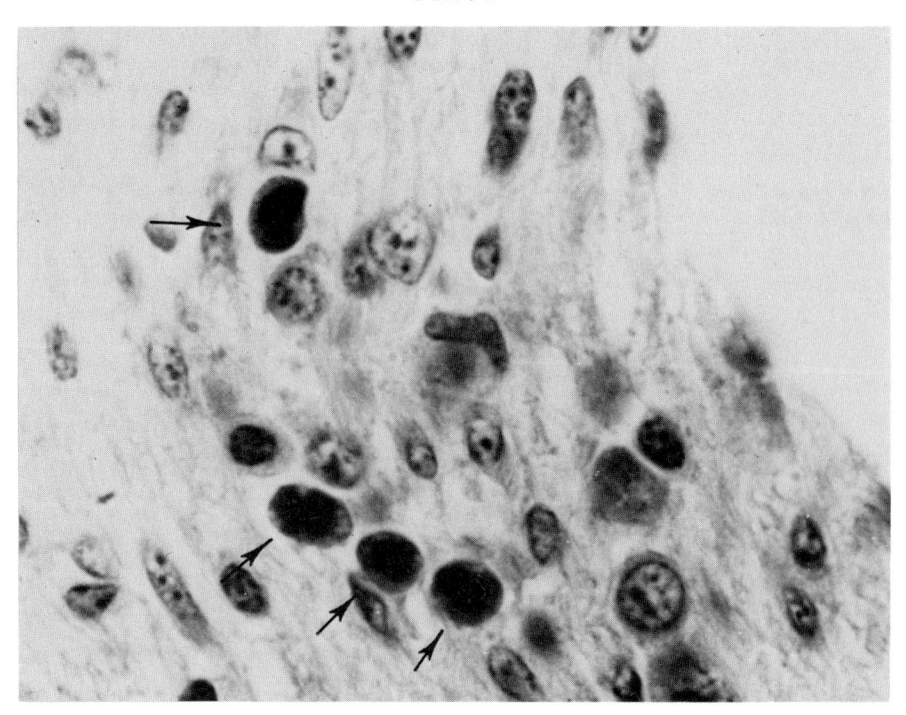

FIG. 31.

the lymphoid cells contained variable amounts of chromatin, and the cytoplasm, which was more abundant with the larger cells, contained many ribosomes, some in the form of polyribosomes, and a few mitochondria. Endoplasmic reticulum was usually sparse. At 21 days and later, nerves contained slight to massive infiltrations of neoplastic-type lymphoid cells (Fig. 32). These lymphoid cells, which were morphologically similar to lymphoid cells seen in the lymphomas that arise in other tissues, were pleomorphic, varied in size, and had sparse endoplasmic reticulum. Some of these cells had nuclear projections. Other (unidentified) cells associated with infiltrations had nuclei of irregular shape containing clumps of chromatin (Fig. 33), and some of these cells appeared syncytial. Very few macrophages with phagocytic vacuoles were present, and very little cell degeneration was observed. Virus particles were seen rarely in infiltrating lymphoid cells at 28 and 35 days post infection; they were usually intranuclear. Particles were not seen in other cell types. These lymphoid cells appeared ultrastructurally similar to those described in type T_{II} lesions by Okada and Fujimoto (1971); these authors also described a "hemocytoblastic large lymphoid cell," the nucleus of which contained unusually large nucleoli, and reticulum cells and a few macrophages were present.

In the type I lesions of Wight (1969) and the type T_I lesion of Okada and Fujimoto (1971), small lymphoid cells predominated, but medium lymphoid cells and reticulum cells were also present. Macrophages were prominent in Wight's material; ribosomes were numerous in the cytoplasm of these cells, and the endoplasmic reticulum was often dilated and filled with granular or flocculent material. Structures resembling lipid inclusions were common in the cytoplasm, although osmiophilic debris, perhaps degenerated myelin, was less common.

In the type III lesion of Wight (1969) lymphoblasts predominated; ultrastructurally they appear to be similar to the large lymphoid cells of our study, with nuclear projections sometimes present. Okada and Fujimoto (1971) did not describe the ultrastructure of their type T_{III} lesion. We suggest that types I and T_I on the one hand, and type III on the other, represent opposite extremes of the mixed cytology of our A-type lesion, and indeed such variants were sometimes observed in our material. It may be speculated that the neoplastic element of the lesion is represented by the lymphoblast, that small lymphocytes are reactive cells, and that the mixture varies according to the equilibrium between proliferating neoplastic cells and host response. It is interesting that our limited ultrastructural studies revealed that A-type lesions induced by the less pathogenic HPRS-B14 virus consisted of small- to medium-sized lymphoid cells, and that neoplastic-type cells with nuclear projections were very rarely seen. The lymphoid cells were fairly uniform in size and morphology and were unlike

---

FIG. 30 (*top*). Mixed population of lymphoid cells in A-type nerve lesion; same case as Fig. 29. × 1600.

FIG. 31 (*bottom*). "MD cells" (arrows) in early A-type nerve lesion in 14-day-old chick infected with HPRS-B14 strain of MDV. × 1600.

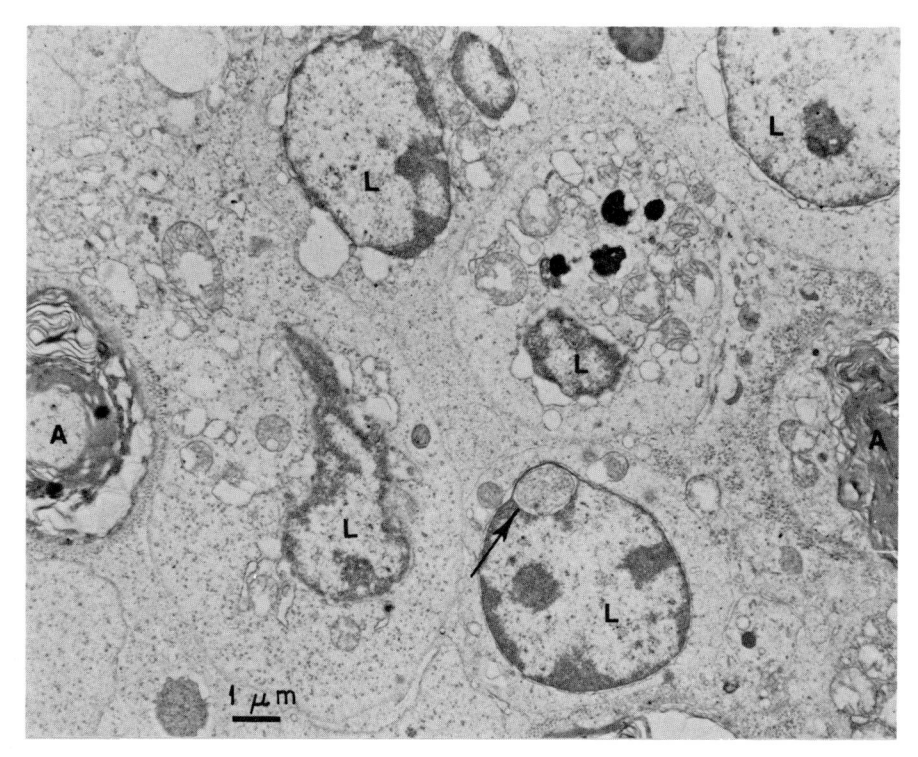

FIG. 32. Lymphoid cells (L), one with a nuclear projection (arrow), and myelinated axons (A), in the sciatic plexus of a 22-day-old chick infected with HPRS-16 strain of MDV. × 6000.

those seen in neoplastic A-type lesions induced with HPRS-16, but resembled those in severe B-type lesions.

The stimulus for the initial migration of lymphoid cells into the peripheral nerves is not known. The two main possibilities are (1) that lymphoid cells are attracted to the nerve by a preceding neural change, or (2) that lymphoid cells in MDV-infected birds have a predilection for some reason to settle in nervous tissue. Support for the first possibility depends on identifying the preceding change; although we believe this is not detectable by light microscopy, preliminary findings discussed below suggest that damage to Schwann cells may be the initiating lesion. There is no direct evidence for the second possibility. Goudie *et al.* (1974) have recently offered explanations for the apparent homing of lymphocytes to nonlymphoid tissues in certain diseases in man. Whatever the nature of the early infiltrating cells in the A-type lesion, it is evident that they rapidly take on a neoplastic character, and morphologically they appear identical to the lymphoma cells that arise in other tissues. Recently analysis of lymphoid cells from A-type nerves for bursal or thymic origin shows that, like lymphomas,

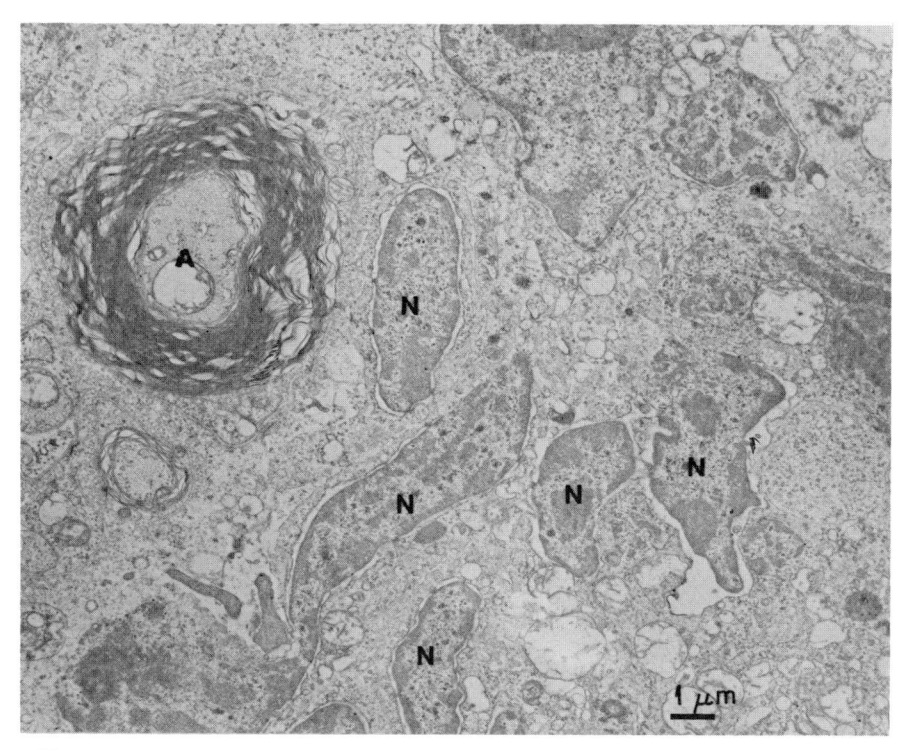

FIG. 33. Apparently syncytial cells with irregularly shaped nuclei (N) and myelinated axon (A) in sciatic plexus of 36-day-old chick infected with HPRS-16 strain of MDV. × 5800.

about 76% of the cells are T cells and 20% B cells (Payne and Rennie, 1976).

ii. *B-type lesion.* Affected nerves typically show interneuritic edema and infiltration by scattered lymphocytes, blast cells, and mature and immature plasma cells (Figs. 34 and 35). The degree of edema and cellularity varies considerably. Demyelination and Schwann cell increase occurs as discussed below (Payne and Biggs, 1967). This type of lesion is more frequently seen with classical strains of MDV than with acute strains, suggesting that it is a response to viruses of limited pathogenicity (Purchase and Biggs, 1967).

Ultrastructural study of B-type nerves induced by HPRS-B14 virus revealed infiltration by small or medium lymphocytes, some larger, mononuclear cells, which were probably macrophages or their precursors, and a few plasma cells. Pleomorphic lymphoid cells with nuclear projections, such as are present in A-type lesions induced by HPRS-16, were observed only very rarely. Occasionally, lymphoid cells were seen in close contact with the Schwann cells and demyelinated axons, and a few appeared to be under the basement membrane of

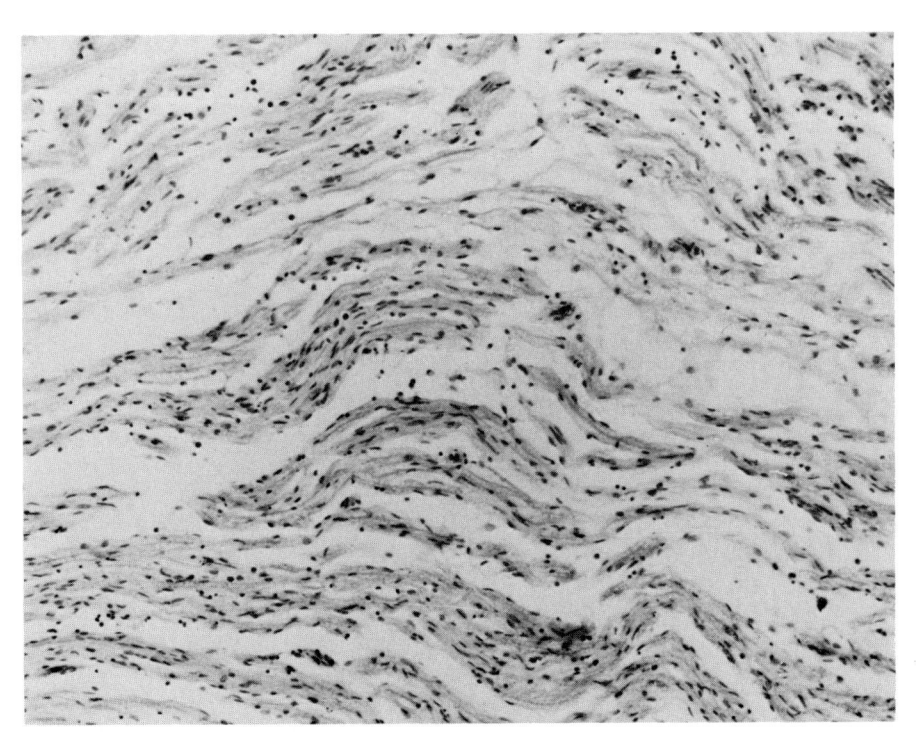

FIG. 34.

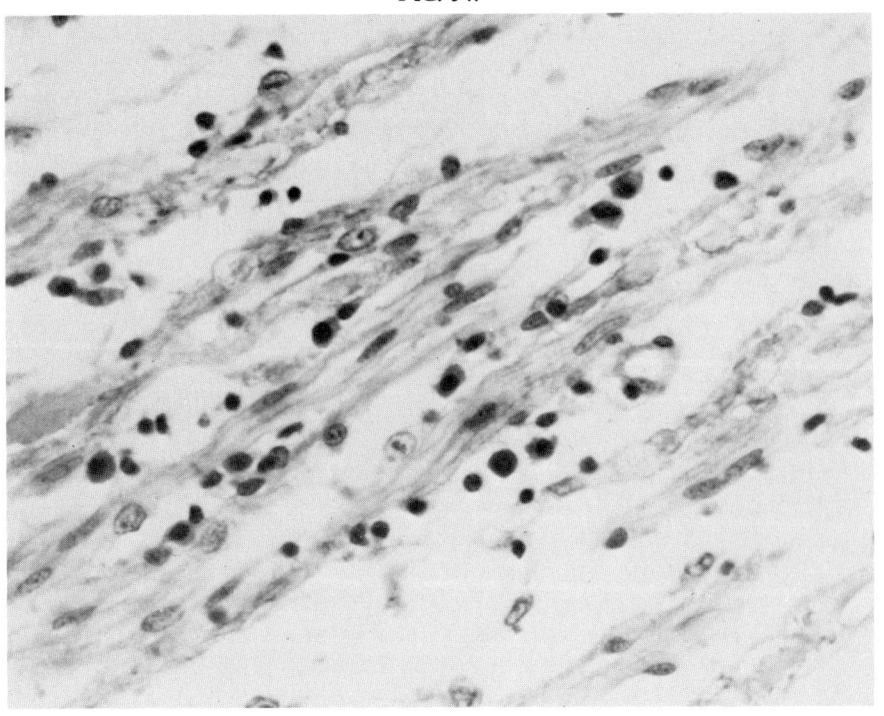

FIG. 35.

the Schwann cells (Fig. 36). Intact, demyelinated axons were commonly observed (Fig. 37). In some lesions, Schwann cells were surrounded by increased amounts of collagen (Fig. 38). The B-type nerve lesion, as mentioned earlier, appears to be identical to the type II lesion of Wight (1962a), who first clearly defined this type of lesion, and to the R-type lesion of Fujimoto et al. (1971). Leaving aside changes in neural elements, which will be considered later, ultrastructural aspects of the infiltrating cells described by Wight (1969) and Okada and Fujimoto (1971) conformed to the findings given above. Macrophages were prominent in Wight's (1969) material, and there was a suggestion of protein elaboration by these cells. These cells were also engaged in phagocytosis of a variety of elements: myelin and cellular debris, lipids, and pigments (Wight, 1969; Okada and Fujimoto, 1971). Okada and Fujimoto commented on the presence of cytoplasmic bridges between macrophages and plasma cells, suggesting a possible interaction in antibody synthesis. Both groups also noted the frequent presence of mast cells in the edematous type of nerve.

Opinion is discordant on the relationship between the A- and B-type lesions (or the equivalent types in other classifications) (Table IV). Because demyelination can occur in the absence of heavy infiltration, and because axon loss (Wight, 1964) and biochemical changes (Heald et al., 1964) were less severe in type II nerves, Wight believed that the type II lesion preceded the type I and type III lesions. However, we suggested that the edematous type nerve lesion was more chronic, and characteristic of birds more resistant to Marek's disease, than was the more lymphoproliferative lesion. Sequential studies suggested that the B-type lesions follow A-type lesions (Payne and Biggs, 1967). Fujimoto et al. (1971) favored this type of sequence (T → R), although they also suggested that a lesion may commence and continue as an R-type. We have not seen early B-type lesions in our experimental material, but it is possible that such lesions are confused with mild A-type or C-type (see below) lesions.

iii. *C-type lesion.* The nerve showing a C-type lesion appears to be normal except for a sparse scattering of plasma cells and lymphocytes (usually small type). There is no edema, nor are there areas of proliferating cells. It is seen particularly in fowl that fail to develop clinical disease following infection with MDV, and it probably represents a mild form of the B-type lesion (Payne and Biggs, 1967).

iv. *Changes in neurites.* In addition to infiltration of peripheral nerves in MD by inflammatory and neoplastic lymphoid cells, degenerative and to a lesser extent regenerative changes occur in the neurites. Early workers considered that axonal and neuritic degeneration was caused by the lymphoid cell infiltration

---

FIG. 34. B-type nerve lesion, showing interneuritic edema and sparse cell infiltration, in peripheral nerve of 70-day-old chicken infected with HPRS-B14 strain of MDV. × 160. From Payne and Biggs (1967).

FIG. 35. Plasma cells and lymphocytes in B-type nerve lesion in peripheral nerve of 70-day-old chicken infected with HPRS-16 strain of MDV. × 640. From Payne (1972).

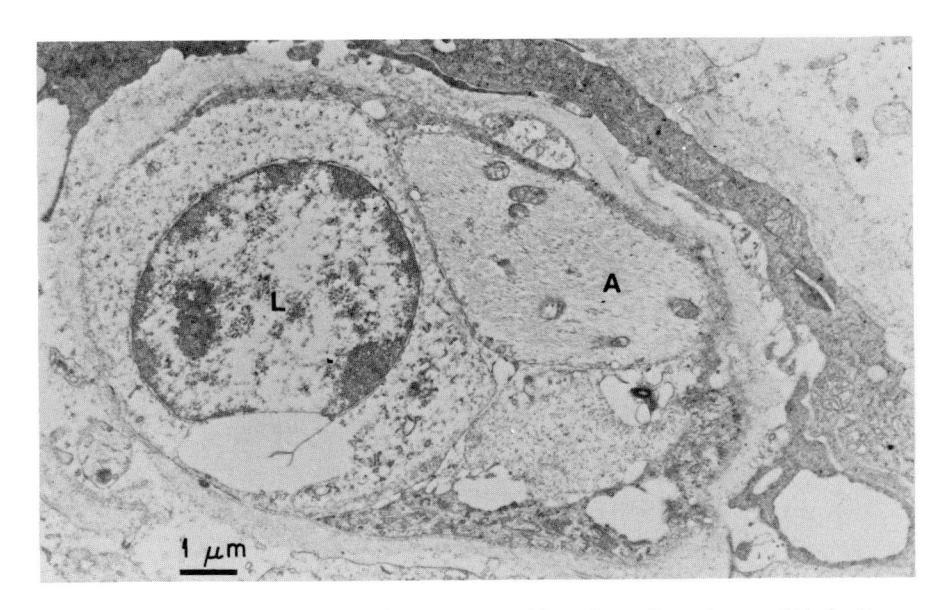

FIG. 36. Lymphoid cell (L) in close contact with a demyelinated axon (A), in B-type nerve lesion in 41-day-old chicken infected with HPRS-B14 strain of MDV. × 7200.

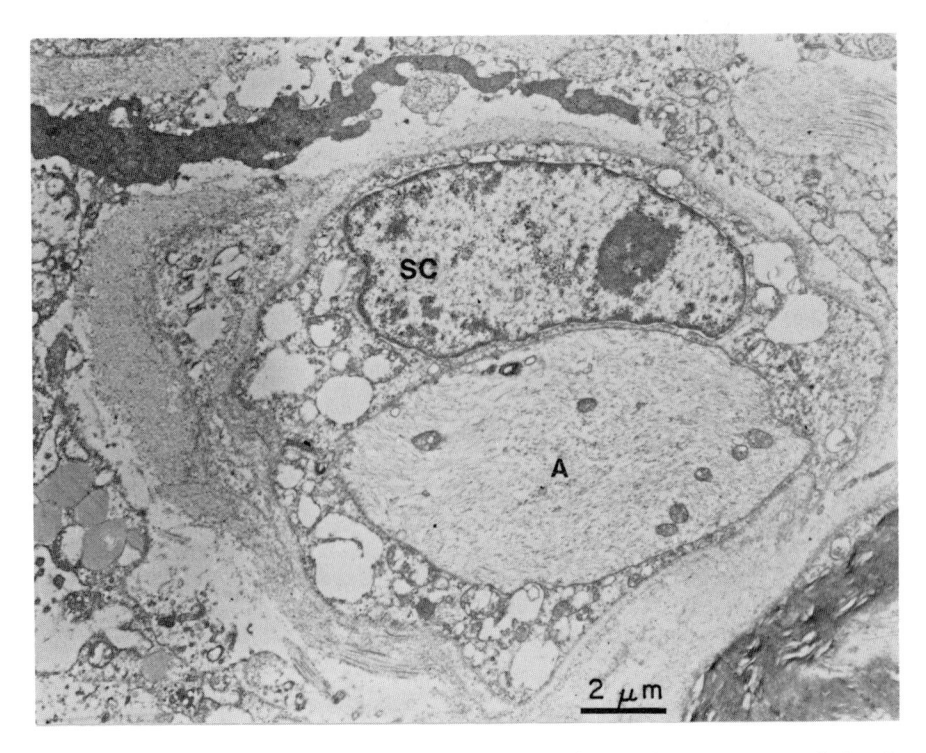

FIG. 37. Demyelinated axon (A), with Schwann cell (SC), in B-type nerve lesion in 41-day-old chicken infected with HPRS-B14 strain of MDV. × 5500.

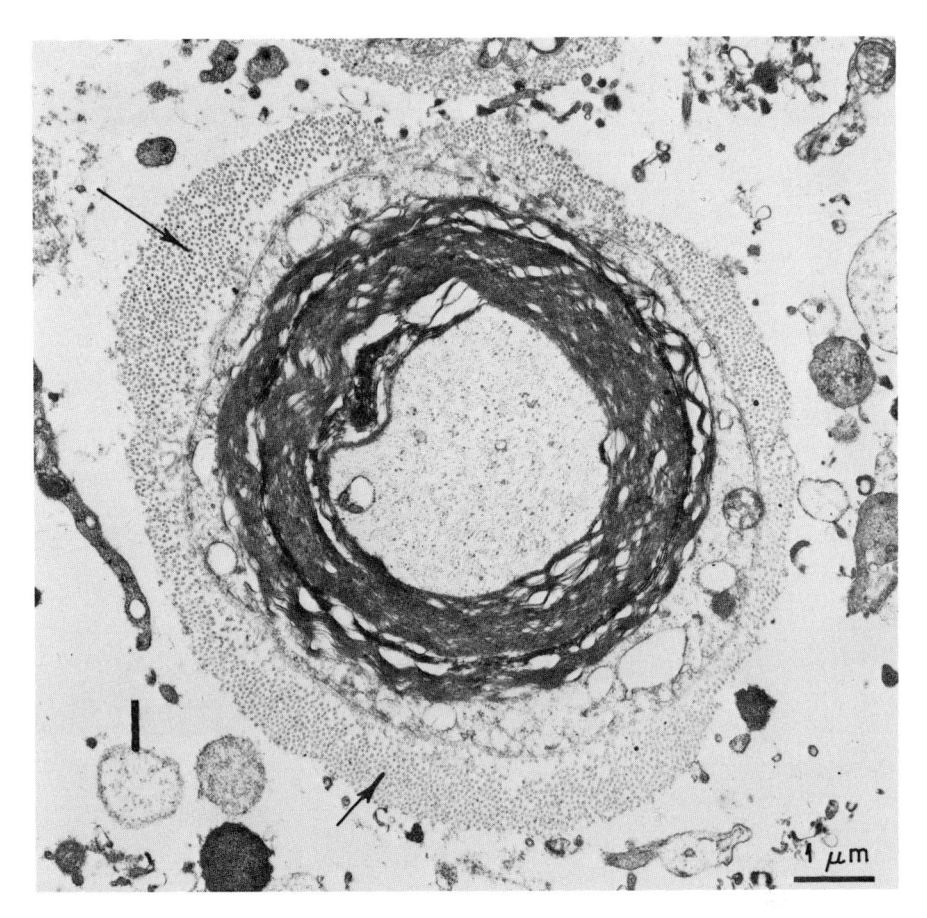

FIG. 38. Increased collagen (arrows) deposition around myelinated nerve from B-type nerve lesion in 41-day-old chicken infected with HPRS-B14 strain of MDV. X 9400.

(Pappenheimer et al., 1926; 1929a, b; Lerche and Fritzsche, 1934; Furth, 1935). Wight (1962a), however, observed that in his type II nerves there was often considerable destruction of neurites but very little cellularity. Subsequently he showed that although demyelination occurred in this type of nerve, the number of axons was not reduced (Wight, 1964). In contrast, axons were reduced in the infiltrative type I and type III lesions. In mild type II nerves Wight (1962a) described demyelination of short segments of unrelated neurites followed in severe cases by axon disruption and formation of digestion chambers containing myelin ovoids. Wight (1964) suggested that the early type II lesion represents a primary demyelination, that this is the initial morphological lesion in the MD nerve, and that in severely edematous or cell infiltrated nerves secondary,

Wallerian, degeneration occurs owing to compression of neurites. Wight (1962a, 1965) showed that neurites in MD had some regenerative capacity.

Although we have questioned the concept that the type II (B-type) lesion precedes the infiltrative lesions, recent ultrastructural studies support the idea that primary and secondary demyelinative processes may be occurring. The two main publications dealing with the ultrastructure of peripheral nerve lesions, including changes to neurites, are those of Wight (1969) and Prineas and Wright (1972). Although Okada and Fujimoto (1971) described the infiltrating cells, they did not describe neuritic changes. Wight (1969) and Prineas and Wright (1972) agreed that heavy lymphoid cell infiltration was associated with typical Wallerian degeneration of axons and myelin. They disagreed, however, about the nature of the primary demyelination they observed. Wight (1969) considered that changes in the Schwann cell, including Schwann cell activation, was prominent and occurred early in the disease, suggesting that this cell is a primary target for MDV or is particularly susceptible to its subsequent effects. Apart from Wallerian degeneration occurring in more severe type I and type III nerves, he considered that a more subtle process occurs in less severe type I and type II nerves which results in degeneration of myelin lamellae but sparing of axons. Wight considered that the latter changes were similar to those seen in experimental diphtheritic neuritis (Webster et al., 1961; Weller, 1965) and lead neuropathy (Lampert and Schochet, 1968), where degenerative changes in myelin sheaths are unrelated to the presence of infiltrating cells, and Schwann cells are the major cells involved in myelin disintegration.

Prineas and Wright (1972) disagreed that myelin degeneration occurred without the participation of infiltrating cells. They found that the appearance of invading inflammatory cells preceded myelin breakdown, and that these cells actually participated in the process of demyelination. No morphological alteration was observed in the myelin until the basement membrane (neurolemma) had been breached and the Schwann cell cytoplasm had been displaced away from the myelin sheath by invading mononuclear cells. Two types of invading cell were seen, frequently within the neurolemma. One was a lymphocyte with more cytoplasm than a typical small lymphocyte, and numerous free ribosomes. The other cell, which was related to overt myelin breakdown, was a macrophage containing moderate amounts of endoplasmic reticulum. Focal lysis of superficial myelin lamellae appeared where the macrophage contacted the sheath and macrophage processes extended through these gaps into the sheath along minor dense lines, and stripped away and engulfed successive layers of myelin. The Schwann cell was displaced away from the myelin sheath and did not participate in myelin breakdown or take up myelin debris, although it was often enlarged and rich in ribosomes and granular endoplasmic reticulum. After removal of the myelin sheath, mononuclear cells disappeared from within the neurolemma leaving an axon of normal appearance surrounded by Schwann cell cytoplasm. Remyelinating and demyelinated fibers were sometimes surrounded by concentrically arranged Schwann cells, mononuclear cell processes, and redundant basement membrane to form "onion bulbs." These structures had previously been observed by light and electron microscopy by Wight (1962a, 1969) in type II nerves and are believed to arise from repeated degeneration and proliferation of Schwann cells (Lampert and Schochet, 1968). Prineas and Wright observed that this type of demyelination was similar to that seen in experimental allergic neuritis, in which a cell-mediated autoimmune response occurs directed against peripheral myelin (Lampert, 1969; Wisniewski et al., 1969a), and they suggested that a similar mechanism was operating in the MD.

There is thus a conflict of opinion from these studies as to whether or not primary demyelination in MD is cell-mediated. Furthermore, the studies were made in field cases in which cellular infiltration of nerves had occurred, so that it is not possible to deduce whether there were neural changes preceding lymphoid cell infiltration. In order to clarify these differences and to identify the primary nerve lesion a sequential study of nerves and dorsal root ganglia of chicks infected with HPRS-16 MDV was carried out, as detailed above. The following descriptions refer mainly to sciatic plexus and celiac nerve, although similar changes were observed in dorsal root ganglia.

Most of the tissues examined at 7 days did not differ significantly from the controls. However, some areas of peripheral nerve were observed in which spaces between the nerve fibers showed increased numbers of profiles consisting of a membrane containing cytoplasmic organelles (Fig. 39) such as was noted by Wight (1969). Wight attributed these structures to cross sections of macrophage or Schwann cell processes. Macrophages were not seen in the 7-day nerves, however, and such profiles may have been an indication of early Schwann cell hypertrophy. In addition, unbound cytoplasmic organelles were observed between nerve fibers, suggesting that Schwann cell disruption occurred. This early change which preceded lymphoid cell infiltration suggests that the initial lesion affects neural tissue. No virions were seen in Schwann cells or in neurons in the dorsal root ganglia.

At 14 days slight lymphoid cell infiltrations in a few areas were seen in most specimens under the light microscope. The cells were usually medium to large lymphoid cells, some of which had nuclear projections. Subsequently they increased in number to give rise to the A-type lymphoproliferative lesion already described. In many specimens at 14 days, including those in which infiltrating cells were absent, large degenerating and disorganized masses of myelin were observed within Schwann cells (Fig. 40). Axons were usually relatively unaffected, although occasionally these too were degenerate. The spaces between nerve fibers were sometimes greater than usual, indicating edema, and increases in endoneurial collagen were occasionally observed. Collagen increase was also observed by Deutsch and Siller (1961) and Prineas and Wright (1972). Some Schwann cells showed increased vesiculation, probably due to increases in endoplasmic reticulum and hypertrophy. As far as could be ascertained the basement membranes around the Schwann cell were intact.

At 21 days some specimens were similar to those at 14 days, with increased

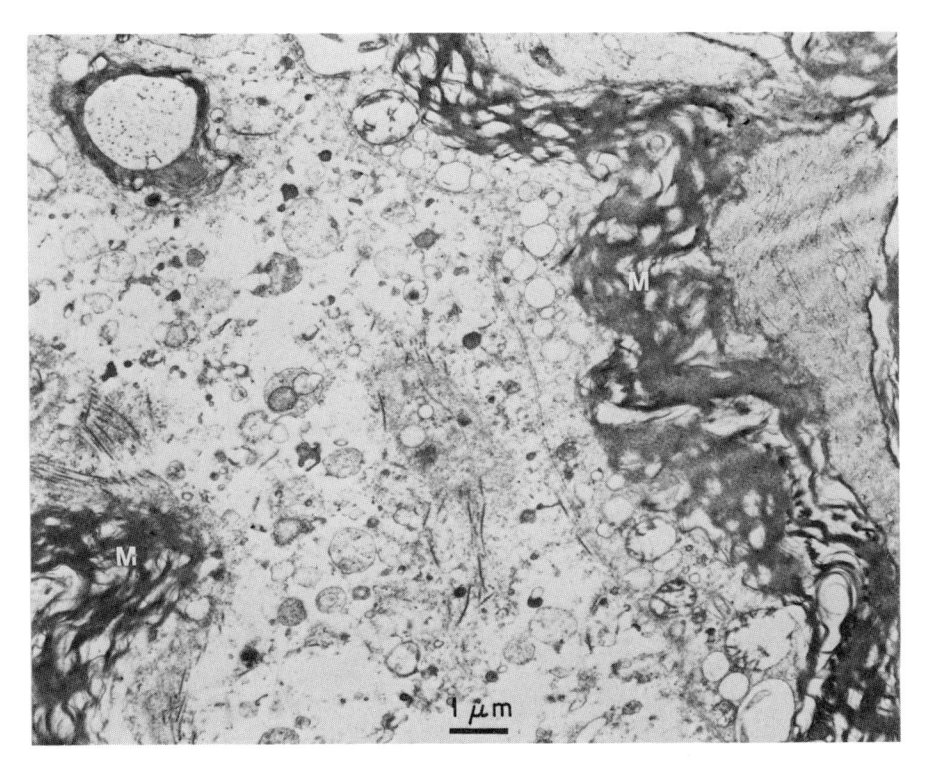

FIG. 39. Cytoplasmic profiles lying between two myelin sheaths (M) in sciatic plexus of 8-day-old chick infected with HPRS-16 strain of MDV. × 7600.

Schwann cell hypertrophy and myelin disorganization and degeneration, while others contained slight to massive infiltrations of neoplastic-type cells. Very few macrophages with phagocytic vacuoles were present in the infiltrations, and very little cell degeneration was observed apart from some myelin degeneration within Schwann cells. Some infiltrating cells appeared to be intimately associated with Schwann cells, although the participation of these cells in primary demyelination could not be identified. Many of the Schwann cells, axons, and myelin with which massive infiltrations were associated appeared normal with intact basal laminae. Degenerating masses of myelin were sometimes seen in heavily infiltrated areas; however, axons were often relatively unaffected. Basement laminae were usually intact.

Samples taken at 28 and 35 days varied in degree of infiltration but were similar to those at 21 days. Occasionally, some areas that were usually associated with either very few or no infiltrating cells contained axons that were almost totally demyelinated or with myelin present only on one side of the axon (Fig. 41). "Onion bulb" formation, as discussed earlier, was occasionally noted.

v. *Proposal for the pathogenesis of MD neuropathy.* On the basis of these various findings it is possible to propose pathogenetic sequences for the neural and lymphoproliferative changes in MD nerves. We suggest that several interdependent pathogenetic processes are occurring.

The results suggest, in agreement with Wight (1969), that the initial demyelination follows a pattern similar to that seen in diphtheritic neuropathies (Webster et al., 1961; Weller, 1965) and lead neuropathy (Lampert and Schochet, 1968), where demyelination with axon sparing proceeds in the absence of infiltrating cells. In these examples myelin breakdown is presumably an indirect or direct reaction to toxins. In MD an acute reaction occurs in lymphoid and other organs at 5–7 days after infection (see Section IV, D, 2). In the absence of evidence for virus infection of Schwann cells or other neural cells at this time, it is possible that the Schwann cell reaction and subsequent myelin damage seen is a response to a toxic factor produced by the acute reaction. Alternatively, these initial changes may arise from a mainly nonproductive infection of Schwann cells or other neural elements by MDV. It is well known that other herpesviruses do replicate in the nervous system. For example, herpes simplex virus replicates in cells of the central and peripheral nervous systems including neurons and

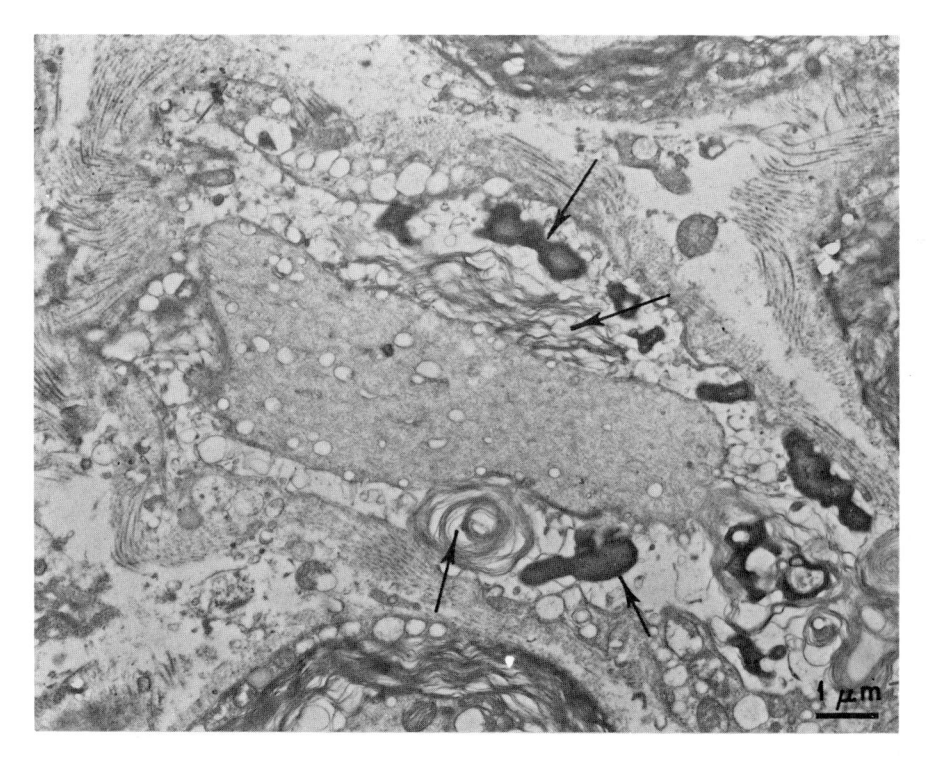

FIG. 40. Degenerating and disorganized myelin (arrows) in Schwann cell from sciatic plexus of 15-day-old chick infected with HPRS-16 strain of MDV. × 8000.

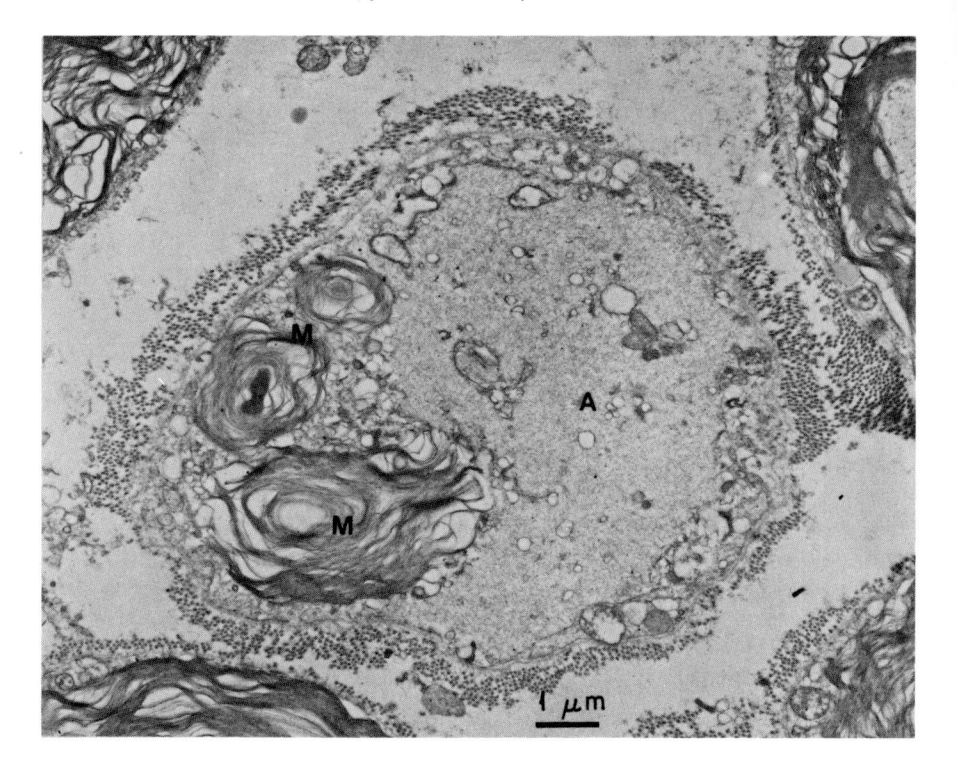

FIG. 41. Demyelinated neurite with disorganized myelin (M) to one side of axon (A) in sciatic plexus of 29-day-old chick infected with HPRS-16 strain of MDV. × 8000.

satellite cells, Schwann cells and axons, astrocytes, glial cells and oligodendrocytes (Rabin *et al.*, 1968; Severin and White, 1968; Baringer and Griffith, 1970; Kristensson, 1970; Hill *et al.*, 1972; Yamamoto *et al.*, 1973). The virus readily replicates with productive infections in the cells of the central and peripheral nervous systems, although it is rarely or never observed in infiltrating inflammatory cells, such as lymphocytes or macrophages (Baringer and Griffith, 1970; Kristensson, 1970; Cook and Stevens, 1973). This is in contrast to MD, where there is little evidence to support the view that MDV replicates to any extent in neural cells. When MDV is seen in peripheral nerves it is usually present in infiltrating lymphoid cells. Ubertini and Calnek (1970) observed herpesvirus particles in the nuclei of Schwann cells in the brachial nerve of a chicken with MD, but this seems to be a very rare occurrence. Herpes simplex virus has been found to establish persistent latent infections in nervous tissue (Knotts *et al.*, 1973; Cook *et al.*, 1974), and it is possible that MDV can enter into a similar relationship and bring about myelin changes.

Demyelination arising from Schwann cell damage could stimulate two trains of events. First, lymphoid cells could become exposed to and sensitized to peripheral myelin, leading to an autoimmune cell-mediated attack on normal myelin. This would explain the similarity between the cell-mediated primary demyelination seen in MD by Prineas and Wright (1972) and that seen in experimental autoimmune disease (Lampert, 1969; Wisniewski et al., 1969a). This type of demyelination was not seen in our study, but it may be relevant that the lesions examined by Prineas and Wright were from classical cases of MD, and therefore probably milder and more longstanding. The idea of an autoimmune disease in MD is not new. Siller (1960) first drew attention to the similarity at the light microscope level between the neural lesions of MD and experimental allergic encephalomyelitis, and Petek and Quaglio (1967), by inoculating chicken and guinea pig nerves in Freund's adjuvant, produced an allergic neuritis indistinguishable from Wight's (1962a) type I and type II lesions. Wight and Siller (1965) found that allergic encephalomyelitis was suppressed in fowl with spontaneous neural MD, and, unexpectedly, that the incidence of spontaneous MD in fowl rendered "tolerant" to allergic encephalomyelitis was not reduced, but rather that there was an apparent increase. Further studies on the interaction between MD and experimental allergic neuritis and encephalomyelitis would be worthwhile.

Recently, the occurrence in cases of MD of allergic skin reactions against myelin of peripheral nerves has been reported (Schmahl et al., 1975). This constitutes the first direct evidence for autoimmune responses to myelin in MD.

The second train of events that may arise from the preinfiltrative change in Schwann cells is the attraction of lymphoid cells into the peripheral nerves and the subsequent proliferation of these cells. Viral or tissue antigens may attract lymphoid cells into the nerve. Among these may be some that are infected with MDV, and some of these may already be transformed into tumor cells or may be transformed later. Proliferation of these cells would then result in the lymphomatous infiltrations of the nerves already described.

Compression of axons by the proliferating lymphoid cells may subsequently give rise to secondary, or Wallerian, demyelination as observed by Wight (1969) and Prineas and Wright (1972).

It must be stressed that this view of the pathogenesis of the MD neuropathy is a speculative and composite one based on observations of workers on tissues of diverse origin. There is need for further sequential studies on nerves of fowl with experimental infections by both acute and classical strains of MDV.

Finally, the possible relationship between MD neuropathy and the Landry–Guillain–Barré syndrome (acute infective polyneuritis) in man should be mentioned. This later disorder is characterized by an acute ascending paralysis, with peripheral nerve changes consisting of edema, demyelination, and axonal degeneration, Schwann cell activation and lymphocytic infiltration (Greenfield et al., 1958), similar to the B-type nerve lesion in MD. Immunological (Caspary et al., 1971; Rocklin et al., 1971) and ultrastructural evidence (Wisniewski et al., 1969b; Prineas, 1971) indicates that a primary cell-mediated demyelination is involved, as is suggested for MD (Prineas and Wright, 1972). The Landry–Guillain–Barré syndrome may follow a variety of virus infections, including two caused by herpesviruses, varicella and infectious mononucleosis. Recurrent polyneuropathy is a disease of man possibly related to acute infective polyneuritis, and similarities between this disease and MD were commented on by Borit and Altrocchi (1971). Current knowledge suggests that MD neuropathy may provide a close model for the Landry–Guillain–Barré syndrome in man.

  b. Central Nervous System. The most detailed account of the histopathology of the central nervous system in MD is that of Wight (1962b), who also reviewed the earlier literature (Marek, 1907; Doyle, 1926; Pappenheimer *et al.*, 1926, 1929a, b; Lerche and Fitzsche, 1934; Lee *et al.*, 1937). Wight's study showed that the central nervous system is often histologically normal in MD, and that when lesions do occur they are usually minimal. The most frequent abnormality was perivascular cuffing by usually mature lymphocytes, occurring in the white and gray matter of the brain and cord. Minimal to mild cuffing was seen in 64%, moderate in 4%, and severe in 7%, of field cases of MD, with 25% showing no cuffing. The severe cases were in birds with type III ("neoplastic") peripheral nerve infiltrations; less severe cuffing was associated mainly with type I and type II nerve lesions. Neuronal degeneration was rare, even in motor neurons supplying heavily infiltrated nerves. There was no specific or general involvement of glia, but microgliosis and astrocytosis could occur, particularly adjacent to severe perivascular cuffing. Primary demyelination did not occur, but severe perivascular cuffing or mechanical distortion caused secondary demyelination. Cuffing of meningeal vessels and lymphoid cell infiltration into the meninges were sometimes seen. In a recent survey of field cases, Fujimoto *et al.*, (1971) recorded perivascular cuffing in 76%, lymphoreticular cell proliferation in 13%, and astrocytic proliferation in 33%.

  Study of experimentaly produced cases of MD reveal that central nervous changes occur early in the course of the disease. Sevoian and Chamberlain (1964) reported hyperplasia of primitive mesenchymal cells of the tunica adventitia of blood vessels in the brain, cord, and meninges as early as 10 days after infection with JM virus, just as they found in other tissues. Vickers *et al.* (1967) observed perivascular cuffing in the corpus striatum and cerebellum 2 weeks after infection with Conn-A strain virus, which reached a peak of severity in these and other central nervous sites 5 weeks after infection. In our study cuffing was first seen 7 days after infection with HPRS-16 strain virus (Payne and Rennie, 1973). These studies add little to those of Wight (1962b) on the details of the histological changes in the central nervous system, and no ultrastructural studies have been undertaken.

  The stimulus for mild perivascular cuffing in MD, which is suggestive of a mild encephalitis in most instances, is unknown. Viral antigen, as detected by fluorescent antibody tests, is absent or extremely rare in brain (Purchase, 1970; Adldinger and Calnek, 1973; Payne and Rennie, 1973). Nevertheless, cell-associated virus can be found in brain as early as 3 days after infection (Phillips and Biggs, 1972), and viral antigen has been detected by the agar gel diffusion test (Adldinger and Calnek, 1973). Further understanding depends on localization of virus or antigen in the brain.

Transient paralysis. Recently MDV has been incriminated in the etiology of an encephalitis of adolescent fowl characterized by sudden paralysis, particularly of the neck and legs, usually lasting only 24–36 hours, followed generally by an uneventful recovery. This syndrome was first described and named "transient paralysis" by Zander (1959), and was subsequently studied by Willemart *et al.* (1967a, b), Walker and Grattan (1968), Wight (1968), and Cho *et al.* (1970). The common features are variable, but usually mild, perivascular lymphocyte cuffing in the central nervous system, mild lymphocytic infiltration of the meninges, and mild focal or diffuse microgliosis. According to Wight (1968), the cerebellum and brain stem are most affected, other brain regions less so, and the spinal cord is rarely affected. According to Willemart *et al.* (1967b), the mononuclear cells in the perivascular cuffs are intermediate between lymphocytes and lymphoblasts and appear to arise by endovascular proliferation and then become perivascular. Wight (1968) also commented on the possible origin of these cells from vascular adventitia. He also observed perivascular cystlike spaces containing pleomorphic material of unknown origin. Neuronolysis, axon degeneration, and demyelination are rarely seen (Willemart *et al.*, 1967a; Wight, 1968). Mild lymphocytic infiltration of peripheral nerves of the C-type occurs (Willemart *et al.*, 1967a, Wight, 1968; Cho *et al.*, 1970). Lesions in other organs are mild and variable: Willemart *et al.* (1967b) reported perivasculitis in some visceral organs and intranuclear inclusion bodies in Langerhans cells in the pancreas; Wight (1968) reported small necrotic foci surrounded by histiocytes in the liver, spleen, and lungs of some birds; and Cho *et al.* (1970) reported atrophy of bursal lymphoid follicles.

Kenzy *et al.* (1973) have been able consistently to produce the transient paralysis syndrome in a proportion of birds inoculated with an acute MDV isolate and to prevent the syndrome by vaccination with turkey herpesvirus or by pretreatment of birds with sera from MD-immune birds. They produced the syndrome 9–10 days after infection with MDV, suggesting that the disease results from an acute encephalitogenic action of the virus in birds which have not yet mounted an immune response to the virus. In this respect it may have similarities to primary herpes simplex encephalitis (Rawls, 1973).

6. *Lymphomagenesis*

a. Pathology. Pappenheimer *et al.* (1926, 1929a, b) were the first to report that visceral lymphomas occur in some cases of MD. The ability of MDV to cause lymphoma formation depends on several factors, most important of which are strain of virus and susceptibility of the host (see Section VI, A and B). In susceptible hosts the acute strains of MDV produce a high incidence of lymphomas in a variety of tissues, whereas the classical strains of MDV produce a lower incidence of lymphomas, mainly in the ovary but occasionally in the other organs commonly affected by the acute strains (see Section IV, B and C).

Our studies on the pathogenesis of MD induced by the classical HPRS-B14 strain (Payne and Biggs, 1967) and the acute HPRS-16 strain (Payne and Rennie, 1973) suggest that the lymphomagenic process is similar for both strains, but that the process is much more vigorous, widespread, and less prone to regression when induced with HPRS-16 strain. With this virus, multifocal lymphoid proliferation is seen as early as 7 days after infection, particularly in the gonads, liver, and proventriculus. Lymphomatous foci are first detectable macroscopically at 14 days after infection, and birds die from advanced lymphomatosis from 21 days (Fig. 42). Cytologically the lymphomatous foci consist, *ab initio*, of a mixture of small and medium lymphocytes, blast cells, primitive and activated reticulum cells, macrophages and Marek's disease cells (Payne and Biggs, 1967; Purchase and Biggs, 1967) (Fig. 43). Lymphoid cells predominate in these foci, but the degree of differentiation they show varies from mainly small lymphocytes to mainly blast cells. Plasma cells and heterophils are rarely seen. A fine

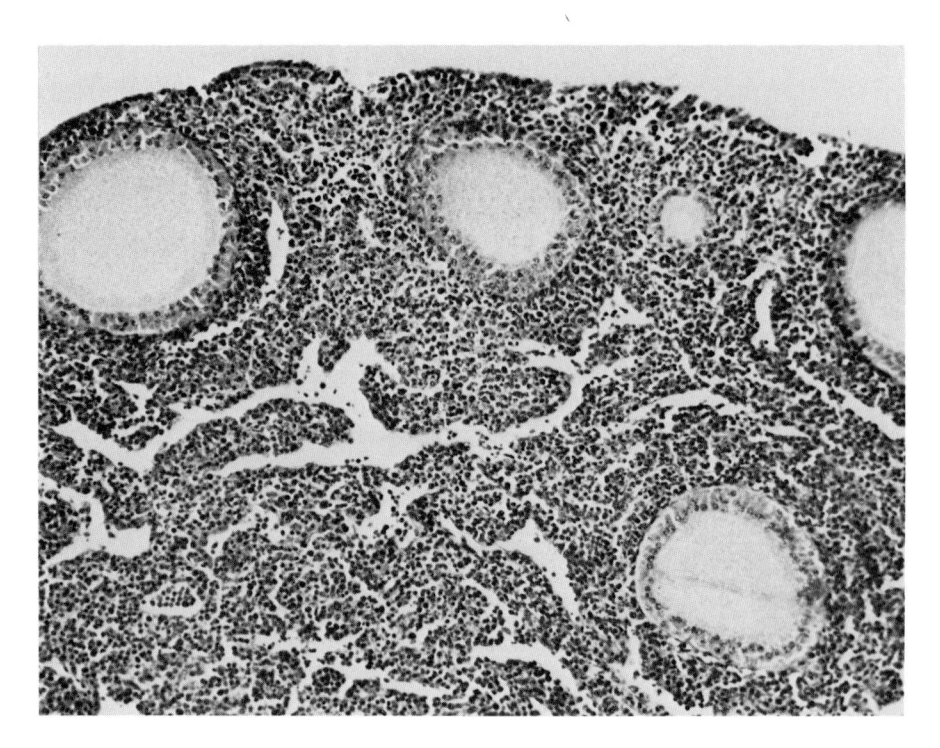

FIG. 42. Ovarian lymphoma in 32-day-old chick infected with HPRS-B14 strain of MDV. X 160. From Payne (1972).

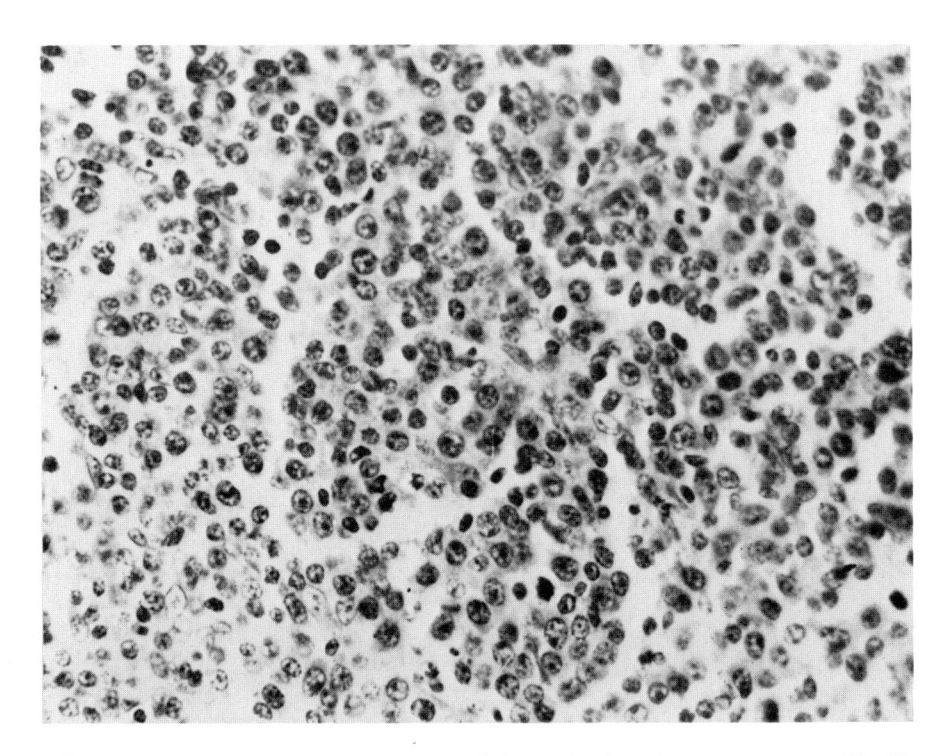

FIG. 43. Mixed population of lymphoid cells in ovarian lymphoma; same case as Fig. 42. × 640. From Payne (1972).

reticulin network is present between the densely packed tumor cells. The cytology of the lymphoma is identical to that of the lymphoproliferative lesion in the A-type nerve. On rare occasions cells containing intranuclear inclusion bodies may be seen among the lymphoid cells, and cell lysis and syncytia are present (Omar et al., 1973); in one such tumor examined by us, scattered large macrophages containing cell debris were present, giving the "starry sky" appearance described for Burkitt's lymphoma (Wright, 1970). Fujimoto et al. (1971) found that visceral tumors could be classified cytologically into three T-types similar to the proliferative nerve lesions (see Section IV, D, 5, a).

Accounts of the tissue distribution of lymphomas following experimental infection with acute strains of MDV are also given by Sevoian and Chamberlain (1964), Horiuchi et al. (1969), Ratz et al. (1972), Szeky and Vanyi (1973), and Kardevan et al. (1973).

The ultrastructure of MD lymphomas has been described by Doak et al. (1973), and our own studies on HPRS-16 strain-induced lymphomas are in agreement (Frazier, unpublished results). The lymphoid cells composing the tumors are pleomorphic and vary in size. The cytoplasm is abundant but contains few cytoplasmic organelles other than mitochondria and ribosomes (usually arranged as polyribosomes). Very little endoplasmic reticulum, and few lysosomes or structures resembling the Golgi apparatus, are observed. The nuclei are fairly large and irregular in shape, and nucleoli are sometimes seen. Chromatin is often arranged around the periphery of the nucleus (Fig. 44).

A notable feature of the tumor cells is the frequent presence of nuclear projections (Fig. 44). These projections have been reported in lymphoid cells of MD tumors, nerve infiltrations, and lymphoid organs of MDV-infected birds (Wight, 1969; Ubertini and Calnek, 1970; Nazerian, 1971; Okada and Fujimoto, 1971; Mladenov et al., 1972; Frazier, 1974a). Lymphoid cells with nuclear projections are rarely seen in the lymphoid organs of normal, healthy birds (Frazier, 1974a). They have been reported in the lymphoid cells in other neoplasms (Achong and Epstein, 1966; Papadimitriou, 1966; Mollo and Stranig-

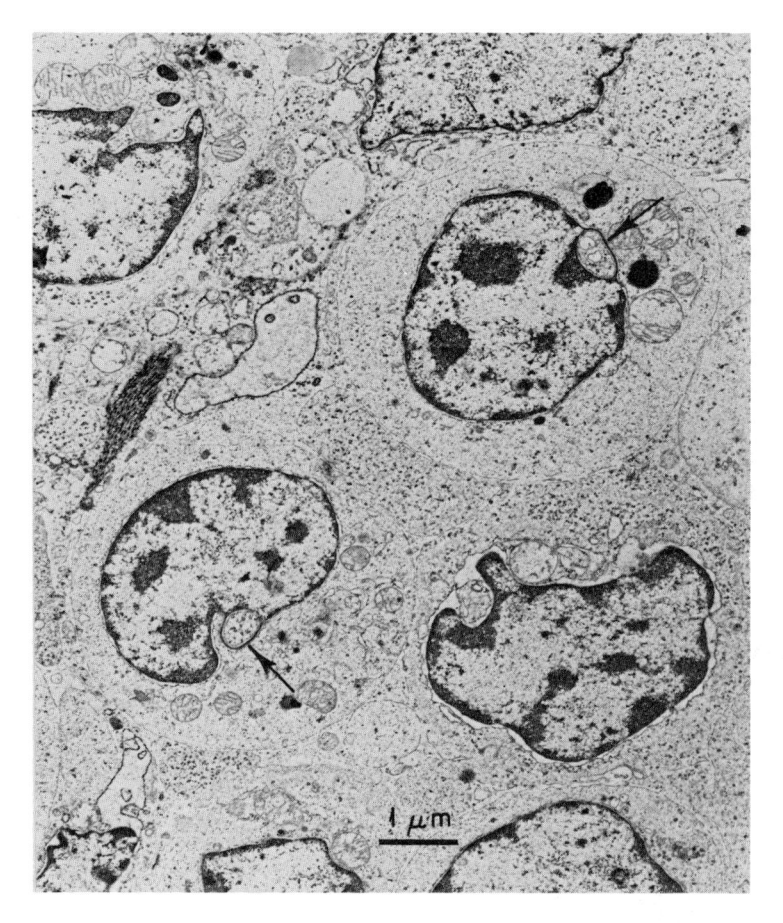

FIG. 44. Ovarian lymphoma induced by HPRS-16 strain of MDV, showing morphology of lymphoid cells, two of which have nuclear projections (arrows). × 10,000.

noni, 1967, Parker et al., 1967; Miller et al., 1969) and also in cultured bovine peripheral blood lymphocytes that were producing C-type virus particles (Weber et al., 1973). However, nuclear projections have also been seen in apparently normal cells (Sebuwufu, 1966; Törö and Oláh, 1966; Huhn, 1967; Smith and O'Hara, 1967) including lymphocytes cultured with phytohemagglutinin (Mollo and Stranignoni, 1967; Frazier, unpublished observations). Thus it appears that nuclear projections can be a feature of normal lymphoid cells, although they are probably associated with increased proliferation. It is not known whether the cells with nuclear projections in MD lymphomas are normal and are produced in response to abnormal tumor cells or viral antigen, or whether the cells with nuclear projections are abnormal and neoplastic. They are present in about 3% of cells from a MD lymphoma cell line (Powell et al., 1974; Frazier and Powell, 1975). Herpesvirus particles are rarely seen in MD tumors, except in maternal antibody-free birds (Schidlovsky et al., 1969; Calnek et al., 1970c; Nazerian, 1971; Kardevan et al., 1973; Frazier, 1974a). The particles are usually intranuclear and unenveloped, indicating an abortive infection, but occasionally enveloped particles are seen in nuclear vesicles (Fig. 45).

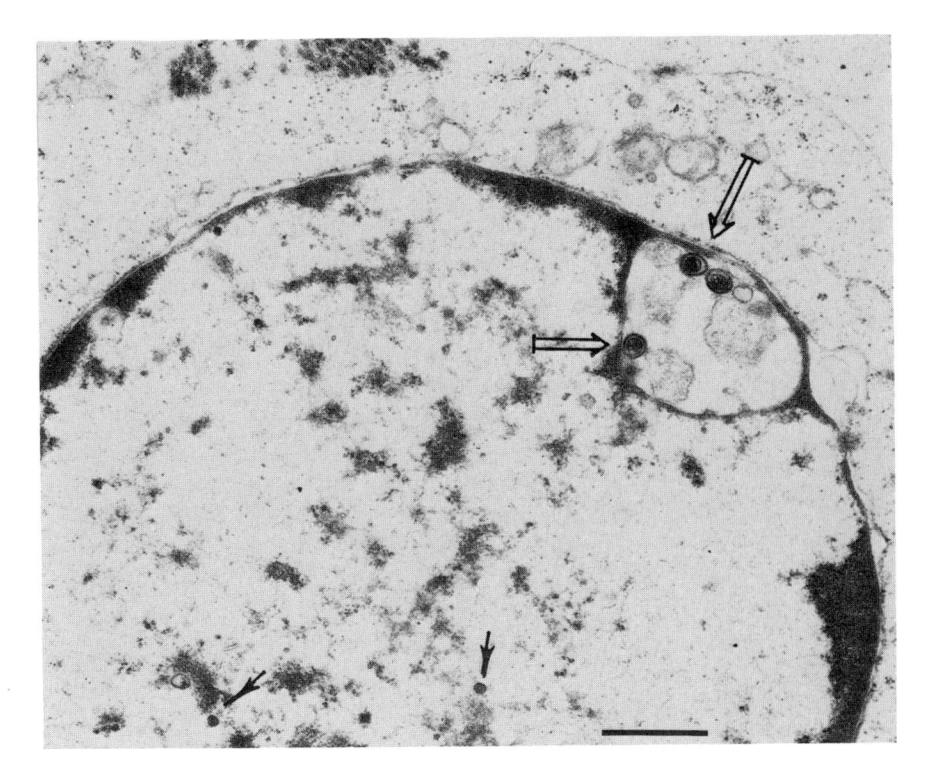

FIG. 45. Part of lymphoma cell, showing unenveloped virions (small arrows) in the nucleoplasm and enveloped virions (large arrows) in a nuclear vesicle. × 14,400.

b. Origin of Lymphoma Cells. The question of the origin of the cells that comprise MD lymphomas has been studied by conventional histological observations, by removal of the bursa or thymus prior to infection, by detection of immunologically competent cells, and most recently by direct straining of B and T cell markers. Sevoian and Chamberlain (1964) were the first to study in detail the pathogenesis of lymphomas. They stated that "sites of earliest cellular activity and proliferation were seen in the tunica adventitia of the small arterioles." The stimulated cell type was identified as a "primitive mesenchymal cell" which appeared to give rise to the mature mononuclear cell, which increased in number with the age of the lesion. This type of response commenced at 4 days after infection and was found to be widespread throughout the tissues. Fujimoto *et al.* (1971), Szeky and Vanyi (1973), and Kardevan *et al.* (1973) also believed that the proliferation starts from vascular adventitial cells, and Fujimoto *et al.* stated: "It may be appropriate to consider that tumorous lesions consisted of proliferated tumor cells which may come from lymphoreticular cell [*sic*] originating from the extracapillary reticular tissue, that is the undifferentiated primitive mesenchymal tissues in the whole body."

This concept of a local origin of lymphoid cells from reticular cells, although long held by classical histologists, goes against recent immunological belief which holds that peripheral lymphoid tissue in the fowl is dependent on and derived from two central lymphoid organs, the thymus and the bursa of Fabricius. The evidence for this was reviewed by Payne (1971). According to this view it should be possible to classify lymphocytes as thymus-derived (T) cells or bursa-derived (B) cells, and it follows that lymphoid neoplasms should be classifiable as thymus- or bursa-dependent and the cells as T or B cells.

Attempts to influence the development of MD by bursectomy met first with equivocal results, but experiments in which bursectomized birds were monitored for bursa-dependent immunological reactivity, i.e., immunoglobulin and antibody production, suggested that the bursa-dependent lymphoid tissue was not essential for MD lymphoma production (Payne and Rennie, 1970; Fernando and Calnek, 1971). Purchase and Sharma (1974) reduced the incidence of MD by treatment with cyclophosphamide, a drug with a depressive effect on B cells, but a possible effect of this drug on T cells cannot be ruled out. Cortisone acetate, 6-mercaptopurine (Foster and Moll, 1968), and prednisolone (Quaglio, 1963) have also been shown to ameliorate MD lesions, but these results throw little light on specific B or T cell involvement, as they are generally active against growing lymphoid cells of either type.

The thymus in MD has received less attention than the bursa, possibly because, for anatomical reasons, complete thymectomy is difficult if not impossible. Payne and Rennie (unpublished, quoted by Payne, 1972) reported that neonatal thymectomy and X-irradiation did not significantly reduce MD mortality in either moderately resistant (HPRS-BrL) or susceptible (HPRS-RIR) strains of birds, but that significant effects on the type of disease were caused. Thymectomy of susceptible fowl (1) decreased the proportion of birds with gross lymphomas, (2) decreased the proportion of birds with lymphoproliferative nerve lesions, and (3) decreased the number of birds with lymphomatous involvement of the bursa. In the genetically more resistant fowl, thymectomy increased the proportion with gross lymphomas (Table V). Payne (1972) suggested that these results indicated that T cells play a duel role in MD: (1) as a source of proliferative target cells, and (2) as the mediators of a cellular immune response against the transformed target cells. In susceptible fowl thymectomy has the effect of removing target cells, and the balance is pushed toward resistance. In resistant fowls, transformed T cells are controlled by a strong cellular immune response by other T cells, and thymectomy reduces the numbers of these cells, thus increasing lymphoma formation.

Identification of immunologically competent B and T cells in lymphomas by means of hemolytic plaque-forming activity and graft-vs-host reactivity suggested that the tumors are composed of both B and T cells (Payne and Roszkowski, 1973). This was confirmed by direct identification of the two cell components by fluorescein-labeled or radioactive isotope-labeled antibody to B or T cells (Hudson and Payne, 1973; Rouse et al., 1973; Payne et al., 1974). Analysis of 10 lymphomas showed that on average (± SEM) they were composed of 75.6 ± 2.8% T cells and 17.1 ± 3.1% B cells (Payne et al., 1974). The sum of these proportions (92.7 ± 2.1%) differs significantly from 100% indicating that cells other than those with B and T markers provide a small component to lympho-

TABLE V

INFLUENCE OF THYMECTOMY ON GROSS LYMPHOMAS, PROLIFERATIVE NERVE LESIONS, AND BURSAL LYMPHOMAS[a]

			\multicolumn{3}{c}{Proportion (%) with}
Strain of fowl	Group[a]	Number of chickens with gross MD	Visceral lymphomas	Proliferative nerve lesion	Bursal lymphomas
HPRS-RIR	SXI	77	72.7	90.9	53.3
	TxXI	61	54.1[c]	75.4[c]	33.3[c]
HPRS-BrL	SXI	83	24.1	53.0	4.8
	TxXI	70	44.3[c]	48.6	12.9

[a]Two experiments with RIR, and two with BrL, were done, and the results within strain were pooled. Chicks were sham-operated or surgically thymectomized at 1–4 days of age, X-irradiated on the day after surgery with 900 R (for RIR) or 500 R (for BrL), and infected at 3–8 days with HPRS-16 strain of MDV. Age at termination was 144–166 days for RIR and 192 days for BrL.

[b]SXI = sham-operated, X-irradiated MDV-infected; TxXI = thymectomized, X-irradiated MDV-infected.

[c]$p < 0.05$.

mas. Occasionally lymphomas were encountered in our other studies (Payne et al., 1974), in which the sum of B and T cells fell far short of 100%. Cells without markers ("null cells," Williams et al., 1973) may represent B or T cells that have lost their markers, or alternatively another cell type.

These results indicate that lymphoma cells are of mixed origin, being derived from both the bursa and the thymus, with some cells, including the reticulum cells, derived from a third, and probably local, source. Further study is required to settle this latter question.

c. Lymphoblastoid Cell Lines Derived from Lymphomas. Until recently an obstacle to *in vitro* investigation of MD was the lack of any MD lymphoma-derived cell lines, although the desirability of such established lines had been recognized for some time (Klein, 1972b). In the case of Burkitt's lymphoma (BL), where, in the absence of suitable experimental animals, priority was given to the long-term culture of BL lymphoblasts, established lines provided continuously available material for a variety of studies, including the histogenesis of the tumors, the nature and functional capabilities of the cells, their genetic makeup, the possible efficacy of chemotherapeutic agents, and the immune responses that might influence the development of disease (Epstein, 1970). In view of Burkitt's epidemiological finding, particular attention was paid to the possibility that the growth of BL cells away from the host defenses might allow the expression of an oncogenic virus whose presence could not be detected *in vivo*; the identification of the Epstein–Barr virus fully justified this approach.

The debate about the nature of the lymphoproliferative stimulus in MD, and of the immune response in resistant birds, emphasized the need for a more satisfactory *in vitro* model. MD lymphoma-derived cell lines have now been established (Akiyama et al., 1973; Powell et al., 1974), by methods similar to those used in the growth of BL lymphoblasts in long-term culture (Epstein and Barr, 1965). Ovarian or splenic lymphomas were used as sources of suspensions of single cells. The cells were incubated, and the cultures were examined for the growth of free-floating, small round cells.

A critical factor in the growth of the cells was the need for incubation at 40°–41°C. The cell lines obtained by these two groups are similar in many respects. They differ, however, in two, perhaps related, aspects. Akiyama and Kato (1974) reported the progressive growth of the cell lines MSB-1 (from spleen) and MOB-1 (from ovarian lymphoma) from the original cell suspensions with very short latent period of between 3 and 5 days. On the other hand, HPRS line 1 and HPRS line 2, both derived from ovarian lymphomas, had latent periods of 31 and 92 days, respectively; a third culture, which failed to establish as a cell line, had a latent period of 90 days (Powell et al., 1975).

The experience of the two groups also differs in the success rate with which tumor cells were grown. MSB-1 and MOB-1 represent a success rate of 2 out of 22 cultures. HPRS line 1 and 2 are 2 from over 200 cultures. These differences may be due to variations in the interactions between the virus strains and the chicken strains used by each group. The difference is reminiscent of the differing mode of growth of BL lymphoblasts, and of human peripheral blood lymphocytes from normal (EB seropositive) individuals. In Burkitt's lymphoma, cells malignantly transformed *in vivo* continue to grow when transferred into tissue culture. The identification of these cells as deriving from the malignant elements of the tumors is supported on cytogenetic (Gripenberg *et al.*, 1969) and morphological (Epstein, 1967) grounds, as well as by the high cloning efficiency of the cells in soft agar (Imamura and Moore, 1968) and the unusual cellular trait of IgM specificity (Nadkarni *et al.*, 1969; Levin *et al.*, 1969). On the other hand, lymphoid cells that grow out from the peripheral blood of normal individuals are probably not already malignantly transformed when removed from the donor (Epstein and Achong, 1973); it would seem that, rather than the culture conditions selecting an already transformed cell, the transformation event takes place *in vitro* (Rickinson *et al.*, 1974). The explantation of the EB genome carrying lymphocytes induces the appearance of transforming virus or factors, in the same way that explanted ganglia release hitherto latent herpes simplex (Stevens and Cook, 1971; Stevens *et al.*, 1972). It is possible that the

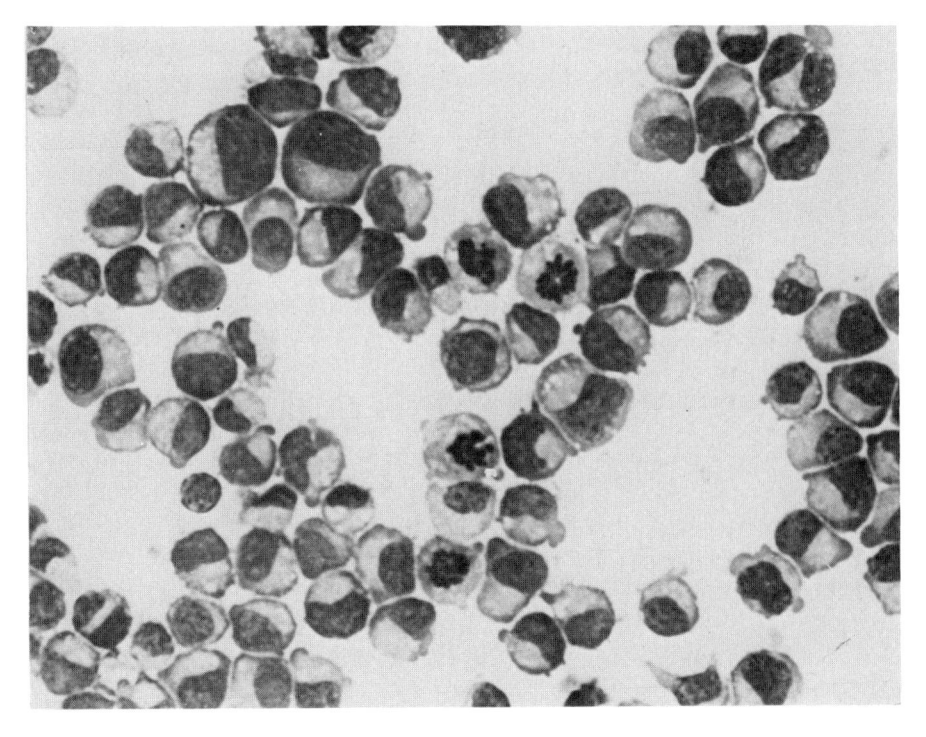

FIG. 46. Impression smear of HPRS line 1 of MD lymphoblastoid cells. X 640. From Frazier and Powell (1975).

combination of virus strain and chicken genotype used by Akiyama *et al.* favored the continuous growth of transformed cells; the combination used in producing the HPRS cell lines may have required transformation *in vitro*.

The MSB-1 and HPRS cell lines are morphologically similar. They are typical lymphoblasts with large nuclei and basophilic cytoplasm containing a small number of vacuoles (Fig. 46). In common with avian lymphoblasts in other situations, produced, for example, by stimulation with phytohemagglutinin *in vitro*, nucleoli are not distinct. In this they differ from human lymphoblasts. MSB-1 cells, however, frequently contain one or two nucleoli (Akiyama and Kato, 1974).

The cells of the various lines resemble one another ultrastructurally. The HPRS lines have been examined in detail (Frazier and Powell, 1975). The cells have

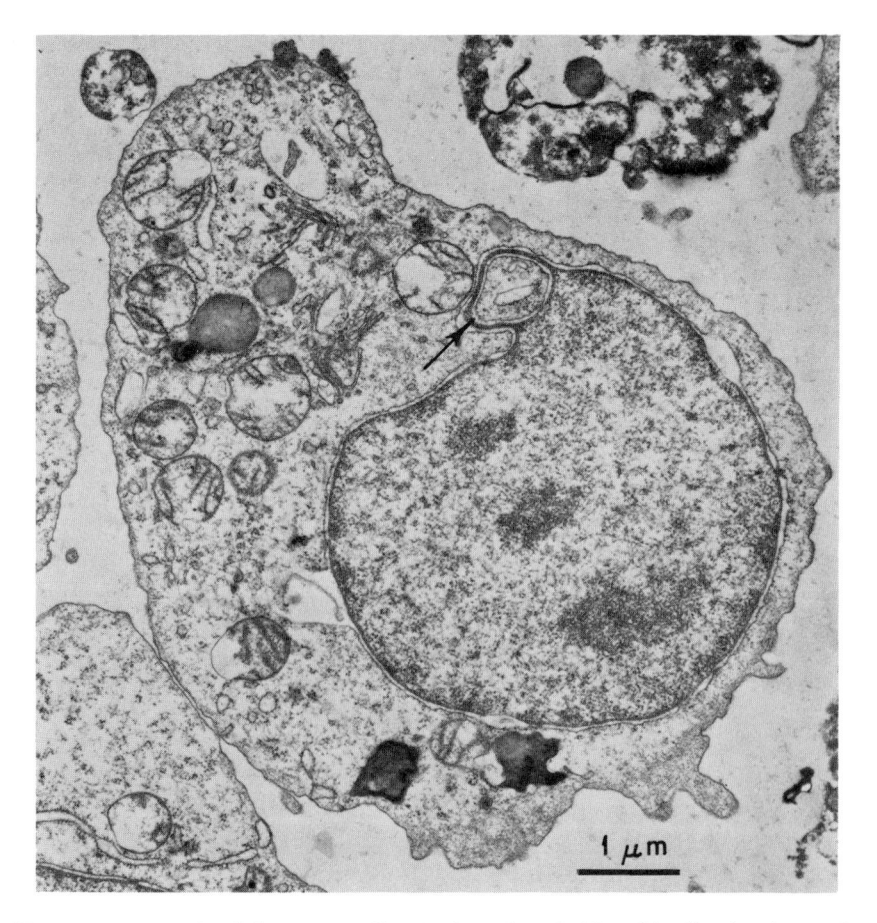

FIG. 47. Lymphoid cell from HPRS line 1 of MD lymphoblastoid cells, showing nuclear projection (arrow). × 13,300.

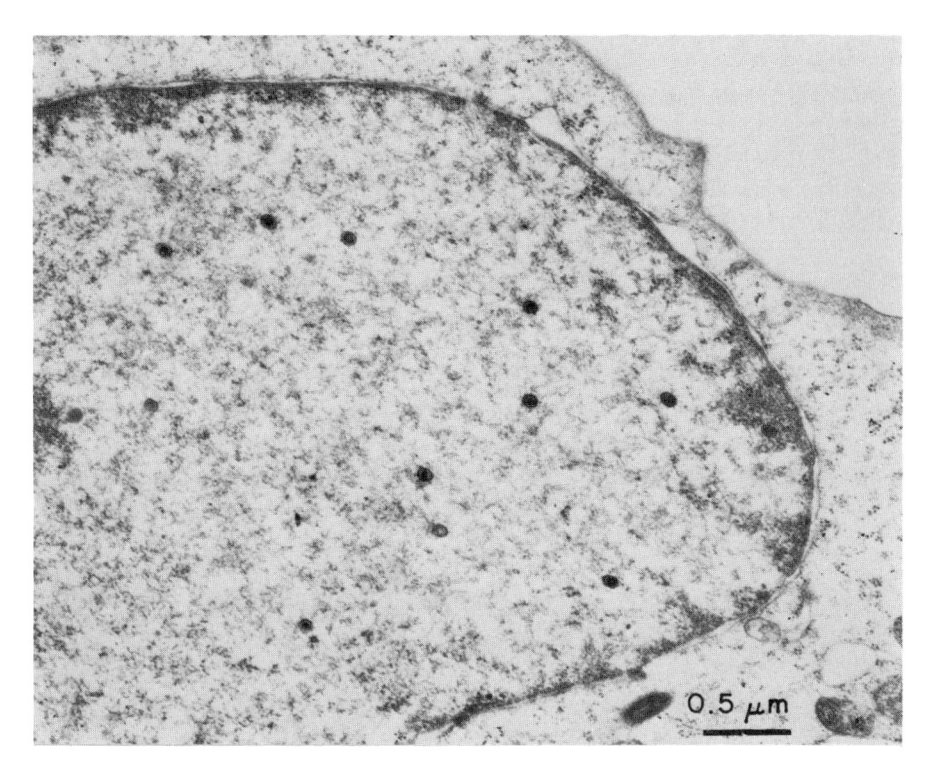

FIG. 48. Unenveloped virions in nucleus of a lymphoid cell from HPRS line 1 of MD lymphoblastoid cells. × 22,200. From Frazier and Powell (1975).

large nuclei with marginated chromatin and occasional nucleoli, and cytoplasm containing several mitochondria, a few small osmiophilic (lipid) bodies, occasional vacuoles, and very sparse, usually rough-surfaced endoplasmic reticulum. Ribosomes and polyribosomes are abundant. Small Golgi apparatuses, centrioles accompanied by spindle tubules, and crystalline structures (Fig. 5) may be observed. The cells generally resemble lymphoblasts from BL; specific points of similarity include annulate lamellae in a small proportion of cells (Fig. 4), and projections of the nuclear membrane, sometimes enclosing portions of cytoplasm in about 3% of the cells (Fig. 47). Scanning electron micrographs reveal the cells to have long, feathery villi, unlike either bursa or thymus cells, but reminiscent of the transformed cells of lymphoid leukosis (Kato and Akiyama, 1975). Cells containing immature intranuclear herpesvirus particles occur very rarely in HPRS line 1 (Fig. 48) are relatively abundant in MSB-1 and MOB-1, but have not yet been seen in HPRS line 2. The percentage of cells with viral antigen demonstrated by immunofluorescence corresponds well with the percentage of cells containing capsids, being undetectably low in the case of the HPRS lines, but in the region of 1–2% in MSB-1 and MOB-1. Some cells of MSB-1 contain many capsids even in the cytoplasm, but none of the cell lines produce cell-free infectious virus. In view of the etiological role of MDV, it would be expected that all the cells harbor the virus genome. This is supported by the results of nucleic acid hybridization studies which have shown that there are many (60–90: Nazerian and Lee, 1974; 54–130: Lee et al., 1975) genome equivalents per cell of MSB-1. However, *in situ* hybridization has yet to be carried out, so that it is not clear whether a few cells contain many genomes, or many or all cells contain few. Expression of viral genome, as measured by immunofluorescence and increase in plaque-forming units, can be induced by placing the cells of MSB-1 in unfavorable conditions, viz. by allowing continued growth in culture without refeeding (Nazerian, 1975).

Induction of viral expression, which is manifest by the appearance of cytoplasmic antigen but does not result in capsid formation, is caused by culture with iodo- or bromodeoxyuridine. Cloning of MSB-1 has produced 10 clones, all of which have a similarly small proportion of virus-expressing cells. It would therefore seem that the virus is associated with all the cells in culture, and it may be essential for the proliferative capacity of the cells. No virus-negative cell lines have, as yet, been produced.

Immunofluorescence studies have allowed the identification of the cells of HPRS line 1 and 2 (Powell et al., 1974) and MSB-1 (Nazerian and Sharma, 1975) as T cells. A transplantable tumor derived from leukemic blood by serial intramuscular injection within a strain of chickens homozygous at the major (B) histocompatibility locus (Jakowski et al., 1974) has been identified as consisting of T cells by a complement-dependent cytotoxic test (Theis et al., 1974). It seems likely that, like herpesvirus saimiri, but unlike Epstein–Barr virus, MDV has a tropism for T cells rather than for B cells. T cells have several characteristics that distinguish them from B cells. They participate in the mixed lymphocyte reaction, respond to phytohemagglutinin *in vitro*, and have splenomegaly-inducing potential in the graft-vs-host reaction *in vivo*. HPRS line 2 has no splenomegaly inducing capacity whereas HPRS line I is intermediate between line 2 and normal blood lymphocytes (Powell et al., 1975). MSB-1, which is a much more rapidly growing line than the HPRS lines, has no graft-vs-host reactivity (Nazerian, personal communication). The HPRS lines do not respond *in vitro* to increasing doses of phytohemagglutinin by incorporating more tritiated thymidine (Powell et al., 1975). Like lymphoma cells (Alm et al., 1972) and leukemic blood cells (Lee, 1972), they show a level of incorporation, in the absence of stimulation, much higher than do normal blood or splenic lymphocytes. This level is not increased in these cases by phytohemagglutinin; the cells may already be fully replicating and unable to incorporate more thymidine—certainly they are totally "blast transformed"—but normal blood cells show a maximum level of incorporation several times greater than lymphoma cells or cells from established lines. These cells may, in the process of malignant transformation, have lost their phytohemagglutinin receptors.

There is some evidence, based on immunofluorescence using antiserum raised against lymphoma cells, for the presence of a tumor-specific antigen on the cells of HPRS lines 1 and 2. The same antiserum stains on average 35% of the cells of freshly explanted tumors. Preliminary observations suggest a specific cytocidal activity of lymphocytes from birds that have recovered from MD against the cell lines (Powell, 1976). The presence of new structures on the cell membranes is supported by the observation that MSB-1 and MOB-1 cells are agglutinated by concanavalin A, whereas normal spleen lymphocytes are not (Akiyama and Kato, 1974). This phenomenon has been reported for cells transformed by a number of agents, including SV40 virus, polyoma virus, chemical carcinogens, and X-irradiation. The studies on the cell membrane need to be extended before the presence of a tumor-specific antigen can be confirmed.

The significance of the cell lines is in supporting the thesis of neoplastic transformation in MD. It appears that interaction between MDV and lymphocytes results in a neoplastic proliferation of T cells. It would be interesting to know whether this is a monoclonal proliferation, as in BL, and how, in this situation, the immune surveillance mechanism functions. Does it lead to civil war among the T cells? (Klein, 1975).

d. The Stimulus for Lymphoma Formation. The argument about whether the lymphomas are inflammatory or neoplastic has recently been restated and extended by asking what is the stimulus for lymphoma formation. The possibilities fall into two groups: (1) those in which the stimulus is extrinsic, lying outside the proliferating lymphoid cells; and (2) those in which the stimulus is intrinsic, i.e., within the cells (Payne, 1972). These might be equated with the inflammatory and neoplastic theories, respectively, although this obviously depends on the nature and definition of neoplasia generally.

i. *Extrinsic stimulation.* In this hypothesis it is suggested that the lymphocytes are proliferating in response to an external antigenic stimulus. The reaction would be essentially immunological, its excessive nature, leading to "lymphoma" formation, perhaps being due to some unusual qualitative or quantitative (perhaps persistent) property of the antigen. Possible antigens could be: (1) virus-infected cells; (2) cell-free virus, viral antigen, or antigen–antibody complexes; (3) host antigens released by virus damage to cells. The extrinsic hypothesis was supported by Rouse *et al.* (1973), who proposed that virus-infected, non-lymphoid cells provided the stimulus, and that the mixed involvement of B and T lymphocytes was indicative of an inflammatory response. Against this explanation are the observations that viral antigen and virions are absent or rare in lymphomas and that there is no clear association between the presence of antigens and virions in other tissues and the predilection of that tissue to lymphoma formation (Payne and Rennie, 1973). For example, feather follicle epithelium and bursa are the sites most often positive for virus and antigen, but they are not the most frequent sites for lymphoma formation.

Failure to detect antigen and virus in lymphoma cells could be explained if antigen or virus were produced at some distant site, e.g., feather follicle, and carried via the blood to sites where sensitized lymphocytes had localized. Continued antigenic stimulation, resulting in cellular proliferation and recruitment of additional lymphoid cells, mediated perhaps by soluble "lymphokine" factors (Dumonde et al., 1969), could give rise to lymphoma formation. If this theory is correct it should be possible to detect specifically sensitized lymphoid cells in lymphomas and to reproduce tumors by continued antigenic stimulation. The possibility of antigen–antibody complexes being specifically involved would appear to be ruled out by the production of lymphomas in agammaglobulinemic fowl (Payne and Rennie, 1970).

Lymphomas could also result from stimulation by normally segregated host antigens, which have not been recognized as "self" (Burnet, 1969), released as a result of viral damage to cells. The possibility that autoimmune mechanisms are involved in the MD neuropathy has already been discussed; there is no evidence to date that they are involved in lymphoma formation, but they should be looked for particularly in view of the strong evidence for autoimmune responses in infectious mononucleosis in man (Davidson and Lee, 1969).

ii. *Intrinsic stimulation.* In this theory, virus infection of the lymphocyte leads to a change in the properties of the infected cell, endowing it with neoplastic capacity. Discussion of the various ways in which the virus might bring this change about is beyond the scope of this review, but one obvious possibility is that persistent virus or viral genome is responsible. Evidence derived from conventional techniques for the presence of virus in MD lymphoma cells is meager: only one cell in 10^2 to 10^5 lymphoma cells can form infective plaques in tissue culture (Churchill and Biggs, 1967; Calnek and Madin, 1969), fluorescent viral antigen is either absent from tumor cells or present in only a few scattered cells, which could be stromal cells rather than lymphoid cells (Calnek and Hitchner, 1969; Spencer and Calnek, 1970; von Bulow and Payne, 1970; Purchase, 1970), and under the electron microscope virions are only occasionally seen (Schidlovsky et al., 1969; Nazerian and Witter, 1970; Frazier, 1974a). The majority of tumor cells therefore do not contain replicating virus. Nevertheless, it is possible, as Calnek and Hitchner (1969) pointed out, that viral genomes exist in many or all tumor cells. Campbell and Woode (1970) found that virions and viral antigen appeared in lymphocytes from MD cases after they had undergone blastoid transformation under the influence of phytohemagglutinin. More direct evidence for viral genome in tumor cells was provided by Nazerian et al. (1973), who detected by a molecular hybridization technique between 3 and 15 virus genome equivalents per tumor cell. Recently Nazerian and Lee (1974) detected 60–90 viral genome equivalents in an MD lymphoblastoid cell line. These results show that there are large amounts of viral genetic material in tumor cells in the absence of replicating virus, indicative of a nonproductive infection. Whether the viral DNA is integrated into host DNA, and whether all the tumor cells carry viral genome, remains to be determined. The discrepancy between the amounts of genome in lymphomas compared to a lymphoma-derived cell line suggests that not all lymphoma cells *in vivo* carry genome. Consistent with these results, only 35.1 ± 9.6 SEM% of lymphoma cells appeared to carry a tumor-specific antigen compared with 96.3 ± 1.2% of a lymphoma-derived lymphoblastoid cell line (Powell *et al.*, 1974). The occurrence of a MD tumor-associated surface antigen (designated MATSA) has been confirmed by Witter *et al.* (1975b). It seems likely therefore that MD lymphomas consist of a neoplastically transformed T cell resulting from a nonproductive virus infection, together with nontransformed B and T cells which may represent a host inflammatory response to tumor-speific antigens, and perhaps viral and extrinsic stimulation of lymphoid cells. This could explain the observation of Lee *et al.* (1975) that the number of genome equivalents varies significantly between birds but not between lymphomas within one bird, owing to differing balances between transformed cells and host lymphoid responses.

Recently, Peters *et al.* (1973) have questioned whether MDV alone is sufficient to induce MD. They reported an interaction between avian RNA tumor (ART) virus infection and MDV infection *in vivo*, in which mortality and tumor incidence was either dependent on, or enhanced by, dual infection, depending on the strain of chickens used. Furthermore, RNA from tissues of birds with dual infection showed increased hybridization with DNA homologous to ART virus, compared with RNA from monoinfected tissues. These results raised the possibility that infection with MDV might lead to activation and perhaps oncogenic expression of endogenous or exogenous ART virus (see Tooze, 1973).

However, subsequent studies have failed to support this hypothesis. Witter *et al.* (1975a) showed that MD could be induced in chickens free of exogenous avian leukosis virus infection, replicating endogenous leukosis virus, gs antigen, and chick helper factor, and that dual infection with exogenous leukosis virus and MDV did not alter the character of the MD lesions. These results were confirmed by Calnek and Payne (1976), who showed also that induction of MD was not associated with any change in the natural expressions of the endogenous virus. It is concluded that MDV can induce tumors without the participation of endogenous leukosis virus genome.

7. Hematological Changes Including Leukemogenesis

Study of the hematology of MD has been neglected. Early reports are inconsistent and probably unreliable (Johnson and Conner, 1933; Seagar, 1933b). The bone marrow becomes infected with MDV soon after infection (Kottaridis and Luginbuhl, 1968; Adldinger and Calnek, 1973), and this may be responsible for the transient (Sevoian and Chamberlain, 1964) or more lasting (Vickers *et al.*, 1967; Nielson and Anderson, 1971) depression in red blood cell count. Severe marrow aplasia and marked anemia was observed in MDV infection in chicks lacking maternal antibody (Jakowski *et al.*, 1970). Depression of thrombocytes was noted by Sevoian and Chamberlain (1964). These authors also reported a transient leukopenia 2 days post infection. In birds developing lymphoproliferative lesions lymphocytosis is the most striking change, with lymphocyte counts ranging to over 200,000 cells/mm^3 (Sevoian and Chamberlain, 1964; Evans and Patterson, 1971). Evans and Patterson (1971) observed increased numbers of large lymphocytes with cytoplasmic extrusions and of large blast cells; in addition, immature red cells and granulocytes were present. In clinical cases of MD, Payne et al. (1974) found significant increases in total lymphocytes and T cells, and significant decreases of monocytes, eosinophils, and basophils. Heterophils were decreased, but not significantly so. In leukemic birds most of the lymphocyte increase was accounted for by T cells, but in two instances B cells were also considerably increased. Increase in "null" cells (lacking B or T membrane markers) was also observed.

8. *Ocular Changes*

The histopathology of the so-called ocular form of lymphomatosis, regarded by many as an expression of MD, has been described by a number of investigators (Pappenheimer *et al.*, 1926, 1929a; McGaughey and Downie, 1930; Warrack and Dalling, 1932; Nelson and Thorp, 1943; Grundboeck, 1965; Yamagiwa *et al.*, 1967; Fujimoto *et al.*, 1971; Moriwaki and Horiuchi, 1974). The common findings are lymphocytic, plasma cell, and sometimes heterophil infiltration of the iris, ciliary body, and conjunctiva, and less commonly of the choroid membrane, pecten, and retina. In experimental MD, Sevoian and Chamberlain (1964) first noted changes 17 days after infection, consisting of perivascular cuffs and infiltrations by mononuclear cells involving the conjunctiva, ciliary muscle, iris and choroid membrane, and hyperplasia and shedding of cells at the inner surface of the cornea. Smith *et al.* (1974) have recently reported a sequential study of eye changes following intra-abdominal and intraocular inoculation of MDV. In addition to lymphoid cell infiltration in sites implicated by other workers, they also noted increased cellularity of the corneal stroma and retained nuclei at the center of the lens.

Simpson (1969a, b) studied the ultrastructure of changes in natural cases of the ocular disease. He observed necrotic striated muscle, mononuclear cells and granulocytes in the iris, and the presence of numerous mature and budding virus particles morphologically similar to ART virus in muscle cells, epithelial cells, vascular endothelial cells, and Schwann cells of iritic nerves. This result raises the possibility that agents other than MDV may also cause ocular lymphomatosis.

V. Immunity

A. Passively Acquired Immunity

Chickens that are infected with MDV, but do not succumb to the disease, carry the virus for the whole of their lives. This situation leads to a relatively high antibody response to the virus, and the transfer of maternal antibody to chicks via the yolk sac (Chubb and Churchill, 1968), although the virus itself is not egg transmitted (Solomon et al., 1970). In the field the majority of chicks possess maternally derived passive antibody which persists for about 3 weeks. The importance of this passive antibody is in the protective role it may play, and in the possible interference it may cause in vaccination.

The development of MD is influenced by maternal antibody, which gives a significant protective effect against morbidity and mortality caused by both acute and classical strains of MDV (Chubb and Churchill, 1969; Spencer and Robertson, 1972). This protective effect was also found when the maternally derived antibody was directed against the related herpesvirus of turkeys rather than MDV itself (Eidson et al., 1971a, 1972a), and the enhanced resistance to MDV of chicks from dams immunized against MD was believed to be due to the protective influence of passively acquired antibody (Ball et al., 1971). The effect of heterologous antibody is, however, much less than that of homologous antibody, and an effect is not always seen. The administration of immune serum to antibody-negative chicks mimics the effect of maternal antibody (Calnek, 1972a; Burgoyne and Witter, 1973).

Antibody-bearing chicks are not refractory but are more resistant to MD lesion development. Four main effects of maternal antibody have been observed: (1) lower mortality (2) delayed onset and increased latent period to death, (3) a reduction in tumor formation, and (4) a suppression of the acute destructive lesions of lymphoid and hematopoietic tissues, which are sometimes associated with early mortality without tumor formation (See Section IV D).

In the absence of antibody, MDV causes necrosis and an acute inflammatory reaction associated with restrictive virus replication, followed by a virus-induced, nonproductive malignant transformation of lymphoid cells, which leads to gross lymphoma formation. In chicks with maternal or passively administered antibody, the initial productive virus infection and acute inflammation are greatly suppressed. The number of tissues with viral antigen and the amount of antigen in positive tissues is lowered, and fewer infected spleen cells can be detected (Calnek, 1972a; Payne and Rennie, 1973; Frazier, 1974a). Passive antibody prevents bursal atrophy and lengthens the latent period for antigen and cell-free virus production in the feather follicle epithelium (Burgoyne and Witter, 1973). The initial response to infection is a proliferation of lymphoid tissue, containing only a minor reticulum cell element, with no intranuclear inclusion bodies. In ultrastructural studies Frazier (1974a) found that the presence of antibody delayed the disappearance of the dense granular lymphocytes first seen in the lymphoid organs at 3 days, and tended to restrict regressive changes and the appearance of cell debris, pale reticulum cells, and macrophages. The appearance of cells with nuclear projections was delayed, and virus particles were not seen at any time.

It seems clear that maternal antibody exercises its effect upon the development of MD by diminishing the extent of the initial virus infection, but the mechanism of action is not known. The level of infection is reduced, but infection is not prevented. The severe necrotizing infection in the absence of antibody is similar to infections caused by herpesviruses in other species in the absence of antibody (Calnek, 1972a), and maternal antibody to canine herpesvirus, for example, does not prevent infection but does prevent disease (Carmichael, 1970; Huxsoll and Hemelt, 1970). It may be that antibody reduces the challenging dose by eliminating some of the inoculum cells, but antibody administered up to 4 days after virus inoculation was shown to have a protective effect, whereas that given after 7 days was ineffective (Calnek, 1972a). There may, therefore, be some interference with the spread of virus throughout the body. Chen and Purchase (1970) demonstrated the presence of virus-associated antigens on the surface of MDV-infected cells; cytophilic antibodies to these antigens may be demonstrated in the blood of infected chickens. Such antibody may interfere with the cell-to-cell spread of virus, though complement-dependent cytotoxic antibody has not been described. Burgoyne and Witter (1973) inoculated cell-associated and cell-free MDV into passively immunized chickens and described an *in vivo* neutralization phenomenon, whose effect was greater against cell-free virus. A similar effect was noted when MDV-infected cells were injected into antibody-containing yolk of embryonated eggs (Biggs and Milne, 1971) or when MDV-infected cells were mixed with immune sera and inoculated into chick kidney cell cultures (Churchill, 1968). It is known that a reduction in focus-forming units occurs when other cell-associated herpesviruses are inoculated onto cell cultures in the presence of specific antibody (Gold, 1965). Some strains of MDV, e.g., GA, may spread throughout the animal as cell-free virus in the plasma (Eidson and Schmittle, 1968) and would be directly available to neutralizing antibody.

It is possible that cell-mediated host responses might also be brought into play by antibody–antigen reactions. Lodmell *et al.* (1973) have suggested that, in the control of cell-to-cell spread of herpes simplex virus, factors generated by antigen–antibody reactions may attract leukocytes to the site of infection where they exert a nonspecific toxic effect on infected and surrounding cells and thereby interfere with virus spread.

It is not known how maternal antiviral antibody exercises its effect on the development of lymphomas. There is the possibility of a direct effect of antibody on the expression of the virus genome in transformed cells, for virus particles may be seen in the lymphoma cells of chicks without maternal antibody, but have not been seen in lymphomas from antibody-positive chicks (Frazier, 1974a). It is, however, more likely that the effect of maternal antibody on the proliferative response is related to its influence on the earlier virological events. This is supported by the correlation that exists between the "viremia" of leukocyte-associated infectivity and subsequent tumor development (Witter *et al.*, 1971), which was found to apply also to chickens of genetically different tumor susceptibilities (Sharma and Stone, 1972). An early sparing of various lymphoid tissues by maternal antibody could (1) protect the immune surveillance system from damage, or (2) reduce the levels of infection and viremia, thus reducing the chances of interaction between virus and potentially transformed target cells.

The presence of maternal antibody to HVT (from vaccinated dams) is also of importance in vaccination, for there is evidence that such antibody can interfere with the development of vaccinal immunity, presumably by influencing the spread of vaccine virus within the host (see Section V, C).

B. Actively Acquired Immunity

It has been clearly established that after infection of susceptible chicks at 1 day of age there follows a peak of virus activity and reactive inflammation at about 5–7 days, a subsequent restoration of morphological normality, with diminished signs of infection, and a second rise in virus activity (Payne and Rennie, 1973; Adldinger and Calnek, 1973). Although this is most striking in the lymphoid tissues, the biphasic nature of virus activity is seen also in other tissues, including the "viremia" of leukocyte-associated infectivity (Phillips and Biggs, 1972). It may be that a developing host immunity interferes with the extent and spread of virus infection, and it is reasonable to assume that the outcome of infection depends upon a balance between the immune response and the destruction caused by the virus in the tissues mounting this response. It is, however, unlikely that the "negative phase" concerning detectable viral antigens in tissue samples observed between the two peaks of the biphasic curve is an expression of masking by antibodies, as this phase correlates with histological signs of recovery.

Specific immunity against infectious agents may be divided into humoral antibody responses, and cell-mediated immunity. Each type of reaction is mediated by a different population of lymphoid cells, with a varying degree of cellular cooperation in the production of responses to different antigens. In the case of virus infections, a third factor, interferon, must be considered.

1. *Humoral Immunity*

a. Precipitating Antibody. A number of techniques have been described for the detection of antibodies to MDV-associated antigens. Up to six antigens have been described in infected cultures of chick kidney cells (Churchill *et al.*, 1969b) using the agar-gel double-diffusion precipitation technique (Chubb and Churchill, 1968), but only three of these are regularly recognized. These are termed A, B, and C antigens. All these antigens are present in infected cultured kidney cells, but only the A antigen is released into the supernatant fluid. The concentration of A antigen decreased with passage in chick kidney cells and was found to be absent from the highly passaged attenuated MDV (Churchill *et al.*, 1969b). All field isolates examined by Biggs and Milne (1972), whether pathogenic or not, were found to possess the A antigen. Some pathogenic cloned strains have been shown to lack this antigen (Purchase et al., 1971b); the cloning procedure, however, involved growth in chick embryo fibroblasts. This is known to cause a rapid decrease in the concentration of A antigen (Ross et al., 1973).

Precipitating antibodies can be detected between 7 and 14 days after inoculation with MDV (Higgins and Calnek, 1975a). There is no relationship between the development of precipitins and recovery from infection (Calnek, 1972b).

b. *Fluorescing Antibody.* An indirect immunofluorescence test for detecting antibody, using infected tissue cultures as antigen, has been described (Spencer and Calnek, 1970; Purchase, 1969) and has been found to be more sensitive than the agar-gel precipitation test (Purchase and Burgoyne, 1970).

Four different antigens have been observed in cultured cells by immunofluorescence: a diffuse nuclear antigen, a diffuse cytoplasmic antigen, a granular cytoplasmic antigen (Purchase, 1969; Nazerian and Purchase, 1970), and an antigen on the surface of infected cells (Chen and Purchase, 1970; Ishikawa et al., 1972). Nazerian and Purchase (1970) and Ahmed and Schidlovsky (1972) found that the immunofluorescent antigens were present only in cells containing virus particles, and that there were no virus particles in cells free of antigens. The antigens occur in infected cells, but are not necessarily made up of virus particles. The cytoplasmic granular antigen never contains virus particles. All three antigens may nevertheless be related to virus structural proteins. The cytoplasmic granular antigen may be similar to that induced in a MD lymphoblastoid cell line by 5-iododeoxyuridine, which is regarded as being the analog of the EB early antigen. Virus particles were not seen in these cells (Nazerian, 1975).

Purchase (1969) studied eight isolates of MDV by immunofluorescence, and failed to detect any antigenic differences. However, he later described differences between viruses with and without the A antigen (Purchase et al., 1971b). Clones of MDV positive for the A antigen produced bright fluorescence in flattened cells around microplaques, whereas in clones negative for A antigen this fluorescence was not seen.

Fluorescent IgM antibody has been observed between 5 and 12 days after inoculation with MDV (Higgins and Calnek, 1975a). This corresponded to the initial detection of neutralizing antibody. IgG antibody first appeared at 7–8 days, and then gradually increased, paralleling the increase in neutralizing antibody.

c. *Virus Neutralizing Antibody.* The discovery that cell-free virus can be obtained from feather follicle epithelium (Calnek et al., 1970a) has made the use of a virus neutralization test possible (Calnek and Adldinger, 1971). Antibodies detected in this test differ from the precipitins detected in the agar-gel test, and are presumably directed against virus envelope. Higgins and Calnek (1975a) found that neutralizing antibodies peaked between 6 and 12 days, followed by a drop, and then a gradual increase in titer for several weeks. The levels were generally greater in resistant birds. A correlation between neutralizing antibody levels and survival in genetically resistant birds was also observed by Calnek (1972b).

d. Hemagglutinating Antibody. An indirect hemagglutination test using tanned horse erythrocytes sensitized with an antigen prepared from MDV-infected DEF has been described (Eidson and Schmittle, 1969). Hemagglutinating antibodies were first detected 4 weeks after infection, and survival was correlated with high titers. Passive antibodies in young chicks were not detected. This test has not been used extensively, probably because of the difficulty in producing the large quantity of antigen necessary.

e. Complement-Fixing Antibody. Cho and Ringen (1969) have described complement-fixing reactions between sera from hamsters inoculated with MD-affected nerve, ovary or testis, and homologous or heterologous MD-infected and control tissues. However, cross-reactions occurred with infected and control tissues in the heterologous system.

f. Immunological Relationships. Studies using immunofluorescence, precipitation in agar gel, and virus agglutination have shown cross reactions between MDV and EBV, the herpes virus of Lucké renal carcinoma, herpes simplex types 1 and 2, and pseudorabies virus (Naito *et al.*, 1970; Ono *et al.*, 1970; Ross *et al.*, 1972; Kirkwood *et al.*, 1972). These cross-reactions may be due to the presence of a group-specific antigen. Cross-neutralization, immunofluorescence, and precipitin tests have been used to construct a subclassification of the group of MD and turkey herpesviruses into 3 serological subtypes. One is represented by the HPRS-24 strain of apathogenic MDV. The other two subtypes comprise pathogenic strains of MDV and their attenuated variants, and turkey herpesviruses (von Bulow and Biggs, 1975a, b).

g. Artificial Suppression of Humoral Responses Evidence has been presented elsewhere (see Section IV, D, 6, b) that the bursa and humoral immune responses do not play an essential role in the pathogenesis of, or resistance to, MD. There are, however, several reports that an intact bursal system has an ameliorating effect on the disease. Carte *et al.* (1969) found that bursectomy increased the severity of MD in a relatively resistant strain of birds, and Morris *et al.* (1969) reported that bursectomy enhanced the disease in susceptible chickens. Smith and Calnek (1974a) found that bursectomy increased the incidence of disease in chickens infected with low-virulence or high-virulence virus strains. Moreover, the lesion spectrum induced by low-virulence virus in individual birds was increased; visceral tumors occurred in bursectomized birds, but only neural lesions were found in control birds. Cho (1970) also found that gross nerve involvement was increased by dual infection with MDV and infectious bursal agent; the latter has profoundly damaging effects on bursal tissue. On the other hand, bursectomy in resistant birds was shown not to increase their susceptibility to MD (Sharma, 1974; Payne and Rennie, unpublished, quoted by Payne, 1972).

2. Cell-Mediated Immunity

In view of the avidly cell-associated nature of MDV, it is likely that the cellular immune system is important in resistance or, as in murine lymphocytic choriomeningitis, in pathogenesis (Allison, 1972a). Moreover, cell-mediated immunity is of importance in herpes simplex infection (Wilton et al., 1972), and a delayed hypersensitivity reaction to a diagnostic antigen released into cultural fluid by herpes simplex-infected cells was reported in 1962 (Anderson and Kilbourne). Viruses stimulating cell-mediated immunity have antigens that infiltrate the plasma membranes of infected cells, thereby forming the "self plus x" antigenic system, which has the required immunogenicity (Allison, 1972b); depletion of the cell-mediated immune system by experimental thymectomy and antilymphocytic serum aggravates infections caused by herpesviruses and poxviruses. This is consistent with the view that not circulating antibody, but cell-mediated immunity, is required for the resolution of such cell-associated infections. Cell-mediated immunity may confer protection against viruses by the direct cytotoxic action of sensitized T lymphocytes against virus-infected cells, by macrophage activation with an increase in the content of lysosomal enzymes and in the capacity to kill intracellular parasites, or by the interferon production that accompanies the transformation of lymphocytes into blast cells (Glasgow, 1970). It is also involved in the immune responses against tumor cells.

Fauser et al. (1973) have reported evidence for the existence of cell-mediated immunity in MD. This was based on delayed hypersensitivity reactions and migration inhibition factor tests using semipurified A antigen. The chickens used were susceptible RPL line 7 birds which were inoculated with a pathogenic strain of virus at 6 months of age. The tests were carried out 1 to 3 months later, so that it was not possible to determine whether the immune reaction observed was connected with the development of lymphomatous lesions or with their regression. As the attenuated virus that may be used in vaccination lacks the A antigen, and some pathogenic strains also lack this antigen, it is unlikely that cell-mediated immunity to A antigen is essential in either process.

Delayed hypersensitivity reactions to various MDV-associated antigens have been demonstrated in chickens with naturally occurring MD infections (Byerly and Dawe, 1972). Stronger reactions were obtained with an antigen derived from infected cell cultures than with antigens from tissue culture medium, or from feather follicles. Delayed hypersensitivity reactions to the cellular antigens were correlated with the presence of gross lymphomatous lesions. The difficulty in obtaining purified virus-associated antigens is a major disadvantage in investigations of cell-mediated immunity in MD, but it is clearly an area that needs further exploration.

3. Interferon

Interferon has been reported to be produced as a response to infection with some strains of pathogenic MDV (Hong and Sevoian, 1971; Kaleta and Bankowski, 1972a, b). It may be important in the initial host response to MDV infection (see Section VI, B), but in view of the relative insensitivity of herpesviruses to the action of interferon (Lockart, 1973), it is unlikely to play a major part in the mechanism of resistance to MD.

4. *Macrophages*

The role played by macrophages in resistance and pathogenesis has not been resolved, despite the fact that they, or their reticulum cell precursors, appear to be a target cell for the virus. They are thought to be a possible mechanism in the distribution throughout the body of virus inhaled into the respiratory tract (Adldinger and Calnek, 1973). Treatment with macrophage-blocking silica particles had no effect on the course of the disease in genetically resistant birds, but caused a delay in the appearance of clinical signs in susceptible birds. Contrary to expectation, however, silica treatment caused a rise in the numbers of circulating monocytes (Calnek, personal communication). Moreover, macrophages in culture could not be infected with virus, and peritoneal exudate macrophages from infected birds were found to be negative for virus by immunofluorescence (Calnek, Powell; unpublished results).

C. VACCINAL IMMUNITY

The first important vaccine development was made by Churchill *et al.* (1969b), who found that a virulent strain of MDV, after attenuation in tissue culture (Churchill *et al.*, 1969a), could be used to protect chickens against MD. Since then a number of live vaccines have been discovered. These may be classified into three groups, namely: (1) modified MDV, (2) apathogenic MDV, and (3) the herpesvirus of turkeys (Biggs, 1973). In addition, vaccination with killed virus vaccines is feasible.

1. *Modified MDV*

Modified viruses include those which have lost their A antigen and do not spread horizontally from chicken to chicken, and those that have retained the antigen and do spread horizontally. The attenuation process described by Churchill *et al.* (1969a) led to loss of pathogenicity, change in plaque morphology, and loss of the A antigen. This last feature was thought to be associated with the loss of oncogenic properties, but this does not seem to be true since apathogenic viruses with the A antigen, and pathogenic viruses without the A antigen, have been found (Biggs and Milne, 1972; Purchase *et al.*, 1971b). A number of isolates have been attenuated in a similar way, and have been found to be effective and safe in preventing MD (Biggs *et al.*, 1970, 1972a; Eidson and Anderson, 1971; Meulemans *et al.*, 1971; Eidson *et al.*, 1971b; Blaxland *et al.*, 1972; Willemart, 1972). The attenuated viruses have not reverted to virulence.

Chicks inoculated when 1 day old develop viremia rapidly and protection is adequate 1–2 weeks later. Doses in excess of 500 PFU were found to be highly effective in day-old chickens (Biggs et al., 1970). As is the case with the other vaccine viruses, superinfection with virulent MDV may occur, and such dual infection leads to shedding of the virulent virus. The passage level of the virus is critical, because before pathogenicity is lost the virus stock may consist of a mixture of pathogenic and apathogenic viruses. On continued passage, its ability to protect chickens against MD may be lost (Purchase, 1973).

Vaccine viruses that have retained A antigen production and the ability to spread from bird to bird are field isolates of low pathogenicity, which have been further attenuated in tissue culture. CVI 988 is a strain that was isolated from a flock of apparently normal chickens and on initial isolation produced only histological nerve lesions (Rispens et al., 1972a, b). Its low level of pathogenicity was reduced by 20 passages in duck embryo fibroblasts, after which it replicated much faster in tissue culture. This vaccine has been extensively used in Holland. Another modified virus is the VC strain, an isolate of low pathogenicity from a case of classical MD, which was attenuated by passage in chick embryos (von Bulow, 1971). The protective value of these modified low-virulence virus vaccines has been demonstrated under experimental conditions where isolation facilities allowed the proper use of controls (Rispens et al., 1972a). Because the viruses spread horizontally, properly controlled field trials have not been possible, but it appears that they provide a good degree of protection (Rispens et al., 1972b; Vielitz and Landgraf, 1971). Theoretically it should be possible to vaccinate only a proportion of birds in a flock and allow natural spread to the other chickens. Unfortunately, spread would have to be rapid to provide an adequate protection, and Rispens et al. (1972b) found that vaccination of 10% of chickens required approximately 4 weeks for the development of flock resistance; this was not sufficiently rapid under field conditions.

2. *Apathogenic MDV*

Zander et al. (1972) have reported the use of blood from naturally MDV-infected chickens as an immunizing agent. The blood contained an avirulent virus which produced large plaques in tissue culture, but apart from this was similar to the apathogenic virus isolated by Biggs and Milne (1972).

3. *Turkey Herpesviruses*

Several strains of HVT have been isolated from turkeys (Kawamura et al., 1969; Witter et al., 1970; Rispens et al., 1972a; Zygraich and Huygelen, 1972); they appear to be similar in their lack of pathogenicity and their ability to protect against MD. Like MDV, these viruses produce plaques in chick kidney and chick embryo fibroblast cultures.

The HVT does not usually replicate fully in the chicken feather follicle epithelium, and so is not shed into the environment (Nazerian and Witter, 1970). When chickens without maternal antibody are given large doses of HVT, however, virus shedding may occur (Cho et al., 1971; Rispens et al., 1972a). It is regularly shed from the feather follicle epithelium of turkeys, in which the virus behaves epizootiologically in a manner similar to MDV in chickens. Commercial turkey poults are hatched free of infection, but soon acquire virus and the resulting antibody against it.

When day-old chicks received an adequate dose of vaccine virus, they were protected against MDV challenge by inoculation at 3 weeks of age (Okazaki et al., 1970). Experimentally a dose as small as 3 PFU resulted in 50% protection at 3 weeks (Purchase et al., 1972a), but a dose as high as 9000 PFU was not protective against challenge 1 week later (Okazaki et al., 1973); 500 PFU given at hatching was found to be effective in preventing outbreaks of MD in the field (Purchase et al., 1971a, c), but to ensure protection under natural conditions of exposure, it was found to be necessary to vaccinate as soon after hatching as possible (Okazaki et al., 1971; Eidson and Anderson, 1971).

There are a number of factors that influence the choice of vaccine. In field trials all three types have been found to be similarly effective, although direct comparisons have not been possible because of the different vaccine doses used. An important consideration is the possibility that altered viruses from chickens could revert to pathogenicity after a period of time. The appearance of a highly pathogenic strain of MDV (Benton and Cover, 1957) in the United States suggests that mutation or reversion may occur. This danger is of even more significance with those strains that spread horizontally, as natural passage through chickens will occur. Horizontally transmitted vaccines might also seriously complicate any future eradication program, once they were widely distributed in the poultry population, while the slow rate of spread of these viruses is a disadvantage for their use as vaccines.

The HVT is the only vaccine virus that is readily obtainable in cell-free form from infected tissue cultures (Calnek et al., 1970b), and it is now commercially available in lyophilized form. The use of a cell-free virus as a vaccine has some advantages over cell-associated preparations, as the latter require exacting conditions of storage and administration in order to maintain viability. MD vaccines are, however, normally administered at hatcheries so that the facilities for storing virus in liquid nitrogen may be centralized. Furthermore, the lyophilized virus is relatively thermolabile and may be unknowingly destroyed before administration.

Maternally derived homologous antibody in chicks may interfere with vaccination. The neutralization effect is greater against cell-free HVT than against cell-associated virus (Calnek and Smith 1972; Patruscu et al., 1972), but there is some activity against cell-associated HVT and against cell-associated attenuated MDV (Spencer et al., 1974). Eidson et al. (1972b), found that maternal antibody derived from dams vaccinated with HTV at 1 day of age did not interfere with the immunization of the progeny, but repeated inoculations of the breeding stock did lead to interference, presumably by raising the maternal antibody titer. These problems can be overcome (1) by ensuring that immunizing doses are sufficiently high to nullify the effects of maternal antibody, (2) by alternating HVT and attenuated MDV from generation to generation, as there is little interference by heterologous antiserum, (3) by not vaccinating the breeding stock, or (4) by using cell-associated virus rather than cell-free virus.

Failure of establishment of infection by HVT because of neutralization by maternal antibody is believed to be a cause of the vaccination failures that are occasionally encountered. Other causes include failure of development of vaccinal immunity prior to early challenge by MDV, and failure to inoculate an adequate dose of HVT because of faults in vaccine manufacture, storage, or chick inoculation methods. Host genetic factors also influence the efficacy of vaccination (Spencer et al., 1974).

Before the advent of vaccination, the only means available for the control of MD was prevention of infection by good husbandry and selection for genetic resistance. Virulent virus viremia and virus shedding are reduced by vaccination and by selective breeding, so the eventual eradication of MDV may be feasible. It is likely that such an eradication would yield benefits over and above the elimination of MD, as vaccination has been shown to have beneficial effects on production traits, such as egg production and body weight (Biggs et al., 1972a; Honnegar et al., 1972; Purchase et al., 1972b), and to reduce deaths from other causes, such as coccidiosis (Biggs et al., 1970).

4. Killed Vaccines

In addition to live virus vaccines, inactivated vaccines may be used as prophylaxis against MD. They may be crude formalinized preparations of MDV-infected cells (as commercially available in Japan in 1971) or semipurified preparations (Kaaden et al., 1974; Lesnik and Ross, 1975).

5. Mechanism of Vaccinal Immunity

The mechanism of the protective action is not understood, but the successful use of material free of DNA and RNA (Kaaden and Dietzschold, 1975) eliminates the possibility of a virus interference phenomonen, or the blocking by vaccine virus of an interaction between host cell and virulent virus. Moreover, heat and formaldehyde inactivated vaccines have been shown to be protective against another oncogenic herpesvirus, herpesvirus saimiri (Laufs and Steinke, 1975). It seems, therefore, that protection is mediated by a conventional immunological process. Humoral responses do not seem to be primarily responsible for protection in vaccinated chickens, as chicks rendered agammaglobulinemic by surgical bursectomy and X-irradiation at 1 day of age can be protected by vaccination (Else, 1974). On the other hand, chemical bursectomy with cyclophosphamide was found to negate the protection afforded by HVT (Purchase and Sharma, 1974). There are three possible explanations for these contradictory results: (1) Cyclophosphamide is more effective than bursectomy and X-irradiation in eliminating the bursa-dependent system. (2) Cyclophosphamide, although fairly selectively active against the bursa-dependent system, causes a temporary depletion of thymocytes (Linna et al., 1972). Vaccination at this stage of thymus suppression may have produced a state of tolerance to the vaccine virus. In the study made by Purchase and Sharma, vaccination was performed during the suppressed stage, which lasts for some 15 days after cyclophosphamide treatment. (3) The depression of the T immune system was such that the latent period for the development of protection was lengthened, so that the birds were challenged too early with virulent MDV.

If protection is immunologically mediated, and serum antibodies are not necessary, cell-mediated immunity may be involved. Cell-mediated immunity has been reported in MD but it is impossible to conclude that it plays an essential role in resistance. The passive transfer of resistance has been achieved using spleen cells (Feldbush and Maag, 1969), but it is clear that in these experiments virus in the cells was also transferred. Experimental thymectomy in the chicken is technically difficult for anatomical reasons. Else (unpublished results, quoted by Else, 1974) reported a marginal increase in MD mortality in thymectomized and vaccinated birds. It has been suggested that suppressor lymphocytes, which respond immunologically to MD antigens, suppress the activity of reactive T cells, thus preventing lymphoma formation in resistant birds (Rouse and Warner, 1974). On this scheme it is postulated that the vaccine virus antigens stimulate suppressor cells more strongly than they stimulate aggressor cells. It would perhaps be simpler to postulate that the more highly immunogenic apathogenic viruses stimulate a strong resistance against transformed cells.

Whatever the immunological mechanism of action of vaccination, it is clear that preinfection with vaccine virus reduces the subsequent levels of viremia of pathogenic virus, and the proportion of birds from which it may be isolated (Purchase et al., 1972b). Moreover, preinfection with a virus strain of low pathogenicity reduces the multiplication of a highly pathogenic strain administered subsequently, and mortality in dually infected birds is determined by the outcome of the initial infection, independently of the highly pathogenic virus (Smith and Calnek, 1974a). The replication of pathogenic and apathogenic viruses differ in their hosts. Apathogenic viruses rapidly reach a peak of virus multiplication, which then quickly decreases; pathogenic viruses reach their peak more gradually, and the level of viremia is maintained. This may be a reflection of the different immunogenicity of the two viruses (Smith and Calnek, 1974b). There is a correlation between viremia and subsequent MD tumor development (Witter et al., 1971; Sharma and Stone, 1972). It may be the levels of viremia that are critical in determining the development of disease, either by an immunosuppressive mechanism or by a virus—cell interaction leading to neoplastic transformation.

It is possible that resistance to MD may be by a two-step mechanism. First, there is the resistance to virus multiplication that is conferred by the active and inactive vaccine preparations. This reduced level of virus activity may result in a much reduced incidence of malignant transformation of lymphocytes. Second, there may be an immunological rejection of transformed cells, independent of the earlier virological events, although influenced by them in the extent of immunosuppression and of lymphocyte transformation. This two-step mechanism would explain apparently contradictory observations concerning resistance to MD. On the one hand, it is possible to protect against MD mortality using vaccine viruses or non-infective preparations of viral antigens which seem to act primarily by reducing the replication or spread of MDV within the infected bird. On the other hand, there is evidence that the rejection of neoplastically transformed lymphocytes is involved in resistance (see Section VI, B) and direct evidence for an anti-tumor immune response has been provided by the observation that birds may be protected against MD by immunization with glutaraldehyde-fixed Marek's disease lymphoblastoid cell lines (Powell, 1975).

D. Immunosuppressive Effects of Marek's Disease

The degenerative and proliferative changes that occur in the bursa of Fabricius, thymus, and spleen of MDV-infected chickens may be associated with an impairment of the immune response. This impairment may be a direct consequence of MDV infection and thus be a factor in lymphoma formation, or it may be a consequence of lymphoma formation. The most consistently observed effect has been a depression of antibody response, observed for both the primary and secondary responses to bovine serum albumin by Purchase et al. (1968) and for the primary response to *Salmonella typhi* and *Brucella abortus* antigens by Payne (1970). A reduced antibody response has also been noted to sheep red blood cells (Burg et al., 1971; Jakowski et al., 1973), *Salmonella pullorum* antigen (Evans and Patterson, 1971) and *Mycoplasma synoviae* antigen (Kleven et al., 1972). These impaired responses occurred both before and during overt MD, and the severity of impairment correlated with the depletion of bursa-dependent follicles from the spleen rather than thymus or bursa damage (Evans et al., 1971). Evans and Patterson (1972) found that the immunological responsiveness of MDV-infected chickens was related to the γ-globulin levels. Infected birds which were able to mount an antibody response to *S. pullorum* antigen were hypergammaglobulinemic as compared with uninfected controls, whereas unresponsive birds were hypogammaglobulinemic. However, the high concentrations of IgG in responsive birds were not associated with specific activity against the *S. pullorum* antigen, which in these birds stimulated an IgM response.

The median skin graft rejection time in infected birds has been found to be normal or slightly delayed. A significant impairment of graft rejection was found when birds which had been infected at 1 day of age were 22 days old, but no difference was found at 33 days (Purchase et al., 1968). Payne (1970) found no difference 19 days after infection, with a significant delay at 40 days after infection. The delay was, however, in both cases quite small. The graft-vs-host reactivity of blood cells was found to be either normal or increased. This conflicts with the skin graft experiments if it is accepted that both these tests are a measure of T-cell function, but an apparent enhancement of graft-vs-host activity may have occurred because of the MDV infecting some of the injected blood cells. Another measure of T-cell function—the delayed hypersensitivity reaction to tuberculin—was shown to be slightly depressed at 36 days after infection (Payne, 1970).

Immunoglobulin levels have been reported to be normal (Purchase et al., 1968) or raised (Howard et al., 1967; Foster and Moll, 1968; Samadieh et al., 1969). Serum immunoglobulin levels have been examined in some detail by Higgins and Calnek (1975a). Up to 9 days after infection an increase in IgM and IgA was noted, but from 10 to 20 days, IgM and IgA levels were lower than in control chickens. After 21 days the IgA level returned to normal, IgG increased to levels about 8 times higher than in control birds, and IgM levels were increased 2-fold in a resistant strain of birds, but were normal in a susceptible strain. The functional capabilities of the high levels of IgG are unknown, but such an elevated level indicates a severe dysfunction of the IgG system.

The activity of splenic T cells from chickens in various stages of the disease has been examined in some detail. The cells from chickens bearing gross tumors showed a reduced response to phytohemagglutinin (PHA) *in vitro*, as compared with cells from controls and nontumor-bearing infected birds (Burg et al., 1971). MD lymphoma cells were unresponsive to PHA (Alm et al., 1972), which is perhaps surprising in view of the presence of immunologically uncommitted bursa and thymus-dependent lymphoid cells in the lymphomas (Payne and Roszkowski, 1973). These observations were confirmed by Lu and Lapen (1974), who also demonstrated a correlation between mitogenic depression and the presence of gross MD tumors. The impaired mitogenic response of MDV infected chickens may be due to the elimination of mitogen responsive cells from the spleen, the reduction of functional mitogen receptors on individual cells, or the dilution of functional cells by the influx of nonreacting tumor cells. Splenomegaly and reduction in mitogen response were found to be associated, so that the depression was probably due to the invastion of the spleen by nonreacting lymphoid cells. This is confirmed by the results of a sequential study on the response of blood lymphocytes to PHA during the development of MD (Powell, unpublished results). No difference was found between the lymphocytes from control birds, infected birds, and vaccinated infected birds. As none of the birds became leukemic, it was assumed that functional T cells were not diluted out by circulating transformed cells. Interestingly, the response of splenic cells to concanavalin A was found to be impaired less than that to PHA and pokeweed mitogen (Lu and Lapen, 1974). It may be that the effect of tumor cell anergy was compensated by an increase in concanavalin A receptors as occurs in Burkitt's lymphoma cell lines (Salle et al., 1972) and is known to occur in the MD cell line MSB-1 (see Section IV, D, 6, c).

The immunosuppressive effects of Marek's disease seem to be related to the lymphoproliferation leading to a reduction in the numbers of immunocompetent cells rather than to the primary immunodepression that is seen in other virus infections (Notkins et al., 1970). The practical effect of the immunosuppression, however, is to increase the susceptibility of the fowl to other diseases. Biggs et al. (1968) found that MD-infected birds were more susceptible to certain coccidial infections as measured by oocyst production. Birds with MD tumors were less able to regress Rous sarcomas than were MDV-infected but clinically normal birds; this suggests impairment of the cell-mediated immune response only in the case of clinical MD (Calnek et al., 1975).

VI. Factors Affecting Pathogenesis and Immunity

A. Virus Strain

Field isolates of MDV differ in their ability to produce clinical disease. Some produce acute MD and some classical MD, as discussed in Section IV, B, and still others appear to be nonpathogenic (Rispens et al., 1969). Biggs and Milne (1972) classified 25 isolates into three categories: acute (12 strains), classical (5 strains), and apathogenic (8 strains). Clearly these different types are well represented in nature; mixed infections occur within flocks, and it has been suggested that mixed infection within an individual may influence the outcome of infection. Apathogenic infections provide an immunity to the effects of pathogenic virus, as shown by the use of such virus for artificial vaccination (Rispens et al., 1972a, b), and such an effect may also occur naturally (Biggs et al., 1972b). HVT is a naturally occurring apathogenic virus whose precise relationship to MDV remains to be determined, and apathogenic variants of pathogenic virus may be obtained by tissue culture attenuation (Churchill et al., 1969b). Von Bulow and Biggs (1975a, b) reported that pathogenic and attenuated MDV, apathogenic MDV, and HVT comprise three serotypes.

The attribute of these strains that is responsible for their differing pathogenicity is still unknown, but several biological differences have been observed. In tissue culture the naturally apathogenic viruses form smaller plaques and spread from cell to cell more slowly than do the classical and acute strains (Biggs and Milne, 1972), and grow to lower levels in the tissue of infected chickens (Phillips and Biggs, 1972). On the other hand, HVT and attenuated HPRS-16 acute MDV formed large plaques in tissue culture and spread more rapidly from cell to cell than did pathogenic virus, but grew to *lower* levels in infected chickens than did pathogenic virus (Biggs and Milne, 1972; Phillips and Biggs, 1972). These findings suggest that pathogenicity is more related to growth *in vivo* than *in vitro*. Theoretically, failure of a virus strain to produce lymphomatous transformation could occur at three levels: (1) failure to infect lymphoid tissue, (2) failure to transform lymphoid cells, and (3) failure of transformed cells to develop into a lymphoma. Smith and Calnek (1974a, b) found that a MDV strain of low virulence did infect the bursa, spleen, and thymus early after infection in a similar manner to high-virulence virus. Bursectomy enhanced lymphoma formation, suggesting that in normal birds transformation with low-virulence virus does occur, but that gross lymphomatosis is prevented by humoral antibody (Smith and Calnek, 1974a). This is consistent with the observation that birds infected with nonpathogenic viruses develop stronger virus neutralizing antibodies than do birds with pathogenic virus (Smith and Calnek, 1973). Cell-associated infectivity peaked early with low virulence virus and then diminished, whereas with virulent virus levels increased more slowly but were progressive (Smith and Calnek, 1974b).

Although the apathogenic viruses normally fail to induce clinical signs or gross lesions, they may induce mild lymphoid cell infiltration in peripheral nerves (Biggs and Milne, 1972; Cho and Kenzy, 1972). Smith and Calnek (1974b) found the infiltrating cells to be transient. These findings suggest that lack of lymphomagenesis with low virulence virus is a post-transformational event mediated by a strong immune mechanism, probably humoral at least. This superior immune response could be related to better immunogenicity of low virulence virus or to its lesser immunosuppressive properties.

Studies on the early events following infection of 1-day-old maternal antibody-free susceptible chicks with 500 PFU of HVT and attenuated HPRS-16 virus are not in complete accord with the findings of Smith and Calnek. Early inflammatory and degenerative changes in the bursa, spleen, and thymus were minimal, little fluorescent antigen was seen, and virions were not seen except in one thymus 6 days after infection with attenuated HPRS-16. Lymphocytes with nuclear projections were not observed at any time between 3 and 28 days post infection (Bradley, Frazier, and Payne, unpublished observations). These findings raise the possibility that with these viruses lack of pathogenicity could be due to failure of virus to infect lymphoid tissue, or failure of transformation. Comparative studies are needed to settle this question.

The type of immune response stimulated by viruses of differing pathogenicity is crucial to the question of mechanism of vaccinal immunity; this is discussed in Section V, C, 5.

B. Genetic Constitution of Host

The genotype of the host is an important factor in determining the outcome of infection by MDV. Response differences due to genotype include incidence, distribution of lesions among tissues and organs, and type of lesion. These differences can be shown within and between commercial strains of fowl, and between inbred lines. The occurrence of genetic differences can be exploited as a means of controlling MD: resistance is a dominant trait and susceptible and resistant strains can be developed by sib and progeny testing using natural (Cole and Hutt, 1973) or artificial exposure to MDV (Cole, 1968, 1972). Genetic control of MD is discussed more fully by Payne (1973b). The effect of genotype on MD incidence is also seen in vaccinated stock (Spencer *et al.,* 1974).

The mechanism of genetic resistance is unknown. It does not lie at a general cellular level because Spencer (1969) and Sharma and Purchase (1974) showed that cultured kidney cells and fibroblasts from genetically susceptible or resistant strains replicated MDV equally well. Rather, resistance is expressed at the level of the entire organism. In discussion of where this may occur the three levels mentioned in connection with oncogenicity of different strains of MDV may be considered, namely (1) failure to infect lymphoid tissues, (2) failure to transform lymphoid cellsnd (3) failure of transformed cells to develop into a lymphoma. It is known that viremia and levels of tissue infection are much lower in genetically resistant birds than in susceptible birds, as early as 1 week after infection (Calnek and Hitchner, 1969; Sharma and Stone, 1972).

More than one mechanism may be involved in limiting virus levels: one early mediator of resistance may be interferon, for Hong and Sevioan (1971) reported higher peak interferon levels in plasma in resistant fowl infected with acute MDV, compared to infected susceptible fowl, 2 days post infection. A protective effect of interferon in MD was shown by Vengris and Maré (1973). Depression of virus levels could simply decrease the probability of infection and transformation of a lymphoid target cell. This explanation is unlikely, however, since Sharma (1973) found that there was no threshold to resistance; i.e., increase of dose of MDV by a factor of 10^6 did not induce a neoplastic response in resistant chicks. Furthermore, there is evidence that the initial early productive virus infection of lymphoid tissues is similar in maternal antibody-free resistant chicks as in antibody-free susceptible chicks (Calnek, 1973). This suggests that resistance is due either to failure of lymphoid cells to undergo transformation, or to failure of transformed cells to proliferate.

Nothing is known of the intrinsic susceptibility of lymphoid cells from resistant birds to transformation; the development of a method for studying *in vitro* transformation of lymphoid cells by MDV would clearly be valuable. No evidence for a strain difference in response to MDV at the chromosomal level has been adduced (Bloom, 1970). It remains possible, and indeed probable, that genetic resistance represents a failure of transformed cells to maintain themselves and propagate, and likely that host immune mechanisms are responsible for this failure. Genetically resistant birds differ from susceptible birds in producing high levels of virus-neutralizing antibody to MDV (Calnek, 1972b; Sharma and Stone, 1972). Precipitating antibodies are at best only poorly correlated with resistance (Spencer *et al.*, 1973). At first it seemed possible that virus neutralizing antibody in some way mediated resistance to tumor formation, but Sharma (1974) failed to abrogate genetic resistance by bursectomy, suggesting that the antibodies reflect rather than cause resistance.

Cell-mediated immunity is a good candidate for an alternative resistance mechanism, particularly as this type of response is known to be important in other herpesvirus infections (see Section V, B, 2). Further evidence against a primary role of antibody is the observation that the low virus neutralizing antibody levels in susceptible strains is not due to an inherent incapacity to produce these antibodies, but is a consequence of the immunosuppressive effects of MDV (Smith and Calnek, 1973; Higgins and Calnek, 1975a). The increase in lymphoma formation in moderately resistant birds following thymectomy (Table V), discussed in Section IV,D,6,b, provides further evidence for a thymic role in resistance.

Sharma and Stone (1972) examined the chronological distribution of lesions in resistant birds and concluded that regression of lesions was not a major factor, but that lesions failed to develop. This does not rule out the possibility that transformed cells are rejected, as they develop, by immunological surveillance. If transformation is followed by cell-mediated immunological rejection, then abrogation of the thymus-dependent lymphoid system would be expected to enhance tumor production in resistant birds. According to these suggestions, birds would be resistant to MD by virtue of possession of genes that control superior cell-mediated immune responses. Such dominant genes could be comparable to the "immune response (Ir)" genes discovered in mice and guinea pigs (McDevitt and Benacerraf, 1969).

The report that resistance to MD and Rous sarcoma virus (RSV) tumor regression are correlated (Carte et al., 1972) suggested the attractive hypothesis that resistance to MD is due to superior immune surveillance which is exercised in a nondiscriminatory fashion. Calnek et al. (1975) have shown, however, that this correlation does not always occur. Nevertheless the possibility remains that certain genetic strains lack genes important at a general level in immune responsiveness, and these birds are unable to mount a strong immune response against either RSV tumors or MD tumors. On the other hand, other strains may possess the necessary genes enabling response at the general level, but lack genes necessary for response to specific MD or RS antigens. These individuals would not necessarily show any correlation between their responses to the two tumors.

We have assumed that neoplastically transformed lymphoid cells occur in MD, that is, that the intrinsic theory (see Section IV, D, 6, d) is true. If, on the other hand, an extrinsic mechanism occurs in lymphoma formation, and the lymphoma represents the immune response (Rouse et al., 1973), then reinterpretation of some of the experimental findings would be necessary. Rouse and Warner (1974) speculated that susceptible strains might be the possessors of strong Ir genes, but this is not compatible with the dominance of genetic resistance. To avoid this objection, and arguing from indirect experimental evidence, they suggested that Ir genes may control suppressor regulator cells that limit the extrinsically stimulated proliferation of T lymphocytes. Demonstration of suppressor cells in MD and further study of the nature of MD lymphomas are needed to settle this conflict.

C. Age of Host

Increase in resistance to clinical MD with age, suspected for many years, has recently been confirmed in well controlled experiments. Witter et al. (1973) found that age resistance developed between 4 and 8 weeks of age, the level being at least 10^4 times that of 1-day-old chicks. Incidence and levels of viremia were higher, and viremia more persistent, in day-old compared with age-resistant chickens (Sharma et al., 1973; Calnek, 1973). Like genetic resistance, age resistance seems to be correlated with ability to make virus neutralizing antibody (Sharma et al., 1973; Calnek, 1973). In resistant birds, the early productive infection of the lymphoid organs occurred apparently to the same extent whether infection took place at 3 days or at 38 days of age, suggesting that the mechanism of age resistance operates at a later stage (Calnek, 1973). Sharma et al. (1973) found that age resistance was associated with ability to regress the quite marked proliferative lymphoid lesions that developed in the nerves of birds infected at 12 weeks of age. Regression was characterized by disappearance of gross nerve lesions which appeared in 50% of the chickens 4 weeks after infection, and transformation of proliferative lesions to nonproliferative lesions. The nature of the age resistance regression has not yet been determined. Calnek (1973) regarded age resistance as being at least partly dependent on genetic resistance, because age resistance failed to develop in genetically susceptible birds and conversely maternal antibody-free chicks from a supposedly genetically resistant strain were not resistant to infection at hatching. However, there is some question as to whether age and genetic resistance are identical, because whereas age resistance seemed to depend on lesion regression (Sharma et al., 1973), genetic resistance did not (Sharma and Stone, 1972).

Sharma et al. (1975) abolished age resistance to MD by neonatal thymectomy, whereas neonatal bursectomy was without effect (Sharma and Witter, 1975). These results suggest that T-cell mediated immune surveillance is an important factor in age resistance.

D. Sex

Sex influences the distribution of MD lesions and the incidence of gross lesions and mortality. The ovary is more prone than the testis to lymphoma formation (Biggs and Payne, 1967; Purchase and Biggs, 1967), and females are more susceptible to clinical disease than are males, by up to 2 times (Purchase and Biggs, 1967; Cole, 1968; Morris et al., 1970). The sex effect is not always seen (Crittenden et al., 1972); according to Morris et al. (1970) it is seen less at extremes of susceptibility or resistance. These latter authors found that males had a higher incidence of involvement of nerve tissue than did females whereas females had more gonadal involvement. Differences between other tissues in their study were not significant; however, Purchase and Biggs (1967) found significantly more liver lesions in females in one strain of bird.

Sex affects mortality more than total gross lesions, indicating that males survive longer than females. The basis for this effect is not known. The effect of sex on the three levels of resistance considered above in relationship to virus strain and genotype should be investigated.

Acknowledgments

We are indebted to Dr. P. M. Biggs and Dr. B. W. Calnek for reading the manuscript and making many helpful suggestions, and to Dr. H. G. Purchase for making a literature search in the Famulus collection of references on avian tumors and avian tumor viruses.

References

Abodeely, R.A., Lawson, L.A., and Randall, C.C. (1970). *J. Virol.* 5, 513.
Achong, B.G., and Epstein, M.A. (1966). *J. Nat. Cancer Inst.* 36, 877.
Adldinger, H.K., and Calnek, B.W. (1973). *J. Nat. Cancer Inst.* 50, 1287.
Ahmed, M., and Schidlovsky, G. (1968). *J. Virol.* 2, 1443.
Ahmed, M., and Schidlovsky, G. (1972). *Cancer Res.* 32, 187.
Akiyama, Y., and Kato, S. (1974). *Biken J.* 17, 105.
Akiyama, Y., Kato, S., and Iwa, N. (1973). *Biken J.* 16, 177.
Allison, A.C. (1972a). *In* "The Scientific Basis of Medicine," Ann. Rev. for 1972, pp. 49–73. Athlone Press, London.
Allison, A.C. (1972b). *Int. Rev. Exp. Pathol.* 10, 182.
Alm, G.V., Siccardi, F.J., and Peterson, R.D.A. (1972). *Acta Pathol. Microbiol. Scand., Sect. A* 80, 109
Anderson, W.A., and Kilbourne, E.D. (1962). *J. Invest. Dermatol.* 37, 25
Anonymous (1941). *Amer. J. Vet. Res.* 2, 116.
Ball, R. F., Hill, J.F., Lyman, J., and Wyatt, A. (1971). *Poult. Sci.* 50, 1084.
Bankowski, R.A., Moulton, J.E., and Mikami, T. (1969). *Amer. J. Vet. Res.* 30, 1667.
Baringer, J.R., and Griffith, J.F. (1970). *J. Neuropathol. Exp Neurol.* 29, 89.
Beasley, J.N., Patterson, L.T., and McWade, D.H. (1970). *Amer. J. Vet. Res.* 31, 339.
Benton, W.J., and Cover, M.S. (1957). *Avian Dis.* 1, 320.
Biggs, P.M. (1961). *Brit. Vet. J.* 117, 326.
Biggs, P.M. (1968). *Curr. Top. Microbiol. Immunol.* 43, 92.
Biggs, P.M. (1971). *In* "Poultry Disease and World Economy" (R.F. Gordon and B.F. Freeman, eds.), BEMB Symp. No. 7, pp. 121–133. British Poultry Science Ltd., Edinburgh.
Biggs, P.M. (1973). *In* "The Herpesviruses" (A.S. Kaplan, ed.), pp. 557–594. Academic Press, New York.
Biggs, P.M., and Milne, B.S. (1971). *Amer. J. Vet. Res.* 32, 1795.
Biggs, P.M., and Milne, B.S. (1972). *In* "Oncogenesis and Herpesviruses" (P.M. Biggs, G. de Thé, and L. N. Payne, eds.), pp. 88–94. International Agency for Research on Cancer, Lyon.
Biggs, P.M., and Payne, L.N. (1963). *Vet. Rec.* 75, 177.

Biggs, P.M., and Payne, L.N. (1964). *Nat. Cancer Inst. Monogr.* **17**, 83.
Biggs, P.M., and Payne, L.N. (1967). *J. Nat. Cancer Inst.* **39**, 267.
Biggs, P.M., Purchase, H.G., Bee, B.R., and Dalton, P.J. (1965). *Vet. Rec.* **77**, 1339.
Biggs, P.M., Long, P.L., Kenzy, S.G., and Rootes, D.G. (1968). *Vet. Rec.* **83**, 284
Biggs, P.M., Payne, L.N., Milne, B.S., Churchill, A.E., Chubb, R.C., Powell, D.G., and Harris, A.H. (1970). *Vet. Rec.* **87**, 704.
Biggs, P.M., Jackson, C.A.W., Bell, R.A., Lancaster, F.M., and Milne, B.S. (1972a). *In* "Oncogenesis and Herpesviruses" (P.M. Biggs, G. de Thé, and L.N. Payne, eds.), pp. 139–146. International Agency for Research on Cancer, Lyon.
Biggs, P.M., Powell, D.G., Churchill, A.E., and Chubb, R.C. (1972b). *Avian Pathol.* **1**, 5.
Blaxland, J.D., Macleod, A.J., Baxendale, W., and Hall, T. (1972). *Vet. Rec.* **90**, 431.
Bloom, S.E. (1970). *Avian Dis.* **14**, 478.
Borit, A., and Altrocchi, P.H. (1971). *Arch. Neurol.* **24**, 40.
Burg, R.W., Feldbush, T., Morris, C.A., and Maag, T.A. (1971). *Avian Dis.* **15**, 662.
Burgoyne, G.H., and Witter, R.L. (1973). *Avian Dis.* **17**, 824.
Burnet, F.M. (1969). "Self and not-self." Cambridge Univ. Press, London and New York.
Byerly, J.L., and Dawe, D.L. (1972). *Amer. J. Vet. Res.* **33**, 2267.
Calnek, B.W. (1972a). *Infect. Immunity* **6**, 193.
Calnek, B.W. (1972b). *In* "Oncogenesis and Herpesviruses" (P.M. Biggs, G. de Thé, and L.N. Payne, eds.), pp. 129–136. International Agency for Research on Cancer, Lyon.
Calnek, B.W. (1973). *J. Nat. Cancer Inst.* **51**, 929.
Calnek, B.W., and Adldinger, H.K. (1971). *Avian Dis.* **15**, 508.
Calnek, B.W., and Hitchner, S.B. (1969). *J. Nat. Cancer Inst.* **43**, 935.
Calnek, B.W., and Madin, S.H. (1969). *Amer. J. Vet. Res.* **30**, 1389.
Calnek, B.W., and Payne, L.N. (1976). *Int. J. Cancer* (in press).
Calnek, B.W., and Smith, M.W. (1972). *Avian Dis.* **16**, 954.
Calnek, B.W., and Witter, R.L. (1972). *In* "Diseases of Poultry" (M.S. Hofstad, ed.), 6th ed., pp. 470–502. Iowa State Univ. Press, Ames.
Calnek, B.W., Adldinger, H.K., and Kahn, D.E. (1970a). *Avian Dis.* **14**, 219
Calnek, B.W., Hitchner, S.B., and Adldinger, H.K. (1970b). *Appl. Microbiol.* **20**, 723.
Calnek, B.W., Ubertini, T., and Adldinger, H.K. (1970c). *J. Natl. Cancer Inst.* **45**, 341
Calnek, B. W., Higgins, D.A., and Fabricant, J. (1975). *Avian Dis.* **19**, 473.
Campbell, J.G. (1956). *Vet. Rec.* **68**, 527.
Campbell, J.G. (1961). *Brit. Vet. J.* **117**, 316.
Campbell, J.G. (1969). "Tumours of the Fowl." Heinemann, London.
Campbell, J.G., and Woode, G.N. (1970). *J. Med. Microbiol.* **3**, 463.
Carmichael, L.E. (1970). *J. Amer. Vet. Med. Ass.* **156**, 1714.
Carte, I.F., Weston, C.R., and Smith, J.H. (1969). *Poult. Sci.* **48**, 1793.
Carte, I.F., Smith, J.H., Weston, C.R., and Savage, T.F. (1972). *Poult. Sci.* **51**, 15.
Caspary, E.A., Currie, S., Walton, J.N., and Field, E.J. (1971). *J. Neurol. Neurosurg. Psychiat.* **34**, 179.
Chen, J.H., and Purchase, H.G. (1970). *Virology* **40**, 410.
Cho, B.R. (1970). *Avian Dis.* **14**, 665.
Cho, B.R. (1974). *Avian Dis.* **18**, 267.
Cho, B.R., and Kenzy, S.G. (1972). *Appl. Microbiol.* **24**, 299.
Cho, H.C., and Ringen, L.M. (1969). *Amer. J. Vet. Res.* **30**, 847.
Cho, B.R., Kenzy, S.G., and Matley, W.J. (1970). *Avian Dis.* **14**, 587.
Cho, B.R., Kenzy, S.G., and Haider, S.A. (1971). *Poult. Sci.* **50**, 881.
Chomiak, T.W., Luginbuhl, R.E., Helmboldt, C.F., and Kottaridis, S.D. (1967). *Avian Dis.* **11**, 646.
Chubb, R.C., and Churchill, A.E. (1968). *Vet. Rec.* **83**, 4.
Chubb, R.C., and Churchill, A.E. (1969). *Vet. Rec.* **85**, 303.

Churchill, A.E. (1968). *J. Nat. Cancer Inst.* **41**, 939.
Churchill, A.E., and Biggs, P.M. (1967). *Nature (London)* **215**, 528.
Churchill, A.E., and Biggs, P.M. (1968). *J. Nat. Cancer Inst.* **41**, 95.
Churchill, A.E., Payne, L.N., and Chubb, R.C. (1969a). *Nature (London)* **211**, 744.
Churchill, A.E., Chubb, R.C., and Baxendale, W. (1969b). *J. Gen. Virol.* **4**, 557.
Cole, R.K. (1968). *Avian Dis.* **12**, 9.
Cole, R.K. (1972). *In* "Oncogenesis and Herpesviruses" (P.M. Biggs, G. de Thé, and L.N. Payne, eds.), pp. 123–128. International Agency for Research on Cancer, Lyon.
Cole, R.K. and Hutt, F.B. (1973). *Anim. Breed. Abstr.* **41**, 103.
Cook, M.K., and Sears, J.F. (1970). *J. Virol.* **5**, 258.
Cook, M.L., and Stevens, J.G. (1973). *Infect. Immunity* **7**, 272.
Cook, M.L., Bastone, V.B., and Stevens, J.G. (1974). *Infect. Immunity* **9**, 946.
Crittenden, L.B., Muhm, R.L., and Burmester, B.R. (1972). *Poult. Sci.* **51**, 261.
Dales, S., and Silverberg, H. (1969). *Virology* **37**, 475.
Dalling, T., and Warrack, G.H. (1936). *Vet. J.* **92**, 310.
Darlington, R.W., and Moss, L.H. (1968). *J. Virol.* **2**, 48.
Davidson, I., and Lee, C.L. (1969). *In* "Infectious Mononucleosis" (R.L. Carter and H.G. Penman, eds.), pp. 177–200. Blackwell, Oxford and Edinburgh.
Davis, W.C., and Sharma, J.M. (1973). *Amer. J. Vet. Res.* **34**, 873.
Deutsch, K., and Siller, W.G. (1961). *Res. Vet. Sci.* **2**, 19.
Doak, R.L., Munnell, J.F., and Ragland, W.L. (1973). *Amer. J. Vet. Res.* **34**, 1063.
Doyle, L.P. (1926). *J. Amer. Vet. Med. Ass.* **68**, 622.
Dumonde, D.C., Wolstencroft, R.A., Panayi, G.A., Matthew, M., Morley, J., and Howson, W.T. (1969). *Nature (London)* **224**, 38.
Eidson, C.S., and Anderson, D.P. (1971). *Avian Dis.* **15**, 68.
Eidson, C.S., and Schmittle, S.C. (1968). *Avian Dis.* **12**, 467.
Eidson, C.S., and Schmittle, S.C. (1969). *Avian Dis.* **13**, 774.
Eidson, C.S., Anderson, D.P., and King, D.D. (1971a). *Amer. J. Vet. Res.* **32**, 2071.
Eidson, C.S., Anderson, D.P., Kleven, S.H., and Brown, J. (1971b). *Avian Dis.* **15**, 312.
Eidson, S.C., Kleven, S.H., Lacroix, V.M., and Anderson, D.P. (1972a). *Avian Dis.* **16**, 139.
Eidson, C.S., Kleven, S.H., and Anderson, D.P. (1972b). *Progr. 109th Annu. A.V.M.A. Meeting* p. 178.
Ellerman, V. (1921). "Leucosis of Fowls and Leucemia Problems." Gyldendal, London.
Else, R. W. (1974). *Vet. Rec.* **95**, 182.
Epstein, M.A. (1967). *In* "Treatment of Burkitt's Tumour" (J.H. Burchenal and D.P. Burkitt, eds.), UICC Monogr. 8, p. 29. Springer-Verlag, Berlin and New York.
Epstein, M.A. (1970). *In* "Burkitt's Lymphoma" (D.P. Burkitt and D.H. Wright, eds.), pp. 148–157. Livingstone, Edinburgh and London.
Epstein, M.A., and Achong, B.G. (1973). *Ann. Rev. Microbiol.* **27**, 413.
Epstein, M.A., and Barr, Y.M. (1965). *J. Nat. Cancer Inst.* **34**, 231.
Epstein, M.A., Achong, B.G., Churchill, A.E., and Biggs, P.M. (1968). *J. Nat. Cancer Inst.* **41**, 805.
Evans, D.L., and Patterson L.T. (1971). *Infect. Immunity* **4**, 567.
Evans, D.L., and Patterson, L.T. (1972). *J. Reticuloendothelial Soc.* **11**, 325.
Evans, D.L., Beasley, J.N., and Patterson, L.T. (1971). *Avian Dis.* **15**, 680.
Fauser, I.S., Purchase, H.G., Long, P.A., Velicer, L.F., Mallmann, V.H., Fauser, H.T., and Winegar, G.O. (1973). *Avian Pathol.* **2**, 55.
Feldbush, T.L., and Maag, T.A. (1969). *Avian Dis.* **13**, 677.
Fernando, W.W.D., and Calnek, B.W. (1971). *Avian Dis.* **15**, 467.
Foster, A.G., and Moll, T. (1968). *Amer. J. Vet. Res.* **29**, 1831.
Frazier, J.A. (1973). *Z. Zellforsch. Mikrosk. Anat.* **136**, 191.
Frazier, J.A. (1974a). *J. Nat. Cancer Inst.* **52**, 829.

Frazier, J.A. (1974b). *Acta Anat.* **88**, 385.
Frazier, J.A., and Biggs, P.M. (1972). *J. Nat. Cancer Inst.* **48**, 1519.
Frazier, J.A., and Powell, P.C. (1975). *Brit. J. Cancer* **31**, 7.
Fujimoto, Y., Nakagawa, M., Okada, K., Okada, M., and Matsukawa, K. (1971). *Jap. J. Vet. Res.* **19**, 7.
Furlong, D., Swift, H., and Roizman, B. (1972). *J. Virol.* **10**, 1071.
Furth, J. (1935). *Arch. Pathol. (Chicago)* **20**, 379.
Glasgow, L.A. (1970). *Arch. Intern. Med.* **126**, 125.
Gold, E. (1965). *J. Immunol.* **95**, 683.
Goodchild, W.M. (1969). *Vet. Rec.* **84**, 87.
Goudie, R.B., Macfarlane, P.S., and Lindsay, M.K. (1974). *Lancet* **1**, 292.
Greenfield, J.G., Blackwood, W., McMenemy, W.H., Meyer, A., and Norman, R.M. (1958). "Neurology." Arnold, London.
Gripenberg, U., Levan, A., and Clifford, P. (1969). *Int. J. Cancer* **4**, 334.
Grundboeck, M. (1965). *Bull. Vet. Inst. Pulawy* **9**, 137.
Haider, S.A., Lapen, R.F., and Kenzy, S.G. (1970). *Poult. Sci.* **69**, 1654.
Hamdy, F., Sevoian, M., and Holt, S.C. (1974). *Infection Immunity* **9**, 740.
Heald, P.J., Badman, H.G., Frunival, B.F., and Wight, P.A.L. (1964). *Poult. Sci.* **43**, 701.
Higgins, D.A., and Calnek, B.W. (1975a). *Infect. Immunity* **11**, 33.
Higgins, D.A., and Calnek, B.W. (1975b). *Infect. Immunity* **12**, 360.
Hill, T.J., Field, H.J., and Roome, A.P.C. (1972). *J. Gen. Virol.* **15**, 253.
Hlozanek, I. (1970). *J. Gen. Virol.* **9**, 45.
Hochberg, E., and Becker, Y. (1968). *J. Gen. Virol.* **2**, 231.
Hong, C.C., and Sevoian, M. (1971). *Appl. Microbiol.* **22**, 818.
Honnegar, K.A., McMuarry, B.L., Gledhill, R.H., and Purchase, H.G. (1972). *Avian Dis.* **16**, 78.
Horiuchi, T., Tezuka, A., Shoya, S., and Yuasa, N. (1969). *Nat. Inst. Anim. Health Quart.* **9**, 203.
Howard, E.B., Jannke, C., Vickers, J., and Kenyon, A.J. (1967). *Cornell Vet.* **57**, 183.
Hudson, L., and Payne, L.N. (1973). *Nature (London), New Biol.* **241**, 52.
Huhn, D. (1967). *Nature (London)* **216**, 1240.
Huxsoll, D.L., and Hemelt, I.E. (1970). *J. Amer. Vet. Med. Ass.* **156**, 1706.
Imamura, T., and Moore, G.E. (1968). *Proc. Soc. Exp. Biol. Med.* **128**, 1179.
Ishikawa, T., Naito, M., Osafune, S., and Kato, S. (1972). *Biken J.* **15**, 215.
Jakowski, R.M., Fredrickson, T.N., Luginbuhl, R.E., and Helmboldt, C.F. (1969). *Avian Dis.* **13**, 215.
Jakowski, R.M., Fredrickson, T.N., Chomiak, T.W., and Luginbuhl, R.E. (1970). *Avian Dis.* **14**, 374.
Jakowski, R.M., Fredrickson, T.N., and Luginbuhl, R.E. (1973). *J. Immunol.* **111**, 238.
Jakowski, R.M., Fredrickson, T.N., Schierman, L.W., and McBride, R.A. (1974). *J. Nat. Cancer Inst.* **53**, 783.
Johnson, E.P., and Conner, B.V. (1933). *J. Amer. Vet. Med. Ass.* **83**, 325.
Jungherr, E. (1937). *Storrs Agr. Exp. Sta. Bull.* **218**, 1.
Kaaden, O-R., Dietzschold, B., and Ueberschär, S. (1974). *Med. Microbiol. Immunol.* **159**, 261.
Kaaden, O-R., and Dietzschold, B. (1975). *Proc. Int. Symp. Oncogenesis Herpesviruses, 2nd, Nuremberg, 1974.* **2**, 337.
Kaleta, E.F., and Bankowski, R.A. (1972a). *J. Nat. Cancer Inst.* **48**, 1303.
Kaleta, E.F., and Bankowski, R.A. (1972b). *Amer. J. Vet. Res.* **33**, 573.
Kaplan, A.S. (Ed.) (1973). "The Herpesviruses." Academic Press, New York.
Kardeván, K., Thakur, H.N., Masztis, Sz., and Tóth, B. (1973). *Magyar Állatorvosok Lapja* **28**, 234.

Kato, S., and Akiyama, Y. (1975). *Proc. Int. Symp. Oncogenesis Herpesviruses, 2nd, Nuremberg, 1974.* **2**, 101.

Kawamura, H., King, D.J., and Anderson, D.P. (1969). *Avian Dis.* **13**, 853.

Kenzy, S.G., McLean, G., Mathey, W.J., and Lee, H.C. (1964). *Nat. Cancer Inst. Monogr.* **17**, 121.

Kenzy, S.G., Cho, B.R., and Kim, Y. (1973). *J. Nat. Cancer Inst.* **51**, 977.

Kirkwood, J., Geering, G., and Old, L.J. (1972). *In* "Oncogenesis and Herpesviruses" (P.M. Biggs, G. de Thé, and L.N. Payne, eds.), p. 479. International Agency for Research on Cancer, Lyon.

Klein, G. (1972a). *Proc. Nat. Acad. Sci. U.S.* **69**, 1056.

Klein, G. (1972b). *In* "Oncogenesis and Herpesviruses" (P.M. Biggs, G. de Thé, and L.N. Payne, eds.), pp. 501–515. International Agency for Research on Cancer, Lyon.

Klein, G. (1975). *Proc. Int. Symp. Herpesvirus and Oncogenesis, 2nd, Nuremberg, 1974.* **2**, 365.

Kleven, S.H., Eidson, C.S., and Anderson, D.P. (1972). *In* "Oncogenesis and Herpesviruses" (P.M. Biggs, G. de Thé, and L.N. Payne), pp. 45–47. International Agency for Research on Cancer, Lyon.

Knotts, F.B., Cook, M.L., and Stevens, J.G. (1973). *J. Exp. Med.* **138**, 740.

Kottaridis, S.D., and Luginbuhl, R.E. (1968). *Avian Dis.* **12**, 383.

Kristensson, K. (1970). *Acta Neuropath (Berl.)* **16**, 54.

Lampert, P.W. (1969). *Lab. Invest.* **20**, 127.

Lampert, P.W., and Schochet, S.S. (1968). *J. Neuropathol. Exp. Neurol.* **27**, 527.

Lapen, R.F., Piper, R.C., and Kenzy, S.G. (1970). *J. Nat. Cancer Inst.* **45**, 941.

Lapen, R.F., Kenzy, S.G., Piper, R.C., and Sharma, J.M. (1971). *J. Nat. Cancer Inst.* **47**, 389.

Laufs, R., and Steinke, H. (1975). *Proc. Int. Symp. Herpesviruses and Oncogenesis, 2nd, Nuremberg, 1974.* **2**, 345.

Lee, C.D., Wilcke, H.L., Murray, C., and Henderson, E.W. (1937). *J. Infect. Dis.* **61**, 1.

Lee, L.F. (1972). *J. Virol.* **10**, 167.

Lee, L.F., Nazerian, K., and Boezi, J.A. (1975). *Proc. Int. Symp. Oncogenesis and Herpesviruses, Nuremberg, 2nd, 1974.* **2**, 199.

Lerche, F., and Fritzsche, K. (1934). *Z. Infekt. - Kr. Haustiere* **45**, 89.

Lesnik, F., and Ross, L.J.N. (1975). *Int. J. Cancer*, **16**, 153.

Levin, A.G., Friberg, S., and Klein, G. (1969). *Nature (London)* **222**, 997.

Linna, T.J., Frommel, D., and Good, R.A. (1972). *Int. Arch. Allergy* **42**, 20.

Lockart, R.Z. (1973). *In* "The Herpesviruses" (A.S. Kaplan, ed.), pp. 261–269. Academic Press, New York.

Lodmell, D.L., Niwa, A., Hayashi, K., and Notkins, A.L. (1973). *J. Exp. Med.* **137**, 706.

Lu, Y-S., and Lapen, R.F. (1974). *Amer. J. Vet. Res.* **35**, 977.

McDevitt, H.O., and Benacerraf, B. (1969). *Advan. Immunol.* **11**, 31.

McGaughey, C.A., and Downie, A.W. (1930). *J. Comp. Pathol.* **43**, 63.

Marek, J. (1907). *Deut. Tieraerztl. Wochenschr.* **15**, 417.

Matsui, T. (1973). *Jap. J. Vet. Res.* **21**, 101.

Melnick, J.L., Midulla, M., Wimberly, I., Barrera-Oro, J.G., and Levy, B.M. (1964). *J. Immunol.* **92**, 596.

Meulemans, G., Halen, P., Schyns, P., and Bruynooghe, D. (1971). *Vet. Rec.* **89**, 325.

Miller, J.M., Miller, L.D., Gillette, K.G., and Olson, C. (1969). *J. Nat. Cancer Inst.* **43**, 719.

Mladenov, Z., Bozhkov, S., Todorov, T.O., and Kirev, T. (1972). *Bull. Inst. Gen. Comp. Pathol.* **14**, 73.

Mollo, F., and Stranignoni, A. (1967). *Brit. J. Cancer* **21**, 519.

Morgan, C., Rose, H.M., and Medris, B. (1968). *J. Virol.* **2**, 507.

Moriwaki, M., and Horiuchi, T. (1974). *Nat. Inst. Anim. Heath Quart.* **14**, 72.

Morris, J.R., Jerome, F.N., and Reinhart, B.S. (1969). *Poult. Sci.* **48**, 1513.
Morris, J.R., Ferguson, A.E., and Jerome, F.N. (1970). *Can. J. Animal Sci.* **50**, 69.
Nadkarni, J.S., Nadkarni, J.J., Clifford, P., Manalov, G., Fenyö, E.M., and Klein, E. (1969). *Cancer* **23**, 64.
Naito, M., Ono, K., Tanabe, S., Doi, T., and Kato, S. (1970). *Biken J.* **13**, 205.
Nazerian, K. (1971). *J. Nat. Cancer Inst.* **47**, 207.
Nazerian, K. (1973). *Advan. Cancer Res.* **17**, 279.
Nazerian, K. (1974). *J. Virol.* **13**, 1148.
Nazerian, K. (1975). *Proc. Int. Symp. Oncogenesis Herpesviruses, 2nd, Nuremberg, 1974.* **1**, 345.
Nazerian, K., and Burmester, B.R. (1968). *Cancer Res.* **28**, 2454.
Nazerian, K., and Chen, J.H. (1973). *Arch. Ges. Virusforsch.* **41**, 59.
Nazerian, K., and Lee, L.F. (1974). *J. Gen. Virol.* **25**, 317.
Nazerian, K., and Purchase, H.G. (1970). *J. Virol.* **5**, 79.
Nazerian, K., and Sharma, J.M. (1975). *J. Nat. Cancer Inst.* **54**, 277.
Nazerian, K., and Witter, R.L. (1970). *J. Virol.* **5**, 388.
Nazerian, K., Solomon, J.J., Witter, R.L., and Burmester, B.R. (1968). *Proc. Soc. Exp. Biol. Med.* **127**, 177.
Nazerian, K., Lee, L.F., Witter, R.L., and Burmester, B.R. (1971). *Virology* **43**, 442.
Nazerian, K., Lindahl, T., Klein, G., and Lee, L.F. (1973). *J. Virol.* **12**, 841.
Nelson, N.M., and Thorp, F. (1943). *Amer. J. Vet. Res.* **4**, 294.
Nielson, K.H., and Anderson, G.W. (1971). *Poult. Sci.* **50**, 1518.
Nii, S., Morgan, C., and Rose, H.M. (1968a). *J. Virol.* **2**, 517.
Nii, S., Morgan, C., Rose, H.M., and Hsu, K.C. (1968b). *J. Virol.* **2**, 1172.
Notkins, A.L., Mergenhagen, S.E., and Howard, R.J. (1970). *Ann. Rev. Microbiol.* **24**, 525.
Okada, K., and Fujimoto, Y. (1971). *Jap. J. Vet. Res.* **19**, 64.
Okada, K., Fujimoto, Y., Mikami, T., and Yonehara, K. (1972). *Jap. J. Vet. Res.* **20**, 57.
Okazaki, W., Purchase, H.G., and Burmester, B.R. (1970). *Avian Dis.* **14**, 413.
Okazaki, W., Purchase, H.G., and Burmester, B.R. (1971). *Avian Dis.* **15**, 753.
Okazaki, W., Purchase, H.G., and Burmester, B.R. (1973). *Amer. J. Vet. Res.* **34**, 813.
Omar, A.R., Lo, H.S., and Teoh, K.C. (1973). *Aust. Vet. J.* **49**, 319.
Ono, K., Tanabe, S., Naito, M., Doi, T., and Kato, S. (1970). *Biken J.* **13**, 213.
Papadimitriou, J.M. (1966). *Proc. Soc. Exp. Biol. Med.* **121**, 93.
Pappenheimer, A.M., Dunn, L.C., and Cone, V. (1926). *Storrs Agr. Exp. Sta. Bull.* **143**, 186.
Pappenheimer, A.M. Dunn, L.C., and Cone, V. (1929a). *J. Exp. Med.* **49**, 63.
Pappenheimer, A.M., Dunn, L.C., and Seidlin, S.M. (1929b). *J. Exp. Med.* **49**, 87.
Parker, J.W., Wakasa, H., and Lukes, R.J. (1967). *Lancet* **1**, 214.
Patruscu, I.V., Calnek, B.W., and Smith, M.W. (1972). *Avian Dis.* **16**, 86.
Patterson, F.D., Wilcke, H.L., Murray, C., and Henderson, E.W. (1932). *J. Amer. Vet. Med. Ass.* **81**, 747.
Payne, L.N. (1970). *Proc. Roy. Soc. Med.* **63**, 16.
Payne, L.N. (1971). In "Physiology and Biochemistry of the Domestic Fowl" (D.J. Bell and B.M. Freeman, eds.), Vol. 2, pp. 985–1037. Academic Press, New York.
Payne, L.N. (1972). In "Oncogenesis and Herpesviruses" (P.M. Biggs, G. de Thé, and L.N. Payne, eds.), pp. 21–37. International Agency for Research on Cancer, Lyon.
Payne, L.N. (1973a). *Proc. Int. Symp. Princess Takamatsu Cancer Res. Fund, 3rd, Tokyo, 1972* p. 235.
Payne, L.N. (1973b). *Avian Pathol.* **2**, 237.
Payne, L.N., and Biggs, P.M. (1967). *J. Nat. Cancer Inst.* **39**, 281.
Payne, L.N., and Rennie, M. (1970). *J. Nat. Cancer Inst.* **45**, 387.
Payne, L.N., and Rennie, M. (1973). *J. Nat. Cancer Inst.* **51**, 1559.

Payne, L.N., and Rennie, M. (1976). *Proc. Int. Symp. Comp. Leukemia Res.*, *7th, 1975*. To be published.
Payne, L.N., and Roszkowski, J. (1973). *Avian Pathol.* **1**, 27.
Payne, L.N., Powell, P.C., and Rennie, M. (1974). *Cold Spring Harbor Symp. Quant. Biol.* **39**, 817.
Petek, M., and Quaglio, G.L. (1967). *Pathol. Vet.* **4**, 464.
Peters, W.P., Kufe, D., Schlom, J., Frankel, J.W., Prickett, C.O., Groupé, V., and Spiegelman, S. (1973). *Proc. Nat. Acad. Sci. U.S.* **70**, 3175.
Phillips, P.A., and Biggs, P.M. (1972). *J. Nat. Cancer Inst.* **49**, 1367.
Potel, K. (1939). *Z. Infekt. - Kr. Haustiere* **54**, 143.
Powell, P.C. (1975). *Nature (London)* **257**, 684.
Powell, P.C. (1976). *Proc. Int. Symp. Comp. Leukemia Res. 7th, 1975*. To be published.
Powell, P.C., Payne, L.N., Frazier, J.A., and Rennie, M. (1974). *Nature (London)* **251**, 79.
Powell, P.C., Payne, L.N., Frazier, J.A., and Rennie, M. (1975). *Proc. Int. Symp. Oncogenesis Herpesviruses, 2nd, Nuremberg, 1974.* **2**, 89.
Prineas, J.W. (1971). *Acta Neuropathol. (Berl.)* **18**, 34.
Prineas, J.W., and Wright, R.G. (1972). *Lab. Invest.* **26**, 548.
Purchase, H.G. (1969). *J. Virol.* **3**, 557.
Purchase, H.G. (1970). *Cancer Res.* **30**, 1898.
Purchase, H.G. (1972). *Advan. Vet. Sci.* **16**, 223.
Purchase, H.G. (1973). *World's Poult. Sci. J.* **29**, 238.
Purchase, H.G., and Biggs, P.M. (1967). *Res. Vet. Sci.* **8**, 440.
Purchase, H.G., and Burgoyne, G.H. (1970). *Amer. J. Vet. Res.* **31**, 117.
Purchase, H.G., and Sharma, J.M. (1974). *Nature (London)* **248**, 419.
Purchase, H.G., Chubb, R.C., and Biggs, P.M. (1968). *J. Nat. Cancer Inst.* **40**, 583.
Purchase, H.G., Witter, R.L., Okazaki, W., and Burmester, B.R., (1971a). *Perspect. Virol.* **7**, 91.
Purchase, H.G., Burmester, B.R., and Cunningham, C.H. (1971b). *Infect. Immunity* **3**, 295.
Purchase, H.G., Okazaki, W., and Burmester, B.R. (1971c). *Poult. Sci.* **50**, 775.
Purchase, H.G., Okazaki, W., and Burmester, B.R. (1972a). *Vet. Rec.* **91**, 79.
Purchase, H.G., Okazaki, W., and Burmester, B.R. (1972b). *Avian Dis.* **16**, 57.
Purchase, H.G., Ludford, C., Nazerian, K., and Cox, H.W. (1973). *J. Nat. Cancer Inst.* **51**, 489.
Quaglio, G.L. (1963). *20th Conv. Pat. Aviare, Varese.* **2**, 199.
Rabin, E.R., Jenson, A.B., and Melnick, J.L. (1968). *Science* **162**, 126.
Ratz, F., Széky, A., andVányi, A. (1972). *Acta Vet. Acad. Sci. Hung.* **22**, 349.
Rawls, W.E. (1973). *In* "The Herpesviruses" (A.S. Kaplan, ed.), pp. 291–325. Academic Press, New York.
Rickinson, A.B., Jarvis, J.E., Crawford, D.H., and Epstein, M.A. (1974). *Int. J. Cancer* **14**, 704.
Rispens, B.H., van Vloten, J., and Maas, H.J.L. (1969). *Brit. Vet. J.* **125**, 445.
Rispens, B.H., van Vloten, H., Mastenbroek, N., Maas, H.J.L., and Schat, K.A. (1972a). *Avian Dis.* **16**, 108.
Rispens, B.H., van Vloten, H., Mastenbroek, N., Maas, H.J.L., and Schat, K.A. (1972b). *Avian Dis.* **16**, 126.
Rocklin, R.E., Sheremata, W.A., Feldman, R.G., Kies, M.W., and David, J.R. (1971). *New Engl. J. Med.* **284**, 803.
Roizman, B. (1972). *In* "Oncogenesis and Herpesviruses" (P.M. Biggs, G. de Thé, and L.N. Payne, eds.), pp. 1–17. International Agency for Research on Cancer, Lyon.
Ross, L.J.N., Frazier, J.A., and Biggs, P.M. (1972). *In* "Oncogenesis and Herpesviruses" (P.M. Biggs, G. de Thé, and L.N. Payne, eds.), pp. 480–484. International Agency for Research on Cancer, Lyon.

Ross, L.J.N., Biggs, P.M., and Newton, A.A. (1973). *J. Gen. Virol.* **18**, 291.
Ross, R.W., and Orlans, E. (1958). *J. Pathol. Bacteriol.* **76**, 393.
Rouse, B.T., and Warner, N.L. (1974). *J. Immunol.* **113**, 904.
Rouse, B.T., Wells, R.J.H., and Warner, N.L. (1973). *J. Immunol.* **110**, 534.
Salle, D.L., Munakata, N., and Pauli, R.M. (1972). *Cancer Res.* **32**, 2463.
Samadieh, B., Bankowski, R.A., and Carroll, E.J. (1969). *Amer. J. Vet. Res.* **30**, 837.
Schidlovsky, G., Ahmed, M., and Jensen, K.E. (1969). *Science* **164**, 959.
Schmahl, W., Hoffman-Fezer, G., and Hoffmann, R. (1975). *Z. Immunitaetsforsch., Exp. Klin. Immunol* **150**, 175.
Seagar, E.A. (1933a). *Vet. J.* **89**, 454.
Seagar, E.A. (1933b). *Brit. Vet. J.* **89**, 557.
Sebuwufu, P.H. (1966). *Nature (London)* **212**, 1382.
Severin, M.J., and White, R.J. (1968). *Amer. J. Pathol.* **53**, 1009.
Sevoian, M. (1967). *Avian Dis.* **11** 98.
Sevoian, M., and Chamberlain, D.M. (1962). *Vet. Med.* **57**, 608.
Sevoian, M. and Chamberlain, D.M. (1964). *Avian Dis.* **8**, 281.
Sevoian, M., Chamberlain, D.M., and Counter, F. (1962). *Vet. Med.* **57**, 500.
Sharma, J.M. (1973). *Avian Pathol.* **2**, 75.
Sharma, J.M. (1974). *Nature (London)* **247**, 117.
Sharma, J.M., and Purchase, H.G. (1974). *Infect. Immunity* **9**, 1092.
Sharma, J.M., and Stone, H.A. (1972). *Avian Dis.* **16**, 894.
Sharma, J.M., and Witter, R.L. (1975). *Cancer Res.* **35**, 711.
Sharma, J.M., Kenzy, S.G., and Rissberger, A. (1969). *J. Nat. Cancer Inst.* **43**, 907.
Sharma, J.M., Witter, R.L., and Burmester, B.R. (1973). *Infect. Immunity* **8**, 715.
Sharma, J.M., Witter, R.L., and Purchase, H.G. (1975). *Nature (London)* **253**, 477.
Siller, W.G. (1960). *J. Pathol. Bacteriol.* **80**, 43.
Simpson, C.F. (1969a). *Cancer Res.* **29**, 33.
Simpson, C.F. (1969b). *Amer. J. Vet. Res.* **30**, 2191.
Smith, G.F., and O'Hara, P.T. (1967). *Nature (London)* **215**, 773.
Smith, M.W., and Calnek, B.W. (1973). *Avian Dis.* **17**, 727.
Smith, M.W., and Calnek, B.W. (1974a). *J. Nat. Cancer Inst.* **52**, 1595.
Smith, M.W., and Calnek, B.W. (1974b). *Avian Pathol.* **3**, 229.
Smith, T.W., Albert, D.M., Robinson, N., Calnek, B.W., and Schwabe, O. (1974). *Invest. Ophthalmol.* **13**, 586.
Solisch, P. (1972). *Monatsh. Veterinärmed.* **17**, 677.
Solomon, J.J., Witter, R.L., Nazerian, K., and Burmester, B.R. (1968). *Proc. Soc. Exp. Biol. Med.* **127**, 173.
Solomon, J.J., Witter, R.L., Stone, H.A., and Champion, L.R. (1970). *Avian Dis.* **14**, 752.
Spencer, J.L. (1969). *Avian Dis.* **13**, 753.
Spencer, J.L., and Calnek, B.W. (1970). *Amer. J. Vet. Res.* **31**, 345.
Spencer, J.L., and Robertson, A. (1972). *Amer. J. Vet. Res.* **33**, 393.
Spencer, J.L., Grunder, A.A., and Robertson, A. (1973). *Avian Pathol.* **2**, 17.
Spencer, J.L., Gavora, J.S., Grunder, A.A., Robertson, A., and Speckmann, G.W. (1974). *Avian Dis.* **18**, 33.
Spring, S.B., Roizman, B., and Schwartz, J. (1968). *J. Virol.* **2**, 384.
Stevens, J.G., and Cook, M.L. (1971). *Science* **173**, 843.
Stevens, J.G., Nesburn, A.B., and Cook, M.L. (1972). *Nature (London) New Biol.* **235**, 216.
Stoker, M.G.P. (1958). *Nature (London)* **182**, 1525.
Széky, A., and Vanyi, A. (1973). *Acta Vet. Acad. Sci. Hung.* **23**, 369.
Theis, G.A., Schierman, L.W., Fredrickson, T.N., and McBride, R.A. (1974). *Fed. Proc.* **33**, 739.

Tooze, J. (ed.) (1973). "The Molecular Biology of Tumour Viruses." Cold Spring Harbor Laboratory.
Törö, I., and Oláh, I. (1966). *Nature (London)* **212**, 315.
Ubertini, T., and Calnek, B.W. (1970). *J. Nat. Cancer Inst.* **45**, 507.
Vengris, V.E., and Maré, C.J. (1973). *Avian Dis.* **17**, 758.
Vickers, J.H., Helmboldt, C.F., and Luginbuhl, R.E. (1967). *Avian Dis.* **11**, 531.
Vielitz, E., and Landgraft, H. (1971). *Deut. Tierarztl. Wochschr.* **78**, 617.
von Bülow, V. (1971). *Amer. J. Vet. Res.* **32**, 1275.
von Bülow, V., and Biggs, P.M. (1975a). *Avian Pathol.* **4**, 133.
von Bülow, V., and Biggs, P.M. (1975b). *Avian Pathol.* **4**, 147.
von Bülow, V., and Payne, L.N. (1970). *Zbl. Vet. Med.* **17**, 460.
von Bülow, V., Biggs, P.M., and Frazier, J.A. (1975). *Proc. Int. Symp. Oncogenesis and Herpesviruses, 2nd, Nuremberg, 1974.* **2**, 329.
Walker, D., and Grattan, D.A.P. (1968). *Vet. Rec.* **82**, 43.
van der Walle, N., and Winkler-Junius, E. (1924). *Tijdschr. Vergelijk. Geneesk.* **10**, 34.
Warrack, G.H., and Dalling, T. (1932). *Vet. J.* **88**, 28.
Weber, A., Fahning, M., Hammer, R.H., and Jessen, C. (1973). *J. Nat. Cancer Inst.* **51**, 81.
Webster, H., Spiro, D., Waksman, B., and Adams, R.D. (1961). *J. Neuropathol. Exp. Neurol.* **20**, 5.
Weller, R.O. (1965). *J. Pathol. Bacteriol.* **89**, 591.
Wight, P.A.L. (1962a). *J. Comp. Pathol.* **72**, 40.
Wight, P.A.L. (1962b). *J. Comp. Pathol.* **72**, 348.
Wight, P.A.L. (1964). *Res. Vet. Sci.* **5**, 46.
Wight, P.A.L. (1965). *Brit. Vet. J.* **121**, 278.
Wight, P.A.L. (1966). *J. Comp. Pathol.* **76**, 333.
Wight, P.A.L. (1967). *Experientia* **23**, 836.
Wight, P.A.L. (1968). *Vet. Rec.* **82**, 749.
Wight, P.A.L. (1969). *J. Comp. Pathol.* **79**, 563.
Wight, P.A.L., and Siller, W.G. (1965). *Res. Vet. Sci.* **6**, 324.
Willemart, J.P. (1972). *Rec. Med. Vet.* **148**, 203.
Willemart, J.P., Moutlaur, D., Verger, M., and Labrousse, F. (1967a), *Rec. Med. Vet.* **143**, 253.
Willemart, J.P., Verger, M., and Alberge, F. (1967b). *Rec. Med. Vet.* **143**, 953.
Williams, R.C., DeBoard, J.R., Mellbye, O.J., Messner, R.P., and Lindstram, F.D. (1973). *J. Clin. Invest.* **52**, 283.
Wilton, J.M.A., Ivanyi, L., and Lehner, T. (1972). *Brit. Med. J.* **1**, 723.
Wisniewski, H., Prineas, J., and Raine, C.S. (1969a). *Lab. Invest.* **21**, 105.
Wisniewski, H., Terry, R.D., Whitaker, J.N., Cook, S.D., and Dowling, P.C. (1969b). *Arch. Neurol.* **21**, 269.
Witter, R.L., Burgoyne, G.H., and Burmester, B.R. (1968). *Avian Dis.* **12**, 522.
Witter, R.L., Nazerian, K., Purchase, H.G., and Burgoyne, G.H. (1970). *Amer. J. Vet. Res.* **31**, 525.
Witter, R.L., Solomon, J.J., Champion, L.R., and Nazerian, K. (1971). *Avian Dis.* **15**, 346.
Witter, R.L., Sharma, J.M., Solomon, J.J., and Champion, L.R. (1973). *Avian Pathol.* **2**, 43.
Witter, R.L., Lee, L.F., Okazaki, W., Purchase, H.G., Burmester, B.R., and Luginbuhl, R.E. (1975a). *J. Nat. Cancer Inst.* **55**, 215.
Witter, R.L., Stephens, E.A., Sharma, J.M., and Nazerian, K. (1975b). *J. Immunol.* **115**, 177.
Wright, D.H. (1970). *In* "Burkitt's Lymphoma" (D.P. Burkitt and D.H. Wright, eds.), pp. 82–102. Livingstone, Edinburgh and London.
Yamagiwa, S., Ono, T., Ueda, A., Inoue, M., Itakura, C., and Takemura, N. (1967). *Res. Bull. Obihiro Univ., Ser. 1.* **5**, 155.

Yamamoto, T., Otani, S., and Shiraki, H. (1973). *Acta Neuropathol. (Berl.)* **26**, 285.
Zander, D.V. (1959). *Proc. Annu. Western Poult. Dis. Conf. 8th, David, Calif.* 18.
Zander, D.V., Hill, R.W., Raymond, R.G., Balch, R.K., Mitchell, R.W., and Dunsing, J.W. (1972). *Avian Dis.* **16**, 163.
Zygraich, N., and Huygelen, C. (1972). *Avian Dis.* **16**, 735.

The Chalone Concept

TAPIO RYTÖMAA

Second Department of Pathology, University of Helsinki, and Institute of Radiation Protection, Helsinki, Finland

I.	Introduction	156
II.	Strategy of Growth	157
	A. Types of Tissues and Cells in Adult Mammals	158
	B. Growth Potential, Aging, and Death of Cells	159
III.	Chalone Mechanism; Some Theoretical Aspects	162
	A. Chalone Synthesis, Release, and Transport	162
	B. Chalone and the Cell Cycle	165
	C. Biochemical Mechanisms	167
IV.	Impurities in Chalone Preparations	168
	A. Nonphysiological Contaminants	169
	B. Cytotoxic Physiological Impurities	170
	C. Other Physiological Impurities	171
V.	Composition and Effects of Crude Leukocyte Extracts; Some Original Data	173
	A. Composition of Crude Leukocyte Extracts	173
	B. "Cold" Thymidine	176
	C. RNA and Protein Syntheses	177
VI.	Tissue Specificity	179
	A. Degree of Specificity; Is It Absolute?	179
	B. Failure to Find Tissue-Specific Inhibitors	180
	C. Experimental Evidence for Specificity of Action	181
VII.	Putative Chalone Systems	187
VIII.	Regulation of Growth by Factors Other Than Chalone	189
	A. Chemical Substances Influencing Cell Division	189
	B. Density-Dependent Inhibition	192
IX.	Chalones and Cancer	194
	A. What Is Cancer?	194
	B. Role of Chalones	195
X.	Conclusions	198
	References	199
	Note Added in Proof	206

I. Introduction

A central problem in current biomedical research is the manner in which cell proliferation is controlled. This problem is of more than academic interest, for clearly the understanding of control of cell populations is fundamental to the understanding of malignant processes. Cancer cells, however, do not really lie at the heart of the basic problem; for all practical purposes, cancer cells proliferate out of control. The basic features of the growth-regulatory mechanisms are better expressed by phenomena that, at the first glance, may appear to be trivial and unexciting: in adult mammals, tissue and organ mass is maintained at a constant level and regenerated after damage.

In recent years a number of steps have been taken toward an understanding of the problem of growth control. Much of the progress is based on the application of a "new" cybernetic principle to this phenomenon: cell proliferation is regulated, at least in part, by means of negative feedback; i.e., an inhibitory effect is exerted on cell division within a population by the population itself. This general idea has been proposed by numerous authors (e.g., Ribbert, 1895; Weiss, 1952, 1955; Weiss and Kavanau, 1957; Osgood, 1957, 1959; Rose, 1957, 1958; Bullough and Laurence, 1960; Bullough, 1962, 1965, 1967; Mercer, 1962; Iversen and Bjerknes, 1963; Bullough and Rytömaa, 1965; Tsanev and Sendov, 1966; Riley, 1969, 1972; Wheldon et al., 1970; Cone, 1971; Bard, 1973). In such a system the basic assumption is that a (chemical) signal is produced by the cells of each tissue, enabling the mass of the tissue to be gauged and cell proliferation to be regulated accordingly. Experimental evidence for these hormonelike endogenous mitotic inhibitors, which are now commonly known as chalones, is the subject of the present review.

The term chalone comes from a Greek word ($\chi\alpha\lambda\acute{\alpha}\omega$) meaning to slacken a sail and so to slow down a boat. Schäfer proposed in 1916 that this term could be used to describe endocrine products that inhibit or depress activity, to distinguish such substances from hormones that stimulate activity (Schäfer, 1916). This proposal was not commonly accepted and, therefore, Bullough (1962) later adopted the term chalone to indicate putative chemical messengers that are produced within a tissue to inhibit cell proliferation within that same tissue.

Application of the negative feedback principle to the autoregulation of cell proliferation is, at the level of experimentation, a relatively new development. Less rigorous concepts and experiments of specific homologous regulation of cellular growth are, however, many years older; growth models of this kind are abundant in the literature (e.g., Robertson, 1923; Carrel, 1925; Fischer and Parker, 1929; Baker, 1935; Simms and Stillman, 1937; Tyler, 1946; Lee and Hanson, 1947; Stone and Vultee, 1949; Teir, 1951, 1952; Tardent, 1955; Saetren, 1956; Menkin, 1957; Bertalanffy, 1960; Glinos, 1960; Johnson, 1969). Consequently, a very large number of different established and hypothetical factors have been suggested to be operational in the physiological regulation of cell proliferation; some of these factors will also be briefly discussed in the present review. Much of the extreme complexity of the field seems to arise from the often vaguely recognized fact that, although many factors do influence cell proliferation, they do not control it (Bullough, 1962).

It is possible that the control of cell proliferation in multicellular organisms is a complex network system that is not adequately described in terms of a single linear cause-effect relation. Nevertheless, it is convenient to distinguish between cell-line specific factors directly involved in the autonomous control of cell proliferation and the other "secondary" factors and causes of growth. The last-mentioned groups include such factors and conditions as nutrients, exogenous triggers (hypoxia in erythropoiesis, bacteria in granulopoiesis, wounding, etc.), functional load, and a number of substances that modify cell proliferation in a manner of steering (e.g., mitogenic hormones). Even if it turns out that the chalone concept is a gross mental oversimplification of growth control, or rather a compromise between exact and generalized formulation of a complex phenomenon, there are, for the time being, good theoretical and practical reasons for accepting the maxim that, basicallly, growth control is simple. Indeed, it seems unlikely, especially from an evolutionary point of view, that the basic control of cell proliferation would be drastically different in different tissues, i.e., that the regulatory mechanisms of the same phenomenon would be extensively duplicated (Riley, 1969).

One of the main purposes of the present article is to evaluate the extent and conclusiveness of the experimental evidence bearing on the suggestion that chalones are the real agents of negative feedback. During the past decade numerous more or less comprehensive reviews have been written on chalones (e.g., Bullough, 1965, 1967, 1969, 1971a, 1972, 1973a; Bullough and Rytömaa, 1965; Bullough and Laurence, 1966a; Bullough et al., 1967; Iversen, 1969, 1970, 1973b; Rytömaa, 1970, 1973a,b; Laurence et al., 1972; Argyris, 1972; Mathé, 1972; Marks, 1972; Elgjo, 1972; Kirsch et al., 1972; Laurence, 1973a; Simnett and Fischer, 1973; Houck and Hennings, 1973; Paukovits, 1973a,b; Moreau and Bullough, 1973; Kieger, 1974; Houck and Daugherty, 1974). Consequently, it seems at this moment pointless to summarize the chalone concept yet again. However, it may be worthwhile to deal with the chalone literature in a somewhat different manner, with the specific aim of describing and analyzing several contradictory or odd findings and weak points in chalone experimentation. It is hoped that such an approach would help in evaluating the validity of the chalone concept more adequately, and perhaps also in avoiding some of the unnecessary connotations that an enthusiastic presentation of the chalone concept seems to invoke.

II. Strategy of Growth

The purpose of this section is to provide a simplistic background of the general strategy of tissues and cells in normal adult mammals. It is believed that appreciation of some qualitative and quantitative aspects of cell proliferation gives a better basis for an informed judgment on methods of growth control.

A. Types of Tissues and Cells in Adult Mammals

On the basis of mitotic potentialities, tissues and organs may be divided into three different categories, commonly designated as renewing, expanding, and static tissues (Bizzozero, 1894; Messier and Leblond, 1960; Goss, 1967).

Renewing tissues, such as hemic cell lines, are characterized by a "growth zone" (see Goss, 1967), a subpopulation of actively dividing cells from which those of the functional compartment are recruited; the end cells usually have relatively short life-spans. Expanding tissues, such as the liver, undergo cell division only to increase tissue mass, e.g., in keeping pace with somatic growth [hence all tissues may be regarded as being originally of the expanding type; see Goss (1967)], or to replace accidentally lost cells; unlike renewing tissues, expanding tissues do not have "growth zones." Static tissues, such as neurons, lack the capacity for cell division altogether; in general, these cells have the potentiality to live for as long as the organism survives. However, it may be of some interest to note in this context that static tissues have also been suggested to control the total life-span of the individual by means of small groups of essential "pacemaker" cells; the life-span of these cells would be programmed

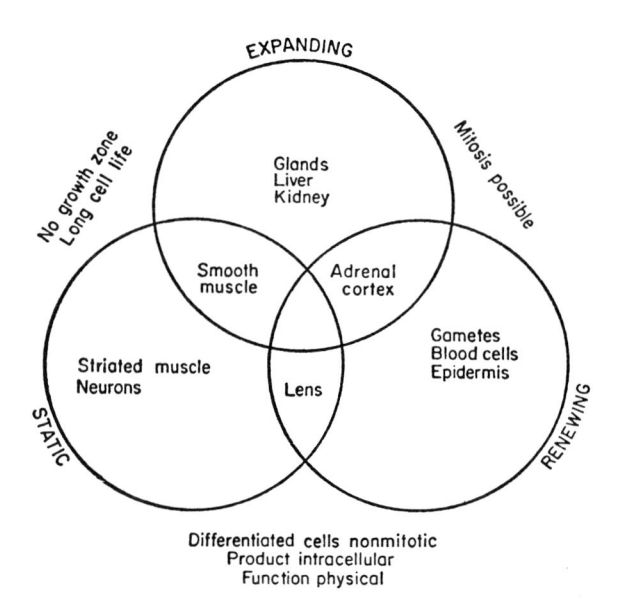

FIG. 1. Classification of tissues. Tissues that do not conform to the simple pattern of renewing, expanding, and static categories are indicated in the overlapping areas. From Goss (1967).

during development as part of the normal process of differentiation (see Bullough, 1971b; Franks, 1974).

A diagram illustrating classification of tissues according to modes of growth and types of differentiation is shown in Fig. 1.

Instead of grouping by tissues, mammalian cells may be classified on the basis of maturation stage and physiological activity. According to these parameters, there are five different categories of cells (cf. Cowdry, 1950): (1) undifferentiated multipotential cells, of which the ovum is the type example; (2) self-maintaining stem cells, such as the pluripotential hematopoietic stem cell which is the ancestor of all hemic cell lines (see, e.g., Lajtha, 1973a); (3) differentiated mitotically active cells, such as the "committed (secondary) stem cells" and the morphologically recognizable precursor cells in the hematopoietic tissues; (4) differentiated "intermitotic" (G_0) cells, which do not normally undergo cell division, but have retained the capacity to do so should the need arise, e.g., liver cells; (5) mature postmitotic end cells, such as neurons and erythrocytes, which have permanently lost their capacity to divide.

Cells of groups 2, 3, and 5 are typical of renewing tissues; expanding tissues, in turn, consist of cells of group 4, and static tissues consist of the cells of group 5. It is clear, however, that all tissues and organs do not conform to this general pattern; in particular, distinction between cells of groups 3 and 4 is somewhat arbitrary, perhaps only a question of semantics.

B. Growth Potential, Aging, and Death of Cells

As already indicated, the renewing tissues of any full-grown mammal undergo continuous cell division; new cells are added to the tissue at a rate that offsets the rate of cell loss. In some tissues, such as the gastrointestinal epithelium, the epidermis, and the hematopoietic cell systems, the normal rate of cell production is high; for instance, each second some two million newborn red cells pour out of the human bone marrow. Owing to this, the total number of cells produced during the lifetime of a normal mammal is huge. Some simple computations may help one to appreciate the quantitative aspects of cell production in renewing tissues.

It can be estimated that an average human adult is made up of approximately 10^{14} cells; of these, 1–2% are lost through cell death each day, and, to maintain the remarkable constancy of tissue mass and function, they must be replaced by new cells. Stated differently, the rate of cell production in a normal human adult would double the body weight in 50–100 days if no cells died; the total cell mass generated in 50 years, in turn, weighs more than 10,000 kilograms.

Owing to the limited interest of these computations in growth control, detailed results or references are not given in this paper. It may be noted, however, that the total cell number in the "standard man" (see Int. Comm. Radiol. Protection (ICRP), 1975) could be estimated from the mass and DNA content of each organ in the adult human body, and from the amount of DNA in a diploid human cell; most of the necessary figures can be found in appropriate textbooks. A simpler way to obtain a rough estimate of the total cell number may be based on the fact that the dry mass of an average mammalian cell is 2 to 4×10^{-10} gm; since the dry mass of the "standard man" is about 20 kg (contents of the gastrointestinal tract and bones excluded), the total cell number should be approximately 10^{14}. The absolute rate of cell production, in turn, may be derived from the mass and renewal time of each tissue; the necessary figures are available with reasonable precision to make the computations meaningful.

Some large tissues in the adult body, such as skeletal muscle, which consists of about 43% of the total body weight in the "standard man," do not produce any new cells; consequently, there must be some other active centers of cell production elsewhere in the body. As already indicated, one such tissue is the bone marrow, a relatively small organ consisting of "only" about 12×10^{11} nucleated cells in man (Donahue et al., 1958; Craddock, 1972); yet, some 2×10^{11} newborn red cells and 1×10^{11} newborn granulocytes are released from the bone marrow to the blood each day. Two other tissues in the mammalian body, the epidermis and the intestinal epithelium, are the other major centers of cell production in the normal human adult.

In the expanding organs, such as the liver, the kidneys, and many of the endocrine and exocrine glands, the normal rate of cell production is low, hardly detectable. However, in these organs most of the cells have retained their ability to proliferate at a fast rate which, if cells are lost by damage, quickly restores the normal tissue mass. The practically unlimited growth potential of these organs is well illustrated by the demonstration that full liver regeneration can occur at least five times in succession following repeated partial hepatectomies (Simpson and Finckh, 1963).

Only a few tissues in the body, the static tissues, such as the skeletal muscle and the nerve cells, irreversibly lose their mitotic potential early in life.

It may be of some interest to note that such a vitally essential tissue as brain has irreversibly lost its regenerative potential. In the light of natural selection, this curious change must confer some advantage, but it is not clear at all what the advantage may be. Nevertheless, the finite life-span of nerve cells and their incapacity to replenish lost neurons sets, in theory, an upper limit to the life-span of the brain owner (see Bullough, 1971b; Franks, 1974). It has been estimated that in the adult human brain some 10,000 nerve cells die every day (Curtis, 1963), a figure that may appear frightening. However, the average brain size of the "standard man" (1500 gm), DNA content of human brain tissue (about 100 mg/100 gm of wet tissue), and the diploid amount of DNA in human cells (about 7×10^{-12} gm per cell) suggest that the "standard man" should have a total of 2×10^{11} brain cells. Although the majority of these cells are glial cells, the total number of neurons in human cerebral cortex may still be as high as 10^{10} [i.e., the proportion of nerve cells would be 5% of the total number of brain cells; in mouse brain this figure has been estimated to be 6.25% (see Franks et al., 1974)]. Thus, if 10^4 nerve cells are lost each day, then the total number of neurons lost in 60 years in human brain would be about 2×10^8, i.e., only some 2% of the full number of brain neurons. The fact that human brain is often found to be smaller in older individuals cannot result from neuron loss; almost always it is a consequence of pathological changes such as arteriosclerosis in the cerebral vessels (see Dayan, 1971; Franks, 1974).

There is no doubt that originally all cells have the inherent tendency to divide; some cell lines also retain an unlimited growth potential indefinitely. Thus, the germ cell line is continuous from generation to generation; i.e., this cell line is able to undergo an indefinite number of generations. Many malignant cell lines can also be propagated indefinitely *in vitro* and, in the case of transplanted tumors, also *in vivo*. Thus, malignant cells express similar inherent and essentially unlimited growth potential as do the germ cells; unlike normal somatic cell lines, the germ cell line and different transformed cell lines know how to avoid senescence.

The mechanism of this immortality is not clear, but an interesting hypothesis has been proposed by Sheldrake (1974). According to this author, accumulation of deleterious breakdown products, such as membrane lipids, is one of the essential causes of cellular senescence; consequently, avoidance of this phenomenon in the nonsenescing cell lines involves cellular rejuvenation by means of asymmetrical divisions, i.e., asymmetrical distribution of deleterious breakdown products between the daughter cells and, hence, unequal mortality of these cells. Sheldrake's hypothesis is taken up here because it has some specific relevance to the theoretical justification of using chalones in the treatment of malignant tumors. This controversial problem (see Iversen, 1970, 1973a) will be discussed later in some detail (Section IX, B), but it may be pertinent to note in this context that the rejuvenation hypothesis predicts that a cell line must ultimately senesce and die out if the cells do not undergo divisions at a rate that keeps pace with the rate of accumulation of deleterious breakdown products or, alternatively, if the cells are prevented from asymmetrical divisions. In view of the current concepts of chalone action, both reactions *may* be achievable by excess chalone.

A unique example of cells' inherent tendency to divide is provided by HeLa cells, the first established human cell line in culture. These cells, derived in 1951 from a woman named Henrietta Lacks, are now grown in hundreds of laboratories around the world; the total number of HeLa cells produced by this time is enormous and, if allowed to grow uninhibited in optimal conditions, they would have taken over the world (see Culliton, 1974). This statement is not as fictitious as it may seem; HeLa cells are already taking over cell cultures in different laboratories (Nelson-Rees et al., 1974). Thus, these cells seem to behave like unicellular organisms (rather than embryonic cells); it is only the quality and quantity of food, the suboptimal growth conditions, which limit cell proliferation. It appears that HeLa cells may have lost their sensitivity to most physiological regulators of cell proliferation which are essential for the orderly behavior of normal cells in multicellular organisms. It has been claimed, though, that HeLa cells respond by mitotic inhibition to the epidermal chalone (Iversen, 1969), but the results from these studies are equivocal, as it has been reported that, contrary to the earlier belief, HeLa cells are not epidermal in nature (i.e., from a squamous cell carcinoma of the cervix) but are cells from a very aggressive adenocarcinoma (Jones et al., 1971).

III. Chalone Mechanism; Some Theoretical Aspects

In this section the chalone concept is considered in a manner that reflects my personal attitude regarding the significance of some theoretical aspects of the chalone mechanism. Experimental evidence, especially that dealing with the reality or nonreality of chalones and their specificity of action, is presented in more detail in the other sections of this chapter; consequently, most of the ideas considered here are relevant only on the assumption that at least some chalones are real.

The discussion is, in part, speculative. I believe that to many researchers it would seem more relevant to stick to hard facts than to present speculative ideas; this is especially so because, in the opinion of many investigators, enthusiastic theoretical considerations have predominated in the chalone literature from the very beginning. There are, in my opinion, two main reasons that make it impossible fully to avoid speculation: first, even most precise and sophisticated measurements are of little, if any, practical value if they are not constructed as hypotheses; second, it seems necessary to oppose some earlier speculation by alternative speculation.

It is almost certain that none of the "new" ideas advanced in this section are original; however, it is perhaps possible to provide a perspective in which the significance of the various experimental findings can be reevaluated.

A. Chalone Synthesis, Release, and Transport

The chalone mechanism has several component parts, such as chalone synthesis, release from cells, transport to other cells, and cellular response to chalone. Regarding synthesis, direct experimental evidence is essentially nonexistent in the chalone literature (see, however, Paukovits, 1971, 1973c); this may not be surprising, as chalone synthesis appears to be a minor problem in the chalone concept. This is not really true, however, because the negative feedback theory as applied to cell populations makes a clear distinction between cells that produce chalone and those that react to it. As will be shown below, a nonbiological application of this general principle could lead to difficulties.

It is commonly suggested that in any tissue the rate of chalone synthesis is probably constant, at least in the postmitotic mature cells (see Bullough, 1973c). In a mathematical simulation of the (epidermal) chalone mechanism, Iversen and Bjerknes (1963), however, had to make the rather critical assumption that the rate of chalone production increases with increasing cell age. This may be true for some parts of a cell lineage (e.g., basal cells in the epidermis may synthesize less chalone than the maturing cells), but clearly the assumption is not generally valid; if it were, erythropoiesis apparently could not be controlled by the chalone mechanism.

The general chalone concept suggests that erythrocytes should regulate erythrocyte production by means of an inhibitor molecule emanating from the mature cells; yet, the nonnucleated erythrocytes are almost certainly unable to synthesize any chalone at all. Nevertheless, these cells *are* the main source of the erythrocyte chalone (see Rytömaa and Kiviniemi, 1967, 1968a; Kivilaakso and Rytömaa, 1970, 1971; Lord et al., 1974; Bateman, 1974), if only because they outnumber their nucleated precursors by a factor of about 30.

The chalone concept thus seems to run up against difficulties: Mitotically active precursor cells must manufacture inhibitor for the mature cells so that these cells, being unable to produce any inhibitor by themselves, could then inhibit the producers of the inhibitor. To put it mildly, this idea does not seem attractive.

Biologically, however, chalone synthesis and the rate of chalone release from cells are two different activities. In particular, the intracellular chalone arising from chalone synthesis may not inhibit the chalone-producing cell itself; it is conceivable, even likely, that chalone acts via the cell membrane, either by activating a second messenger (which is not cyclic AMP, however; see later), or, alternatively, by releasing an "antimitotic" molecule linked to a "carrier" molecule which has recognized the specific receptor on the cell membrane. Thus, it is the chalone escaping from other cells that occupies the surface receptors of the target cell, hence leading to the activation of the inhibitory message. The self-made chalone is inactive and effectively retained within the precursor cell; if it were not retained within these cells, it could not be present in the mature nonnucleated cells. Another possible explanation to the dilemma would be that the immature precursor cells produce an inactive "prochalone," which is later activated and released from mature erythrocytes. Thus, the main suggestion arising from these considerations is that the chalone produced by a cell is nonfunctional as such; for an effect, the molecule must either be activated or it must trigger a second message. Both are, of course, common principles in biology.

Experimental evidence shows that the postmitotic (functional) cells, such as polymorphonuclear granulocytes, continuously release chalone (see, e,g., Rytömaa and Kiviniemi, 1968b), which then affects the mitotically active precursor cells of the same cell line. Sometimes the chalone transport from cell to cell seems to operate within a very short range only, e.g., within about 1 mm in mouse epidermis (Bullough and Laurence, 1960). In pathological conditions, however, chalone escaping from the cells depresses cell proliferation even in distant areas. Thus, it has been observed that in mice and rabbits bearing a large epidermal carcinoma, cell proliferation is inhibited in normal squamous epithelia in different parts of the body (Bullough and Laurence, 1968a; Bullough and Deol, 1971b; Kariniemi and Rytömaa, 1976). Similarly, it has been found that granulocyte chalone is present in excess in rats suffering either from a local chloroma tumor or from a generalized leukemia (Rytömaa and Kiviniemi, 1964, 1967, 1968c,d); even the growth of homologous cells cultured in diffusion chambers in the peritoneal cavity is inhibited in a specific manner (Vilpo et al., 1973; Ferris et al., 1973a).

Effective chalone transport is also clear from the common finding that intraperitoneal or subcutaneous injection of chalone depresses cell proliferation in the appropriate tissue, however distant it may be (e.g., Bullough and Laurence, 1968a; Rytömaa and Kiviniemi, 1968d, 1969a; Hennings et al., 1969; Frankfurt, 1971; Marks, 1971; Laurence and Randers Hansen, 1971; Schütt and Langen, 1972; Kieger et al., 1972; Houck et al., 1973c).

In spite of all this evidence indicating humoral transport of different chalones, it is not certain that chalones carried in the blood have direct biological significance in normal conditions; erythrocyte chalone may be the only exception. In the case of epidermal chalone(s), long-distance humoral "transport" is, in essence, unnecessary; the same seems to be true in most other chalone systems. For instance, although the granulocyte chalone content of blood is relatively high even in normal conditions (see Rytömaa and Kiviniemi, 1968a, 1968c), it may not contribute much to the chalone content of the bone marrow (see also Smeby, 1974). This is suggested by the fact that bone marrow contains a very large number of mature granulocytes; in man the "marrow granulocyte reserve" is some 30 times bigger than the total pool of circulating granulocytes (see Craddock, 1972).

Owing to the large marrow granulocyte reserve, the reactions of this cell system resemble wound healing: granulocyte production may be stimulated even when the chalone content of the total body has not been reduced by any mechanism (death of cells, inactivation by "antichalone," etc.). This would occur in all cases involving acute need for granulocytes in the periphery; in these situations mature cells are rapidly discharged from the bone marrow reserve to the blood, presumably as a response to a blood-borne "leukocytosis inducing factor" (see Gordon et al., 1964; Boggs, 1967; Schultz et al., 1973). As a consequence, chalone content of the bone marrow decreases quickly, and this then leads to an immediate stimulation of granulocyte production. It has been pointed out before (Rytömaa, 1973a) that, without this type of regulation, changes in granulocyte production, i.e., in the output of functional cells, would be extremely sluggish, involving a delay of many days in man. From the teleological point of view, it would indeed be strange if an effective and quick mobilization of large numbers of granulocytes to combat, for example, invading bacteria would automatically lead to a life-threatening and long-lasting shortage of these cells.

B. Chalone and the Cell Cycle

The cyclic nature of the cell division events has long been known; usually the cell cycle is represented in terms of a perfect circle subdivided into different phases (G_1, S, G_2, and M). It is clear, however, that a realistic cell cycle diagram must be made more complex; for one thing, it should illustrate the variation within each of the cycle phases (Fig. 2).

Another complication that should be taken into account in a cell cycle diagram is the apparent fact that when cells traverse through G_1 (or sometimes through G_2) they may stop movement altogether. This behavior has led to the formulation of different concepts expressed in terms such as resting phase (R_1 or G_0), proliferative pool, and growth fraction (see, e.g., Mendelsohn, 1960; Lajtha, 1963). According to these concepts, some fertile cells sit in the state "no cell cycle" from which they can be triggered back into cell cycle after appropriate stimulation. An alternative interpretation of the nature of G_1 "arrest" is the existence of an indeterminate state (between M and S phases) in which a cell may remain for *any* length of time, throughout which its probability of leaving this state remains constant (Smith and Martin, 1973). This concept is fundamentally different from the G_0 concept, and, if true, it would provide a simple mechanistic explanation for chalone action (chalone could alter a cell's probability of leaving the indeterminate state).

Bullough (e.g., 1963, 1973b) has tailored the life "cycle" diagram of cells differently in order to illustrate the apparent points of chalone action (Fig. 3). According to Bullough, after the completion of a mitosis, the two daughter cells enter the dichophase (D), in which the decision is made whether to reenter the

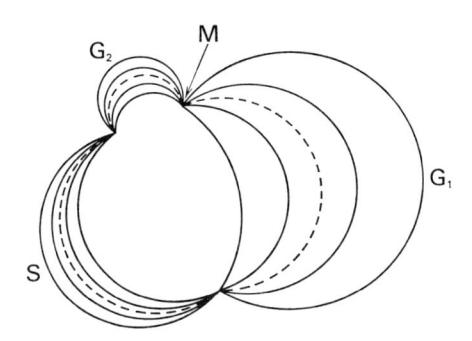

FIG. 2. Representation of the cell cycle which illustrates the variation within each of the phases G_1, S, and G_2. From Balls and Billett (1973).

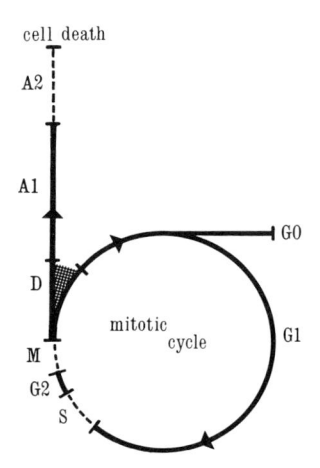

FIG. 3. The course of cell life (in epidermis). In the dichophase, D, the decision is made whether to enter G_1 (low chalone concentration) or the aging pathway, A_1 (high chalone concentration). From Bullough (1973b).

mitotic cycle (= cell cycle) or to prepare for tissue function; if the cell enters the aging pathway (A_1) it can stay there, progress toward death (A_2 phase), or revert to mitotic cycle should the need arise. In Bullough's recent concept of the mechanism of chalone action the (epidermal) chalone determines the behavior of cells as follows (Bullough, 1972, 1973b): (i) chalone delays the passage of cells around the mitotic cycle, presumably by slowing or blocking cells either in G_1 or in G_2, or in both these phases; (ii) chalone diverts cells from dichophase to the aging pathway; and (iii) chalone delays or stops the passage of cells along the aging pathway.

These mechanisms may be, in part, easier to visualize from the cell cycle diagram of Houck and Daugherty (1974) shown in Fig. 4.

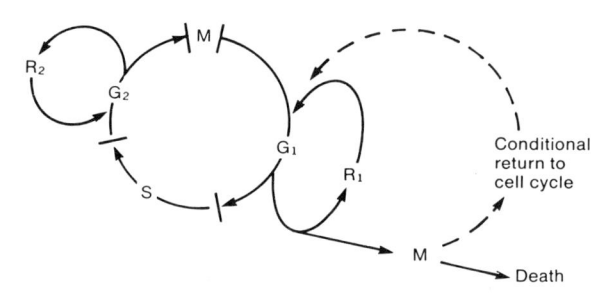

FIG. 4. Cell cycle diagram indicating the accessory components of the basic cycle. There seem to be two resting states in the cell cycle: R_1 (frequently referred to as the G_0 state) and R_2. M = maturation pathway (in the cycle, M is mitosis). From Houck and Daugherty (1974).

Using the terminology adopted in this diagram, a high chalone concentration would divert cells from G_1 to R_1 and M (= maturation pathway), and from G_2 to R_2, and would slow down the passage of cells along M. A low chalone concentration, in turn, would "push" cells from R_1 to G_1 and from R_2 to G_2, allow G_1 cells to progress toward S, revert some cells from M to G_1, and speed up the passage of cells along M. There is no doubt that, if Bullough's chalone concept is correct and applicable to other tissues as well, "the (chalone) control mechanism is not a simple negative feedback mechanism" (Bullough, 1973a).

The already complex picture of the suggested points of chalone action becomes even more complex if we note that some chalones may also prolong the duration of the S phase (Ferris *et al.*, 1973a; Laerum and Maurer, 1973; Bateman, 1974) and even the visible mitosis (Bullough and Laurence, 1964, 1966b). It is quite clear that this multitude of suggested chalone actions—together with the fact that essentially all proposals are either unsupported by *direct* experimental evidence or have not been confirmed by other investigators (see Sections IV and VII)—tends to imply that some findings are artificial and some ideas are wrong; in any case, experimental evidence does not seem to keep pace with theoretical considerations in chalone research.

Perhaps the only plausible conclusion drawn from the observed and suggested actions of tissue extracts is that the chalone mechanism is a cascade effect, probably somewhat similar to the activation of the complement chain or the sequence of blood coagulation reactions. The first step in the "chalone cascade" is unknown; it *could* be the reversion of cells from G_1 to the maturation pathway (see Bullough and Rytömaa, 1965; Laurence *et al.*, 1972).

C. Biochemical Mechanisms

In view of the fact that pure chalone preparations are not available, it is not surprising that virtually nothing is known of the biochemical mechanisms of chalone action. However, several hypotheses have been postulated by different authors (e.g., Bullough, 1965, 1967; Iversen, 1969; Argyris, 1972; Vorhees *et al.*, 1973; Houck and Daugherty, 1974). Among these is the proposal that the well known scheme that holds for bacterial enzyme induction can be carried over into the chalone theory, i.e., that chalone corresponds to the classical repressor and attaches to a gene locus, "chalone receptor," which in turn corresponds to the classical operator. This is an attractive idea but, in my opinion, it cannot be correct without some essential modifications; for instance, in its present form the model is in conflict with the observations made on chalone synthesis (see Section III, A).

As already indicated, another common proposal is that chalone acts at the level of the cell membrane; in addition to obvious logical arguments, experimental evidence supports this idea. Thus, the reversibility of chalone inhibition can be demonstrated simply by washing the inhibited cells (see Houck and

Daugherty, 1974; *Brit. J. Cancer*, 1974). It has also been shown that although neoplastic cells produce chalone and respond to it, their sensitivity to chalone is decreased, owing to inadequate binding of the inhibitor (e.g., Rytömaa and Kiviniemi, 1968c,d; Houck and Irasquin, 1973); because neoplastic cells have altered surface properties, it is tempting to assume that these two phenomena are related.

The suggestion that chalone functions at the cell membrane makes one wonder whether chalone acts via the cyclic AMP (cAMP) system, especially because this popular substance is involved in the regulation of cell proliferation in some assay conditions (e.g., Heidrich and Ryan, 1970; Byron, 1971; MacManus and Whitfield, 1969). The possible role of cAMP in the chalone mechanism was first suggested by Iversen (1969) on the basis of findings indicating that the action of the epidermal chalone *in vitro* required epinephrine as a cofactor (see Bullough and Laurence, 1964). It is now clear that the interpretation of the original *in vitro* results that led Iversen to consider this possibility is wrong; it has been shown that the epidermal chalone (G_2 inhibitor, see later) is fully active *in vivo* in the absence of epinephrine after all (Laurence and Randers-Hansen, 1971; Laurence *et al.*, 1972) and that several other chalones do not use epinephrine as cofactor even *in vitro* (e.g., Rytömaa and Kiviniemi, 1967, 1969b; Garcia-Giralt *et al.*, 1970b; Houck *et al.*, 1971; Dewey, 1973).

In spite of all this, some experimental evidence has been obtained that seems to support the idea that cAMP may play a role in the epidermal chalone mechanism (Powell *et al.,* 1971; Brønstad *et al.,* 1971; Marks and Rebien, 1972; Vorhees *et al.,* 1973); however, the evidence is inconclusive (see also Marks and Grimm, 1972). For instance, exogenous cAMP "mimics" epidermal chalone action only when very high concentrations of the drug are used; in bone marrow cells these concentrations ($> 10^{-5} M$) cause a pharmacological effect (Rytömaa and Kiviniemi, 1975). In some cell systems, such as bone marrow and thymic lymphocytes, *low* concentrations of exogenous cAMP elicit a stimulatory effect on cell proliferation (e.g., MacManus and Whitfield, 1969; Byron, 1973; Whitfield *et al.*, 1973; Tisman and Herbert, 1973; Hovi and Vaheri, 1973), and therefore it seems highly unlikely that cAMP would be a universal second messenger in the chalone-induced inhibition.

IV. Impurities in Chalone Preparations

The presence of impurities in chalone preparations is the major criticism of virtually all chalone experimentation; in fact, it seems likely that some of the observed biological properties of chalones will turn out to be artificial when pure, fully characterized materials are available. Therefore, it may be worthwhile to analyze in some detail the nature and effects of impurities contaminating many chalone preparations.

A. Nonphysiological Contaminants

It is self-evident that cells can be easily inhibited by a wide variety of factors that have nothing to do with the postulated autoregulation of cell proliferation. Some of these artificial inhibitors are trivial, such as those producing crude chemical or physicochemical changes in the growth environment of the target cells; these need not be discussed here. Others, however, are less trivial, and their existence may not even be suspected; some examples of this sort will be given below.

One obvious way to induce nonphysiological inhibition of cell proliferation is to introduce exogenous toxic factors into the test preparation; such factors may originate, for instance, from the preparative techniques used. Usually the possible presence of these contaminants is apparent, and there is no real danger of overlooking this experimental hazard. Sometimes, however, significant amounts of foreign material creep into a test preparation by routes and from sources that are not readily apparent. Such examples have been described in the literature, including an amusing story from Szent-Györgyi (1966): During his attempts to isolate a putative thymic hormone, Szent-Györgyi "made his only brilliant chemical work" by isolating a wonderful fluorescent substance in crystals. Constitution analysis showed that this substance, present in trace amounts in the thymus extracts, originated from the rubber tubings.

Another example, and much less amusing, concerns chalones. It was reported in 1968 by a research team (Mohr *et al.*, 1968) that when extracts of normal skin or of melanomata—both of which contained the melanocyte chalone as judged from the *in vitro* tests (Bullough and Laurence, 1968b, 1968d)—were injected for 5 days into mice and hamsters bearing large malignant melanomata, rapid tumor regression occurred and in some cases led to a complete cure. Later, however, the same research team reported that the striking oncolytic activity was caused not by the melanocyte chalone, but by a few spores of *Clostridium* that had contaiminated some of the test preparations (Mohr *et al.*, 1972a,b). Even if the new evidence is not convincing to the present author (for discussion, see Section IX, B), the results obtained do demonstrate that crude tissue extracts may be contaminated by unexpected and disturbing exogenous factors.

Nonphysiological constituents in crude tissue extracts may, in fact, be more common than is usually believed, although the consequences need not be as grave as in the case of *Clostridium* spores. This statement can be supported by two minor incidents from our own laboratory. Granulocyte chalone is normally obtained from leukocytes by incubating nonhomogenized cells in physiological solutions under aseptic conditions, then separating the conditioned supernatant by centrifugation and purifying it by techniques such as dialysis, Sephadex chromatograhy, and ultrafiltration (see Section V, A). Because the active inhibitor is of small molecular size, it is unlikely that the partially purified preparations would be contaminated by agents such as *Clostridium* spores. Furthermore, owing to the minimal amount of chemistry involved in the commonly used purification processes, the chances of contaminating granulocyte extracts with any sort of foreign material are not particularly great; yet it has happened more than once. Thus, at one time we discovered that all our partially purified test preparations were grossly toxic to bone marrow cells *in vitro*; preparation of new batches of test material did not improve the situation. Solution of the problem was not difficult, however: We had adopted a new commercial infusion apparatus, widely used for fluid therapy in different hospitals, to feed the elution liquid into the Sephadex columns; the plastic of this apparatus released unidentified toxic material into the eluent, which then seriously damaged the bone marrow cells in the *in vitro* assay.

Another case of exogenous contamination was discovered more accidentally, because the factor happened to be silent in the biological assay. For reasons of pure scientific curiosity we analyzed several crude leukocyte extracts by neutron activation analysis and atomic absorption spectrophotometry (for results, see Section V, A); it was discovered that one of the lyophilized extracts contained copper in an amount (0.2% of the solid weight) which exceeded severalfold the total copper content of the leukocyte mass subjected to extraction. The origin of the excess copper was not clarified.

B. Cytotoxic Physiological Impurities

The appearance of toxic exogenous material in chalone preparations is not a remote possibility which can be fully ignored. Clearly, however, the presence of physiological impurities in the tissue extracts is a far more serious problem. This is especially so because extremely crude extracts have been used in most chalone experiments reported so far. In a typical case the chalone is obtained simply by homogenizing the appropriate tissue and extracting it with water; insoluble material is then removed by centrifugation and the lyophilized supernatant is referred to as the chalone.

It is clear that tissue extracts of this type contain many biologically active factors; some of these may be cytotoxic, while others may merely interfere with the assay technique used to monitor cell proliferation. It has been claimed that the most important cytotoxic material present in extracts of many tissues are complement and IgM (Houck and Hennings, 1973). Activation of the complement cascade leads to the activation of different proteases and other cytolytic enzymes similar to phospholipase; consequently, the target cells may be enzymically damaged and this then results in an apparent inhibition of cell proliferation (Houck and Hennings, 1973). It has also been emphasized by Houck (1973) that it is impossible to prove that a cell is not being cytotoxically rendered incapable of normal proliferative activity; there is no need to injure the cell to the point of death.

It may thus appear that the use of tissue extracts that have not been extensively purified is always a serious experimental hazard in chalone research. In principle, this is certainly true; mild cytotoxicity, which would injure the cells only marginally without causing detectable morphological damage, seems to be especially difficult to exclude. However, primary cytotoxic events of any degree are highly unlikely if the following findings can be made:

1. Tissue specificity; it is improbable that the action of any cytotoxic agent would be specific for one cell line only.

2. Reversibility; a strong argument against cytotoxicity is obtained if it can be demonstrated that the inhibition of cell proliferation is reversible.

3. Intact cell metabolism; cytotoxicity is rendered unlikely if the inhibition of DNA synthesis is not associated with general inhibition of RNA and protein syntheses.

4. Activity *in vivo*; cytotoxic injury to the target tissue is a less serious problem *in vivo* than *in vitro*, because the whole organism has effective mechanisms of detoxification, which the isolated target cells evidently do not have.

Briefly, therefore, it is possible, at least in theory, to obtain good experimental evidence with crude tissue extracts regarding the existence of chalones, provided that all necessary control studies have been successfully made. It is unfortunate, perhaps, for the acceptance of the whole chalone concept that the experimental evidence for most chalone systems investigated so far is very limited and, therefore, not convincing in quality.

C. Other Physiological Impurities

Complications arising from the presence of impurities in tissue extracts are not limited to the various cytolytic enzymes, which, besides the activated complement system, may also include lysosomal acid hydrolases (Houck and Hennings, 1973). Tissue extracts are often contaminated by enzymes that do not injure the target cells at all, but interfere with the assay technique used to monitor cell proliferation. Today most investigators examine cell proliferation by determining the incorporation of ^{3}H-labeled thymidine into DNA on the commonly accepted assumption that the rate of thymidine uptake parallels the rate of cell proliferation. Therefore, contamination of tissue extracts by enzymes such as thymidine phosphorylase, or perhaps even by thymidine kinase, which can alter thymidine prior to its entrance into a cell, may lead to spurious inhibition of ^{3}H-labeled thymidine incorporation.

In principle, the possible presence of contaminating enzymes in the tissue extracts which alter the exogenous labeled thymidine would be easy to detect by direct determination of the enzyme activities. However, such analyses are not really needed in practice, because complications of this sort would obviously make it difficult, if not impossible, to demonstrate the most important biological characteristics of an inhibitor deserving the name chalone; for instance, the action of thymidine phosphorylase on labeled exogenous thymidine is not likely to depend on the type of target cells present in the assay system and, therfore, the inhibition of ^{3}H-labeled thymidine incorporation would not display cell-line specificity.

In the case of the low-molecular-weight chalones (see Section VII), possible contamination of tissue extracts by cytolytic or thymidine-catabolizing enzymes is not a serious problem; it is easy to remove the large-molecular enzymes from the small-molecular chalones simply by molecular sieving. On the other hand, the small-molecular-weight chalones are particularly sensitive to another type of complication arising from the presence of small-molecular-weight impurities in the crude tissue extracts. Tissue and cell extracts, even when obtained from nonhomogenized cells, are always contaminated with "cold" nucleosides and nucleotides; even thymidine has been demonstrated in these extracts (Lenfant *et al.*, 1973; Paukovits, 1974).

The presence of "cold" thymidine in a test preparation serves to dilute the specific activity of the added ^{3}H-labeled thymidine, and this leads to spuriously low values of thymidine incorporation and hence to an apparent inhibition of cell proliferation. It has, in fact, been claimed that the most inadequate technique for measuring cell proliferation is the incorporation of ^{3}H-labeled thymidine (Houck, 1973). This is, however, an overstatement, because complications associated with the use of labeled thymidine can be detected by appropriate controls. One simple way to do this is thymidine dilution; if an excess of "cold" thymidine is added to both control and test cultures, the possible small extra dilution of the marker substance by the test extract becomes insignificant. Some original results obtained with the dilution technique will be given in Section V,B.

Inaccuracies arising from the possible presence of thymidine in the chalone preparations can also be detected by a variety of other methods. Thus, it is possible to check the validity of ^{3}H-labeled thymidine uptake as an indicator of cell proliferation by several independent techniques, such as measuring population growth rates directly by cell counting (e.g., in closed *in vivo* cultures in diffusion chambers) or by determining mitotic activity with Colcemid. Furthermore, the number of cells synthesizing DNA at any given time can be determined with radioactively labeled precursor substances other than thymidine, with the aid of specific S-phase killing agents, such as hydroxyurea, or with the aid of a new fluorometric technique that measures the DNA content of single cells (pulse cytophotometry); it is also possible to monitor cell proliferation by a unique new method based on the phenomenon of fluorochromasia coupled with the technique of fluorescence polarization (see, e.g., Cercek *et al.*, 1973). All these techniques have been successfully used in the study of the granulocyte chalone (see Rytömaa and Kiviniemi, 1967; Vilpo *et al.*, 1973; Laerum and Maurer, 1973; Benestad, 1974; Lord *et al.*, 1974). Briefly, therefore, even if the incorporation of ^{3}H-labeled thymidine *can* be—and often is—a completely inadequate measure of cell proliferation in chalone experimentation, this is not always the case in practice.

Complications arising from the presence of other nucleosides and nucleotides in crude tissue extracts are discussed in Section V, A.

V. Composition and Effects of Crude Leukocyte Extracts; Some Original Data

In this section some previously unpublished experimental results will be given which have a direct bearing on several easily criticized aspects of chalone assays. In brief, these experiments deal with the use of ^{3}H-labeled thymidine uptake as the main indicator of cell proliferation and with complications arising from the possible presence of different biologically active impurities in crude tissue extracts. The experiments reported here have been made with leukocyte extracts, usually assaying the effects of the test preparations in short-term bone marrow cultures as described before (see Rytömaa and Kiviniemi, 1967, 1968a; Rytömaa, 1969). Consequently, the findings are not, strictly speaking, relevant to chalones and chalone assays in general; clearly, however, direct evidence of any critical aspect of chalone experimentation is important even if it applies to one particular system only.

Owing to the nature of the present article, exhaustive description of experimental details has been omitted; however, the essential technical procedures should be evident from the presentation of the results. Full accounts of the original work described in this section will be given elsewhere.

A. Composition of Crude Leukocyte Extracts

Most chalone experiments made so far have been performed with crude tissue extracts which, as discussed before, may contain several physiologically active substances. Rarely, if ever, is the composition of these extracts given even in rough terms; therefore, the general composition of a typical leukocyte extract with a strong inhibitory activity will be presented here as an example.

The extracts analyzed for chemical composition were prepared from ox blood leukocytes by Dr. W.A. Jones (Weddel Pharmaceuticals Ltd., London) using a relatively large-scale method capable of providing significant quantities of blood leukocytes. The method is largely based on a previously published technique (Rytömaa and Kiviniemi, 1970) of lysing whole blood with hypotonic saline and collecting the residual cells and cell debris. Two further treatments with hypotonic saline completely destroy the erythrocytes with a 60–85% recovery of the original leukocyte popluation; approximately 60% of the recovered cells are granulocytes. The leukocytes are then "extracted" with Hank's solution for 1 hour at 37°C and the "conditioned" supernatant is lyophilized. Six extractions are usually made with a mean cell viability of about 60%; the cell content of the suspensions is commonly rather high, about 7 × 10^{11} leukocytes per liter of Hank's solution.

The total protein-polypeptide content of the extracts was determined by Dr. Jones from the nitrogen content of sodium tungstate precipitates; the other analyses were made by us with the aid of UV spectrophotometry, thin-layer chromatography, column chromatography on Sephadex, atomic absorption spectrophotometry, and neutron activation analysis (the two last-mentioned techniques were used for the purpose of confirming the elementary composition of the solids and detecting possibly interesting trace elements; these analyses were performed by Dr. E. Häsänen, Reactor Laboratory, Technical University of Helsinki).

The composition of a typical crude leukocyte extract is given in Table I. It is clear that these results do not provide any information on the chemical nature of the granulocyte chalone present in the extract. However, some interesting calculations that are relevant to chalone studies can be made from these data: As shown later in this section, 100 µg of crude extract per milliliter is a potent inhibitor of DNA synthesis in bone marrow cells *in vitro* without

TABLE I

COMPOSITION OF A TYPICAL LEUKOCYTE EXTRACT[a] OBTAINED FROM BLOOD LEUKOCYTES

Constituent	Percent of dry weight
Hank's components and other inorganic compounds	85
Protein/polypeptides	5
Purine/pyrimidine bases and their derivatives[b]	<2
Other organic substances (free amino acids, sugars, etc.)	~8
Trace elements[c]	≪0.1

[a] One milligram of the extract corresponds to about 7 × 10^7 leukocytes; strong inhibition of DNA synthesis is obtained with 100 µg/ml (see Section V, C), i.e. with 5 µg of protein per milliliter.

[b] Thymine base/nucleoside/nucleotide content is <0.05% (see also Section V, B).

[c] Cu, Zn, Fe, and Br are usually present in an amount of about 50 ppm each (Br is a common contaminant of NaCl); e.g., Co, Cr, Mn, Ba, and Pb have not been detected.

detectable action on RNA and protein synthesis; 100 μg of the solid per milliliter corresponds to a total protein/polypeptide content of 5 μg/ml and a total base/nucleoside/nucleotide content of 1–2 μg/ml (i.e., less than 10^{-5} M); these concentrations are evidently very low for a *crude* tissue extract and, therefore, suggestive of a high biological activity of the granulocyte chalone or its effective release from the unbroken cells.

Simple purification of crude leukocyte extracts by ultrafiltration and column chromatography on Sephadex gives active test preparations corresponding to a protein content of 0.1 μg/ml or less. Much higher purification levels may be obtained by more sophisticated biochemical techniques (see Paukovits, 1973c), but even this value compares favorably with almost any tissue extract used in chalone studies so far. It may be noted for comparison that crude tissue extracts are sometimes tested at concentrations of 1–5 mg of protein per milliliter (see Iversen, 1968; Volm et al., 1969; Jones et al., 1970), and only a few extracts seem to be active at concentrations of 5–10 μg/ml (see Verly, 1973; Houck and Daugherty, 1974). The epidermal chalones, however, have been purified more extensively; thus the G_1 inhibitor is active in the mouse when less than 10 μg is injected (Marks, 1973), and the G_2 inhibitor is active *in vitro* at a concentration of 0.15 μg/ml (Hondius Boldingh and Laurence, 1968).

Nucleosides and nucleotides contaminating crude tissue extracts represent a potential experimental hazard that is particularly prominent in studies dealing with low-molecular-weight chalones, especially when the effect of the test material is measured in terms of ^{3}H-labeled thymidine incorporation. Thymidine and the corresponding nucleotides are the most potent nonspecific inhibitors of ^{3}H-labeled thymidine incorporation, but, as shown, for example, by the dilution technique (Section V, B), "cold" thymidine is not a problem in the case of leukocyte extracts (see also Rytömaa, 1973c; Lord et al., 1974). In reality, the other nucleosides and nucleotides are much more critical; significant nonspecific inhibition of ^{3}H-labeled thymidine incorporation into bone marrow cells can be induced by several nucleosides and nucleotides added to the assay cultures at sufficiently high concentrations (about 10^{-4} M; see also Rytömaa and Kiviniemi, 1975).

The results given in Table I indicate (compare the relative amounts of proteins/polypeptides and purine/pyrimidine derivatives) that a critical nucleoside/nucleotide level ($> 10^{-5}$ M) may easily be reached when experimenting with crude tissue extracts; indeed, it is likely that most, if not all, crude extracts prepared from homogenized cells and tissues would contain sufficient amounts of nucleosides and nucleotides to invalidate *direct* testing for chalone activity in our assay system. Because of the problems arising from these impurities, we have actually studied the effect of different purine/pyrimidine bases and their derivatives on rat bone marrow cells *in vitro*. The results have shown that ^{3}H-labeled thymidine incorporation into the cells is not affected by any of these substances when tested at a concentration 10^{-5} M or less; however, several of the substances are strongly inhibitory at higher concentrations.

B. "Cold" Thymidine

As already indicated, thymidine is a constituent of many chalone preparations, and this may seriously complicate the interpretation of ^{3}H-labeled thymidine incorporation data. This hazard is particularly great in the case of chalones of low molecular weight, because thymidine is not readily separated from these chalones by the commonly applied purification procedures.

In order to reevaluate whether the thymidine content in primary granulocyte extracts is a complicating factor in interpreting ^{3}H-labeled thymidine incorporation, experiments were made by adding cold thymidine to the assay cultures; the results are given in Fig. 5 and Table II.

It is clear from these results that in the presence of extra thymidine the crude leukocyte extract inhibited ^{3}H-labeled thymidine uptake much more strongly than would be expected on the assumption that the original 20% inhibition, i.e., the effect in the absence of extra thymidine, had been caused by thymidine contamination of the extract. Addition of extra thymidine up to a concentration of 5×10^{-6} M did not alter the inhibitory power of the test extract at all; even in the presence of 10^{-5} M extra thymidine, the observed inhibition was still much stronger than that "expected," although the power of the extract was now significantly reduced (Table II). This last-mentioned phenomenon is probably due to a toxic action of excess thymidine (Dörmer and Brinkmann, 1970; see also Rytömaa and Kiviniemi, 1975), which may simply mask the action of physiological inhibitors. (Such a result would be another entertaining corollary to Houck's law, which states that "dead cells do not divide" (Houck, 1973)—

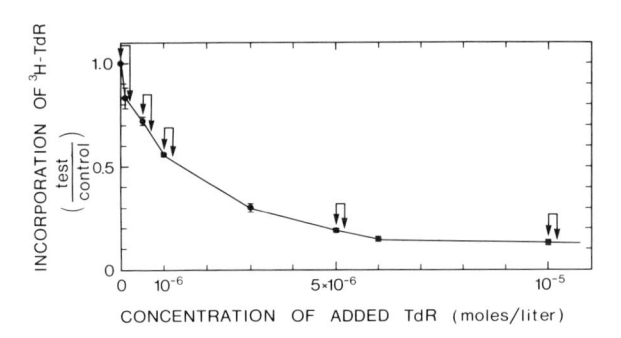

FIG. 5. Inhibition of incorporation of ^{3}H-labeled thymidine into rat bone marrow cells *in vitro* by "cold" thymidine. The arrow pairs indicate the effect of 2×10^{-7} M thymidine when added to cultures already containing different concentrations of extra thymidine. Each filled circle is the mean (±SE) of 16 test cultures.

TABLE II

INHIBITION OF INCORPORATION OF ³H-LABELED THYMIDINE INTO RAT BONE MARROW CELLS *IN VITRO* BY A CRUDE LEUKOCYTE EXTRACT[a] AND BY 2 × 10⁻⁷ M "COLD" THYMIDINE[b] IN THE PRESENCE OF EXTRA THYMIDINE

Concentration of extra thymidine in culture medium (M)	Inhibition of thymidine-³H incorporation (%)[c]	
	Crude leukocyte extract[a]	2 × 10⁻⁷ M "cold" thymidine[b]
None	20 ± 2	20
5 × 10⁻⁷	22 ± 4	9
10⁻⁶	20 ± 4	5
5 × 10⁻⁶	21 ± 3	<4
10⁻⁵	9 ± 3	<1

[a] Lyophilized extract, 100 μg/ml (see Section V, A and Table I). The protein/polypeptide content of this particular extract was 4.4%.
[b] The effects given are computed from the results shown in Fig. 5.
[c] Mean ± SE of 3 experiments.

dead cells do not respond by mitotic inhibition either.) The conclusion is consistent with the finding that if rat bone marrow cells are grossly damaged by cytotoxic material, such as activated complement, the effect of leukocyte extracts is paradoxically "stimulatory"; the crude extracts somehow protect the cultured cells from the action of cytotoxic enzymes.

The results given in Fig. 5 and in Table II also indicate that the thymidine content of the extract used in these experiments must have been less than 0.05% of the solid weight; this is the concentration that would be required for the production of 20% reduction in ³H-labeled thymidine incorporation in the absence of any other inhibitor. Low thymidine content has also been confirmed by chemical analyses which showed that thymine was not detected when 10 mg of crude leukocyte extract were hydrolyzed by perchloric acid and then assayed by thin-layer chromatography for purine/pyrimidine bases (Table I).

C. RNA AND PROTEIN SYNTHESES

The possible presence of cytotoxic materials in crude tissue extracts is another experimental hazard which deserves serious consideration. A strong argument against primary cytotoxic events is obtained if it can be demonstrated that the

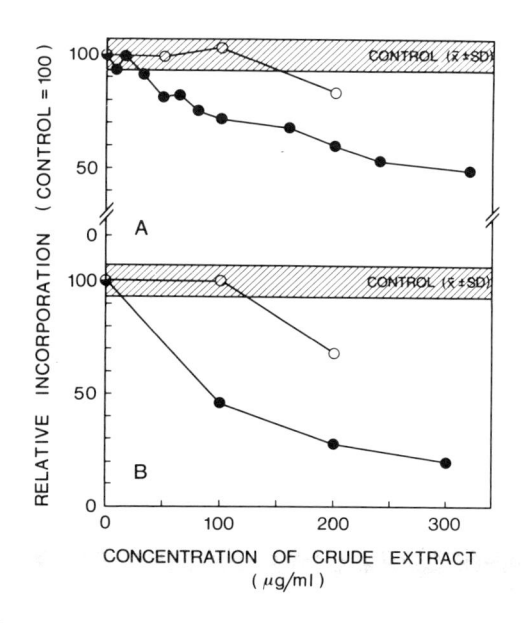

FIG. 6. Effect of a crude leukocyte extract on DNA, RNA, and protein synthesis in rat (A) and human (B) bone marrow cells *in vitro*. At the time of the experiment, human bone marrow cells had been grown on petri dishes for 2 days (RPMI 1640 essential medium supplemented with 20% of fetal calf serum; 95% air–5% CO_2 atmosphere); virtually all proliferating cells were myeloid, as judged from cell morphology. DNA, RNA, and protein syntheses were measured in terms of incorporation of thymidine-^{3}H, uridine-^{3}H, and leucine-^{3}H, respectively; the incorporation times were 4 and 8 hours for rat bone marrow cells, and 6 and 22 hours for human bone marrow cells. Each dot is the mean of at least 8 individual cultures. The composition of the crude leukocyte extract was essentially identical to that shown in Table I; thus, 100 µg of the solid per milliliter corresponds to a protein concentration of about 5 µg/ml. ○, RNA + protein; ●, DNA.

inhibition of DNA synthesis is not associated with general inhibition of RNA and protein synthesis. In order to study the effects of leukocyte extracts on these synthetic activities, experiments were made with human and rat bone marrow cells; the results are given in Fig. 6.

It can be seen from Fig. 6 that RNA and protein syntheses were not inhibited at all when the test extract was used at a concentration of 100 µg/ml or less; in contrast, DNA synthesis was significantly inhibited by even lower concentrations of the solid. Solid contents of 200 µg/ml or higher, however, inhibited RNA and protein synthesis significantly in both types of target cells; this may be indicative of marginal cell injury despite the fact that morphological signs of damage could not be detected even with higher concentrations (cf. Houck and Daugherty, 1974). If this conclusion is accepted as valid, then the dose-response curves obtained with ^{3}H-labeled thymidine are misleading after some threshold concentration of the test extract; consequently, as judged from the response of RNA and protein synthesis, the maximal specific inhibition of DNA synthesis would be 30–50% in the assay conditions used here.

VI. Tissue Specificity

There is no doubt that, within some limits, the growth control of different populations of cells is independent. Therefore, if chalones are considered as autonomous signals emanating from the same cell line on which they act, unequivocal demonstration of cellular specificity of the chalone action is of the utmost importance.

Lack of extensive or convincing experimental evidence of specificity is a commonly criticized aspect of chalone experimentation; essentially all published research on chalones has been considered inadequate in this respect. The four main arguments put forward by the critics are the following (see Kohn and Fuchs, 1970; Metcalf, 1971; Metcalf and Moore, 1971; Lajtha, 1973b; *Brit. J. Cancer,* 1974): (1) the source of cells from which the chalone is extracted is not a pure population; (2) the control extracts have been prepared from completely unrelated tissues; (3) the action of a specific chalone is tested on cell types that have no close relationship to the suggested target population; (4) the comparative tests have not been made in identical assay conditions or with identical assay methods.

The basic relevance of this criticism cannot be questioned and, therefore, if it is not met by experimental evidence, the validity of the chalone concept may be in doubt. In this section the available evidence is presented in some detail.

A. Degree of Specificity; Is It Absolute?

It has been pointed out before (Rytömaa, 1973b) that the specificity of chalone action need not be absolute, and that a certain amout of nonspecificity may even be expected. For instance, highly undifferentiated (embryonic) and pathological (malignant) cells may not be able to recognize the specific chalone with absolute precision; some chalones may also be retained within a short range *in vivo*, which prevents their action on other potentially responsive cell populations; this is, in fact, the case with the epidermal chalone(s) as indicated below. In principle, some degree of "background" responsiveness could be allowed to all cell populations without making the different signaling systems ineffective and nondiscriminative *in vivo*. From an evolutionary point of view it may even seem likely that different cell types recognize some familiarity between different chalones; such a situation would not be entirely different from that existing in immunological reactions. If this speculation is valid, then a small degree of nonspecificity may be expected in chalone experiments performed on isolated cells *in vitro*, especially when high chalone concentrations are used; the situation *in vivo* could be different because of the effective dilution by the other "nonspecific" chalones.

B. Failure to Find Tissue-Specific Inhibitors

Spielhoff (1971) has reported results which fail to demonstrate the presence of tissue-specific inhibitors in liver and kidney extracts; crude tissue extracts, as well as different alcohol precipitates prepared according to the principles adopted for the purification of epidermal chalone, inhibited the incorporation of ^{3}H-labeled thymidine in liver and kidney in young rats, but the effects were not specific either with respect to the source of the extract or to the target of the action. Similarly, Volm *et al.* (1972) and Wayss *et al.* (1973) observed that although liver extracts inhibited ^{3}H-labeled thymidine incorporation in regenerating rat liver, the effect was not specific, as similar extracts from some other tissues exhibited the same degree of effect. Furthermore, these authors (Volm and Wayss, 1971) have also reported that their original conclusion of a chalonelike action of human endometrium extracts on HeLa cells (Volm *et al.*, 1969; Hinderer *et al.*, 1970) is untenable, because the extract also inhibited liver and kidney cells in culture.

There is no doubt that the results obtained in these studies have failed to demonstrate the existence of tissue-specific inhibitors. However, in the opinion of the present author, the experiments do not provide adequate evidence for concluding that chalonelike inhibitors do not exist in liver, kidney, or endometrium. It is self-evident that crude tissue extracts may contain a large number of factors that inhibit incorporation of ^{3}H-labeled thymidine in a nonspecific manner as discussed in detail before; the *established* presence of such factors invalidates conclusions regarding the existence or nonexistence of chalones. Furthermore, the experimental design of these studies may not be adequate; for instance, when regenerating liver was used as the target tissue, 200–400 mg of test extracts (protein) were injected into the animals 2 hours *before* partial hepatectomy (see Volm *et al.*, 1972). If the results obtained (e.g., by Verly, 1973) on liver chalone are relevant, then chalone injections given prior to hepatectomy are likely to be ineffective, or, alternatively, exceedingly large chalone doses are needed; the latter alternative may be impossible to achieve with crude tissue extracts because of the toxicity of the material.

Regarding lymphocyte chalone(s), Garcia-Giralt has recently reported odd results obtained with partially purified spleen extracts (see Garcia-Giralt, 1973; Garcia-Giralt and Macieira-Coelho, 1974; *Brit. J. Cancer*, 1974); according to him, brief treatment with the extracts produces different types of protracted effects including long-term graft-vs-host suppression and an essentially nonspecific long-term inhibition of DNA synthesis. The graft-vs-host suppression was observed despite the finding that the extracts did not inhibit the proliferation of lymphocyte precursors; excessive inhibition of DNA synthesis (up to 90% for 2–4 days), in turn, did not lead to decreased growth rate in rapidly proliferating established lymphoid cell lines. Garcia-Giralt has suggested that the extracts bind to the immune-competent cells, preventing blastic transformation in a specific manner; this may be true, but because the same extracts *also* cause pronounced nonspecific effects (they even inhibit DNA synthesis in an established fibroblastic cell line; see Garcia-Giralt and Macieira-Coelho, 1974), there is no apparent reason why the decreased phytohemagglutinin (PHA) or pokeweed mitogen transformation rate should nevertheless be specific in nature. For the time being, therefore, the only rational explanation for these odd findings seems to be toxicity of the extracts. Furthermore, it may be questioned whether the prevention of blastic transformation is related to direct proliferation inhibition at all (a step is inhibited which *leads* to proliferation, but the affected cells are not really in the cell cycle); thus the reaction seems more like an "anti-poietin" effect, i.e., essentially similar to the effect of those substances that inhibit erythropoietin or colony-stimulating factor (see Section VIII, A).

One more failure should be considered in this context. Jones *et al.* (1970) have reported that lymphoid cell extracts inhibit DNA synthesis in human leukemic cells *in vitro* in an apparently nonspecific manner, because acute myeloblastic leukemia cells also respond by inhibition. There are at least three alternative explanations for these results: (1) the type of leukemia was incorrectly diagnosed as being myeloid (evidently highly unlikely); (2) some pathological cells fail to recognize the specific chalone with absolute precision (possible, but unlikely; see, however, Sections VI, C and IX, B); (3) ^{3}H-labeled thymidine incorporation was inhibited nonspecifically (note that specific inhibition of DNA synthesis cannot then be detected, even if it exists, because the indicator is prevented from monitoring it). This last-mentioned alternative is most probable, because the crude tissue extract was added to the assay cultures at an apparently toxic concentration (1.3 mg of protein per milliliter; see Sections IV and V).

C. Experimental Evidence for Specificity of Action

Absolute cell-line specificity of chalone action is very difficult, if not impossible, to demonstrate in practice; it may not even exist. Among the practical problems are complications arising from the transport of virtually all chalones to different parts of the body (see Section III, A) and the "contamination" of many organs by "foreign" cell types; for instance, many organs are rich in granulocytes and lymphocytes and hence unsuitable as control materials for leukocyte extracts. Another type of complication is based on the fact that only a limited number of cell lines can be assayed in conditions that are virtually identical to those of the supposed target population.

Demonstration of absolute specificity of chalone action would require that control and test extracts be prepared from closely related *pure* populations of cells and assayed on closely related cell types in identical conditions and with identical techniques. In most chalone experiments an attempt to fulfill these requirements has not even been made; in some cases the requirements are not even meaningful, because specificity of the inhibitory action may also be determined on other grounds than the chemical characteristics of the chalones (cf. squamous epithelia; see below).

In three chalone systems the problem of cell-line specificity has been studied rather extensively, and in some of these studies the experimental setup is not far from the ideal mentioned above. Consequently, combined evidence from these three systems provides a basis for an informed judgment on the extent and quality of the existing evidence.

An overview of the assay systems used, parameters measured, control extracts tested, and types of cells used for comparison is given in Table III. It is self-evident that the different extracts have not been tested on all cell types listed, and that different growth parameters have not been studied in all assay conditions.

Information compiled in Table III indicates that each of the three (or four) chalone systems has been studied extensively with respect to the source and target of the chalone.

Erythroid and granulocytic cells provide an almost ideal pair of cell types for the demonstration of absolute specificity of chalone action; the reasons are the following: (1) Erythroid and granulocytic cells develop from a common hematopoietic stem cell and are therefore closely related. (2) Both cell lines share essentially the same anatomical locations in the body and, therefore, secondary mechanisms such as spatial separation cannot be operative in the establishment of cellular specificity. (3) Almost pure populations of cells can be obtained for chalone extraction (the best erythrocyte populations used are absolutely pure, at least for all practical purposes, and the best granulocyte populations are 85—90% pure; if the granulocytes are obtained from peritoneal exudate, the contaminating cells are macrophages, and if the cells are obtained from blood, the contaminating cells are lymphocytes). (4) Erythroid and granulocytic precursor cells can be tested in virtually identical assay conditions. (5) The effects of the test preparations can be compared with the same end points.

In the early studies a strict cell-line specificity of the granulocyte and erythrocyte chalones was demonstrated autoradiographically in short-term bone marrow cultures (Rytömaa and Kiviniemi, 1968a, 1970; Kivilaakso and Rytömaa, 1971). However, doubts were later expressed as to the validity of these data (see Metcalf and Moore, 1971; Lajtha, 1973b; *Brit. J. Cancer,* 1974), the main arguments being that the sources of cells from which the chalones were extracted were not pure, that erythroid cells deteriorate rapidly in most culture conditions, and that small-rodent bone marrow autoradiography is exceedingly difficult. This criticism is justified, at least in principle; nevertheless, subsequent studies by other authors have confirmed the correctness of the original data.

Thus, a physical separation of the bone marrow cells by the Ficoll density step centrifugation revealed that the only subpopulation that responded to partially purified granulocyte chalone was the fraction with the highest enrichment of myeloid precursors (Paukovits, 1973c). Further support for the cell-line specific action of the granulocyte and erythrocyte chalones was obtained by Bateman (1974), who refined the original assay methods in three ways: first, the erythrocyte chalone was extracted from pure erythrocyte populations (granulocyte chalone, however, was extracted from blood leukocytes containing both granulocytes and lymphocytes); second, proliferation of erythroid cells in the short-term cultures was apparently improved by the use of suckling rats as the bone marrow donors; and third, reliable identification of normoblasts in the autoradiograms was made easier with the aid of benzidine staining specific for hemoglobin. The results obtained autoradiographically showed that erythroid cells responded only to erythrocyte extracts, and nonerythroid cells responded only to leukocyte extracts.

Complete specificity of action of partially purified erythrocyte, granulocyte, and lymphocyte extracts on their own precursor cells has also been demonstrated by measuring their effects on the "structuredness" of the cytoplasmic matrix using the unique technique of fluorescence polarization (Lord et al., 1974). Changes in the "structuredness"—which have been shown to be closely related to the proliferative state of the cells (Cercek et al., 1973, 1974)—indicated that lymphocyte extracts affected only lymphoid cell populations, granulocyte extracts affected only granulocyte cell populations, and erythrocyte extracts affected only erythroid cells. Furthermore, in each case the active fractions resided in the molecular weight ranges observed in the earlier studies for cell extracts possessing DNA synthesis inhibiting properties.

Taken together, these studies demonstrated that extracts prepared from mature granulocytes inhibit cell proliferation in an absolutely cell-line specific manner. This conclusion is strongly supported also by a number of other studies based on the cultivation of granulocytic and different nongranulocytic cell lines in diffusion chambers *in vivo* (Benestad et al., 1973; Vilpo et al., 1973; Laerum and Maurer, 1973; Ferris et al., 1973a). In the experiments utilizing the diffusion chamber technique, the effects have been measured in terms of population growth (cell counting), DNA labeling (including determination of the labeled mitosis curves), and distribution of cells between the different cell cycle phases (determination of DNA content of single cells with automatic fluorescence cytophotometry); cell-line specificity of action was invariably demonstrated for the granulocyte chalone.

Owing to the broad spectrum of assay techniques used, the granulocyte chalone seems to be the best studied of all chalones known so far. Nevertheless, specificity of action of the lymphocyte and epidermal chalones (cf. Table III), and even the erythrocyte chalone (see above), is equally well documented and, therefore, the reality of at least some chalone-type inhibitors cannot be ques-

TABLE III
SPECIFICITY OF THE THREE BEST-STUDIED CHALONE SYSTEMS

	Epidermal chalone(s)		Granulocyte Chalone	Lymphocyte Chalone(s), T or B, or both
	G_1 inhibitor	G_2 inhibitor		
Main assay systems	*In vivo*	*In vivo*; tissue explants; epithelial outgrowth	*In vivo*; closed *in vivo* cultures in diffusion chambers; short-term cultures of normal and leukemic bone marrow; long-term cultures of myeloid cells	*In vivo*; PHA-stimulated lymphocytes; "*Monilia*"-stimulated lymphocytes; mixed lymphocyte cultures; established cultures (lymphocytic leukemia)
Growth parameters	Uptake of ^{3}H-TdR; prevention of hyperplasia	Mitotic activity; prevention of hyperplasia	Uptake of ^{3}H-TdR; uptake of different RNA and protein precursors; DNA content of single cells (pulse-cytophotometry); S-phase killing drugs; "structuredness"; population growth (cell numbers)	Uptake of ^{3}H-TdR; uptake of amino acids; "structuredness"; thymus size; graft-vs-host reaction; allograft rejection; xenograft rejection
Control extracts	Liver; kidney; lung; dermis; basal cells	Hair bulbs; hypodermis; lymphocytes; granulocytes; rectum; liver; kidney; lung; brain; melanoma cells; human sweat	Erythrocytes; lymphocytes; liver; skin; HeLa cells[a]; kidney[a]; spleen[b]	Erythrocytes; Granulocytes; fibroblasts; kidney; lung; muscle; brain

184

Control targets	Lung; liver; kidney; spleen[c]; diaphragm; adipose tissue	Sebaceous glands; eccrine sweat glands; small intestine; rectum; melanoma cells; lymphoma cells, bone marrow (G_1 effect)	Erythroid cells; lymphocytes; macrophages; epidermis; body growth; HeLa cells; mastocytoma cells; Ehrlich ascites cells; thymus[a]; spleen[a]	Erythroid cells; myeloid cells; fibroblasts; chorioncarcinoma cells; colon carcinoma cells; HeLa cells
Origin of information	Elgjo et al. (1972); Elgjo and Egdehill (1973) Frankfurt (1971) Hennings et al. (1969) Iversen et al. (1974) Marks (1971, 1973)	Bullough and Deol (1972) Bullough and Laurence (1964, 1968a, b, 1970a) Bullough et al. (1967) Chopra et al. (1972) Frankfurt (1971) Iversen et al. (1974) Laurence (1973a, b)	Balázs et al. (1972) Bateman (1974) Benestad et al. (1973) Ferris et al. (1973a) Laerum and Maurer (1973) Lord et al. (1974) Paukovits (1973c) Rytömaa and Kiviniemi (1967, 1968a, b, c, d, 1970) Vilpo et al. (1973)	Chung and Hufnagel (1973) Lasalvia et al. (1970) Houck and Daugherty (1974) Houck et al. (1971) Kieger et al. (1973)

[a]Inconclusive evidence because the effects were measured in terms of mitotic indices (Balázs et al., 1972).
[b]Inconsistent results: inhibitor was detected by Paukovits (1973c), but not by Balázs et al. (1972).
[c]Short-lasting inhibition was observed (Marks, 1973).

TABLE IV
Chalone Systems Reported in the Literature

Chalone	Observed point of action	Molecular weight	Evidence for stress hormone cofactors	Purification level
Eccrine sweat gland[a]	G_2	—	Yes	—
Epidermis[b]	G_1	100,000	—	50,000-fold
	G_2	30,000–40,000	Yes (*in vitro*)	2,000-fold
Erythrocytes[c]	G_1	2,000?	None	—
Fibroblasts[d]	G_1	30,000–50,000	None	—
Granulocyte[e]	G_1	<1,000–4,000	None	>1,000-fold
Intestine[f]	G_2	—	—	—
Kidney[g]	G_2	—	Yes?	—
Lens[h]	G_2	20,000–30,000	Yes	—
Liver[i]	G_1	1,000	Yes?	450-fold
	G_2	—	—	—
Lung[j]	G_2	—	Yes?	—
Lymphocyte[k]	G_1	30,000–50,000	None	>100-fold?
	G_2	—	Yes	—
Melanocyte[l]	G_1?	≤2,000	None	—
	G_2	—	Yes	—
Sebaceous gland[m]	G_2	—	Yes	—
Spermatogonia[n]	G_1	—	—	—
Stomach[o]	G_2	—	Yes	—
Thyroid[p]	—	—	—	—
Tumor cells	—	See Section IX	—	—

[a] Bullough and Deol (1972).
[b] See Table III; Baden and Sviolka (1968); Bullough and Laurence (1968e); Finegold (1965); Hall (1969); Hondius Boldingh and Laurence (1968); Iversen and Elgjo (1967); Iversen *et al.* (1965); Marrs and Vorhees (1971); Rothberg and Arp (1973).
[c] Bateman (1974); Kivilaakso (1970); Kivilaakso and Rytömaa (1970, 1971); Lord *et al.* (1974); Rytömaa and Kiviniemi (1967, 1968a).
[d] Garcia-Giralt *et al.* (1970a); Houck *et al.* (1972, 1973a).
[e] See Table III; Cross and Barer (1972); Shadduck (1971).
[f] Brugal (1973); Galjaard *et al.* (1972).
[g] Chopra and Simnett (1969, 1970, 1971); Saetren (1956, 1970); Simnett and Chopra (1969).
[h] Voaden (1968); Voaden and Leeson (1970).
[i] Brugal (1973); Lenfant *et al.* (1973); Saetren (1956); Scaife (1970); Verly *et al.* (1971); Verly (1973).
[j] Simnett *et al.* (1969).
[k] See Table III; Bullough and Laurence (1970b); Garcia-Giralt *et al.* (1970); Houck and Irasquin (1973); Jones *et al.* (1970); Kieger (1971); Moorhead *et al.* (1969).
[l] Bullough and Laurence (1968b, d); Dewey (1973); Mohr *et al.* (1968).
[m] Bullough and Laurence (1970a).
[n] Clermont and Mauger (1974).
[o] Philpott (1971).
[p] Garry and Hall (1970).

tioned. Regarding the other chalones reported in the literature (see Table IV), the available experimental evidence of cellular specificity is less conclusive; however, the demonstrated specificity of the inhibitors of epidermal and hematopoietic cell proliferation suggests, that the other tissues also contain specific inhibitors of the chalone type.

In has already been noted that the specificity of action of the epidermal chalone(s) is not absolute in the same sense as the action of granulocyte and lymphocyte chalones; mitotic rate is inhibited not only in epidermis, but also in other squamous epithelia, such as gingiva, tongue, forestomach, and esophagus (e.g., Bullough and Laurence, 1964; Randers Hansen, 1967; Frankfurt, 1971). Biologically, however, the action is completely specific because all normal reactions in surface epithelia are essentially local; consequently, there is no obvious biological need for separate chalones in the different squamous epithelia. Nevertheless, it has been observed that epidermal chalone(s) extracted from different body sites may not be identical; thus, palatal extract depresses mitotic activity in tongue more strongly than skin extract whereas the opposite is true in ear epidermis (Laurence and Randers Hansen, 1972).

VII. Putative Chalone Systems

Chalone has been defined by Bullough (1967) as "an internal secretion produced by a tissue for the purpose of controlling by inhibition the mitotic activity of that same tissue." A useful operational definition of chalones (see Rytömaa, 1970, Laurence, 1973a; Houck and Daugherty, 1974) may also be based on a few biological properties that have been established for the best-studied (see Table III) substances: (1) chalones inhibit cell proliferation; (2) chalone action is cell-line specific; (3) chalones are produced by the same cell line on which they act; (4) chalone action is noncytotoxic and reversible; (5) chalones are species nonspecific.

So far only a few chalones have been shown to fulfill these criteria reasonably well; however, several inhibitors have been described in the literature which satisfy to some extent the two most important discriminative properties of chalones (points 2 and 3 above). These putative chalones are listed in Table IV.

It can be seen from Table IV that several tissues seem to contain two different chalones, the G_1 and G_2 inhibitors. Distinction between these two chalones is based on the assay technique used; G_1 inhibitors, usually determined by measuring the incorporation of labeled DNA precursors into the cells, prevent the transition $G_1 \rightarrow S$ (reduction of continuing DNA synthesis in S phase cells may also be involved) whereas G_2 inhibitors block the entry of cells into visible mitosis (usually determined by trapping cells in metaphase by Colcemid). It is possible, of course, that G_1 and G_2 inhibitors are not different substances but that one inhibitor is acting at two sites; however, at least in the case of epidermis the two inhibitors seem to differ in regard to their chemistry (Marks, 1971, 1973) and also to their origin (G_2 inhibitor has been extracted from the basal cells and G_1 inhibitor from the differentiating cells; see Elgjo and Hennings, 1971a; Elgjo, 1973). G_1 and G_2 inhibitors extracted from JB-1 ascites tumor cells have also been shown to differ "chemically"; the apparent molecular weight of the G_1 inhibitor is between 10,000 and 50,000, and that of the G_2 inhibitor is between 1000 and 10,000 (Bichel, 1973). It thus seems that several tissues may indeed contain two distinct chalones; in fact, the nonexistence of either one has not been convincingly demonstrated in any tissue. However, the results obtained by Laerum and Maurer (1973) by pulse-cytophotometric analysis of (normal) granulocytic cells grown in diffusion chambers suggest that cells in the G_2 and M phases are not inhibited by the granulocyte chalone; on the other hand, the labeled mitosis curves obtained by Ferris *et al.* (1973a) show that the G_2 phase *is* prolonged in leukemic granulocytes (chloroleukemia cells were grown in diffusion chambers in chloroleukemic host animals which have an elevated chalone content in the body; see also Rytömaa and Kiviniemi, 1968c; Vilpo *et al.*, 1973).

Another point worth noting in Table IV is the rather consistent finding that G_2 inhibitors require stress hormones as cofactors for full activity, whereas the G_1 inhibitors appear to be effective in the absence of these hormones. A closer survey of the literature reveals that epinephrine (and often also hydrocortisone) is needed only in the *in vitro* cultures. It is true that adrenalectomy strongly increases mitotic activity *in vivo* and that it also leads to the disappearance of the diurnal mitotic rhythm (e.g., Bullough and Laurence, 1971), but nevertheless, adrenalectomy does not result in a reduced inhibitory power of the epidermal G_2 inhibitor injected into the animals (Laurence and Randers Hansen, 1971). These apparent discrepancies have been explained in terms of an indirect effect of epinephrine by postulating the existence of a dermis-borne "chalone antagonist" whose action is negated by epinephrine (Laurence *et al.*, 1972).

One exception to the general "rule" that stress hormones act as cofactors for G_2 inhibitors *in vitro* has been published by Chopra *et al.* (1972). These authors observed that the epidermal G_2 inhibitor was fully active *in vitro* when tested on human epithelial outgrowths (i.e., dermis-free cultures of epidermal cells). The other "rule" suggested by the available data, i.e., that G_1 inhibitors do not require stress hormones as cofactors, has been challenged by Verly (1973), who reported that inhibition of DNA synthesis of hepatocytes needed the synergistic action of the inhibitor and the stress hormones.

As indicated in Table IV, a few chalones have been extensively purified, e.g., the epidermal G_1 inhibitor by 50,000-fold (Marks, 1973). However, none of the chalones has been chemically fully characterized; insofar as known, the active substances appear to be proteins/polypeptides (or glycoproteins), but in some cases even this is not at all clear in spite of the high purification level reached. This is not really surprising; it has been calculated by Maurer and Laerum (1973) that to purify 100 μg of the granulocyte chalone one would need to start with 1000 kg of granulocytes, i.e., with about 1 million liters of blood.

VIII. Regulation of Growth by Factors Other Than Chalone

A. CHEMICAL SUBSTANCES INFLUENCING CELL DIVISION

Besides chalones, numerous other factors have been found or postulated to affect cell proliferation, and even to control it. Some of these substances are well established, and there is no doubt as to their specific role in the regulation of cell populations. In the past few years major progress in this field has been achieved in the hematopoietic tissues.

The hematopoietic system is a complex tissue consiting of a whole chain of interlinked cell populations starting with a pluripotential stem cell, which, at least in the mouse, is the ancestor of all hemic cell lines, i.e., erythrocytes, granulocytes, platelets, and even lymphocytes (both T and B lymphocytes). The pluripotential stem cell gives rise to several committed cell populations from which cells then further differentiate into the morphologically recognizable precursor cells as a response to specific stimuli. Both the committed and the recognizable cell populations are transit populations; during transit the cells divide, thus amplifying their number. With the exception of lymphocytes, all mature functional cells are end cells, i.e., incapable of proliferative activity; for two cell lines, the red cells and the platelets, the end-cell state is carried to the extreme limit in which the cell lacks a nucleus. For reviews of the hematopoietic cells, see, e.g., Metcalf and Moore (1971) and Lajtha (1973a).

It is clear that this complex system must be controlled by a large number of regulatory signals, and several of these have been well established. Regarding the pluripotential stem cells, the number of cells in the proliferative cycle is probably controlled by a local negative feedback, i.e., by a chalone-type mechanism; however, experimental evidence of this factor is lacking. From the pluripotential stem cell population a small proportion is continuously triggered to differentiate into the committed cell populations; the nature of this mechanism is not clear, but it seems that the signal for differentiation is not really local and that it originates from the committed cell population (see Lajtha, 1973a). The committed cells undergo a varying number of divisions during their transit; these may be under the control of the cell-line specific chalone as suggested by preliminary experimental evidence (Paukovits, 1973c). The second-step differentiation from the committed cell populations into the morphologically recognizable amplifying transit populations requires humoral factors, commonly known as poietins.

One such poietin is the erythropoietin, the specific inducer of hemoglobin synthesis. Erythropoietin is a glycoprotein of about MW 46,000; it is produced by kidney and possibly by some extrarenal sites as a response to hypoxia (for a recent review, see Gordon et al., 1973). It seems that the well established and extensively studied colony-stimulating factor (CSF) is the granulopoietin. CSF, which is produced by most tissues in the body, is a glycoprotein of about MW 45,000 (molecular weights may actually vary within wide limits depending on the source of CSF); it is necessary for the development of granulocyte and macrophage colonies when culturing hematopoietic cells in semisolid agar or methyl cellulose (for reviews, see, e.g., Metcalf and Moore, 1971; Metcalf, 1973). A third poietin, the thrombopoietin, has also been described in the literature. The biological and chemical properties of this substance are less clear than those of erythropoietin and CSF, but it has been suggested that it promotes the differentiation and proliferation of megakaryocyte precursors which result in increased blood platelet production (for a review, see Odell, 1973).

The lymphocyte system may not contain an "endogenous" poietin at all; in this case the specific change in lymphocytic progenitor cells seems to be induced by antigen. According to the current concept, antigen first stimulates the proliferation of antigen-reactive cells derived from thymus (T lymphocytes); these cells, in the presence of antigen and macrophages, then stimulate antibody-forming cell precursors from the bone marrow (B lymphocytes) to generate a clone of antibody-forming cells.

In addition to the poietin-type substances, the hematopoietic cell lines are also influenced by a number of other factors, but none of these substances is likely to be a primary regulator. Among the "secondary" factors are erythropoietin inhibitors (see Lindeman, 1971), a complex of serum lipoproteins and other substances, which seem to modulate the action of the CSF (see Paran et al., 1969; Metcalf, 1973; Moberg et al., 1974), granulocytic "anti-chalone" (see Rytömaa and Kiviniemi, 1967, 1968a), the "leukocytosis-inducing factor," which causes the release of mature granulocytes from the bone marrow (for a review, see Schultz et al., 1973), and a large and heterogeneous group of humoral factors believed to be involved in immune responses.

Besides the hematopoietic system, several other cell lines have also been found to be influenced by specific factors. Some of these growth-stimulating substances have been isolated and fully characterized chemically; evidently the best known is the nerve growth factor (NGF), an essential protagonist in the growth and development of the sympathetic nervous system (for a review, see Angeletti et al., 1973). The fundamental unit of NGF is composed of 118 amino acids with a resultant MW of 13,259; NGF is present in small amounts in several tissues but the highest concentrations appear to be in the male mouse submaxillary gland. Curiously, this same organ also contains large amounts of another fully characterized peptide hormone, the epidermal growth factor (EGF) which enhances proliferation and keratinization of embryonic and neonatal epidermis *in vivo* and *in vitro* (Cohen, 1965; Savage and Cohen, 1972). The physiological role of EGF, however, is not at all clear.

Other established growth stimulators are the different serum mitogens required for the multiplication of diploid and heteroploid fibroblasts (see Houck and Cheng, 1973; Houck *et al.*, 1973c; Gospodarowicz, 1974), putrescine, which similarly stimulates cell proliferation in cultures of fibroblasts (Pohjanpelto and Raina, 1972), and a tripeptide from human serum which stimulates liver cells *in vitro* (Pickart and Thaler, 1973). Several orthodox hormones, such as estrogens, androgens, and thyrotropin also stimulate cell proliferation in a tissue-specific manner, perhaps by "neutralizing" the chalone of the target tissue (see Bullough, 1967; Epifanova, 1971); other hormones, such as epinephrine and hydrocortisone, in turn, inhibit cell proliferation (see Bullough, 1965, 1967; Section VII). In contrast to these well known substances, the existence of so-called "wound hormones" is controversial (see Bullough, 1973c; Ferris *et al.*, 1973b), but if "antichalones"/"chalone antagonists"/chalone-catabolizing enzymes—especially lysosomal enzymes (see Fell, 1973)—are considered as "wound hormones," then even these substances appear to be real (see Laurence *et al.*, 1972; Elgjo and Edgehill, 1973; Iversen *et al.*, 1974).

In contrast to the other growth-influencing factors considered above, "wound hormones," especially if they are chalone-catabolizing enzymes, may not be specific to any particular tissue; however, the action of these factors should at least be local. It has sometimes been implied that humoral regulators of cell proliferation may also exist which have a generalized action within the body. One such substance would be retine, an inhibitor of growth, which was found to be widely distributed in nature in, for example, mammalian thymus and urine, mushrooms, and molluscs (see Szent-Györgyi, 1966). Another substance, promine, was also found in many tissue extracts; promine stimulated growth. It turned out to be exceedingly difficult to isolate these substances in pure form, but the experiments indicated that retine may be a ketoaldehyde, possibly methylglyoxal, and that promine may be glyoxalase, an enzyme system that transforms methylglyoxal to lactic acid (see Szent-Györgyi, 1968). Methylglyoxal interacts with SH groups and thus exerts an inhibitory action on cell division by cutting out protein synthesis (Otsuka and Együd, 1968); synthesis of DNA and RNA is only partially inhibited. The physiological role, if any, of retine in the control of cell proliferation remains to be shown, especially because this simple substance inhibits virtually any type of cell, including bacteria.

The extreme complexity of the field of growth control is apparent. However, the situation may be a little easier to comprehend if it is assumed that the basic parameter of the regulatory mechanism is chalone, and that most of the other substances influence cell proliferation either by providing sufficient conditions for growth or by interfering with some component parts of the chalone mechanism. The few established growth regulators, such as erythropoietin, which exert an essentially inducer-type action, belong in a different category; these substances either are or resemble genuine embryonic inducers.

It seems probable that chalones transmit their inhibitory signal by interacting with specific receptors sited on the cell membrane (see Section III) and, therefore, a second messenger may be involved in the chalone mechanism. If this is the case, then a number of physiological substances may actually influence cell proliferation by interfering with this second step directly or indirectly (e.g., by occupying chalone receptors) rather than "neutralizing" chalone chemically.

B. Density-Dependent Inhibition

In addition to the large and heterogeneous group of established and hypothetical chemical regulators of cell growth, multiplication of normal cells *in vitro* is also believed to be controlled by a somewhat different mechanism, often referred to as contact inhibition of growth (Abercrombie and Heaysman, 1954). In this process, now more adequately termed density-dependent inhibition (Stoker and Rubin, 1967) or topoinhibition (Dulbecco, 1970), the proliferation of normal cells stops when the cultures have formed confluent monolayers; transformed cells do not display this phenomenon, and therefore it has even been suggested by some investigators that contact inhibition holds the key to the solution of the cancer problem.

According to a popular theory, density-dependent inhibition of normal cells is a reflection of some specific property of the cell surface that allows the establishment of lateral cell-to-cell contacts (see Pontén, 1971). Normal cells can in fact be temporarily released from the density-dependent inhibition by a variety of factors that act on cell surface; among these are proteolytic enzymes and neuraminidase (Burger, 1971; Vaheri *et al.*, 1972). This reinitiation of growth seems to be a direct consequence of temporarily altered cell membrane, possibly involving sialic acid residues (Vaheri *et al.*, 1972).

Although altered membrane properties evidently play an important role in the loss of density-dependent inhibition, convincing experimental evidence has never been obtained in support of the concept that intimate cell-to-cell contacts are essential for the cessation of growth. Perhaps the best evidence in favor of this idea has been the finding that cell multiplication can be activated in stationary cultures by wounding (Todaro *et al.*, 1965). In contrast to the nonlocalized effects induced by factors such as serum, insulin, trypsin, and neuraminidase, wounding results in short-range topographical effects only; the behavior of the nongrowing cells in the confluent sheet and the growing cells in the wound is quite different despite the fact that both cells are in the same medium and also very close to each other.

Recently, however, much new evidence has been obtained that indicates that intimate cell-to-cell contacts are not mandatory for density-dependent inhibition (Holley and Kiernan, 1968; Kruse *et al.*, 1969; Dulbecco and Elkington, 1973;

Stoker, 1973). For instance, the original concept has been made untenable by the work of Dulbecco and Elkington (1973), who demonstrated that the multiplication of epithelial cells in culture is limited by the amount of plastic surface available per cell, and that of fibroblastic cells by the availability of medium factors; intimate contacts between cells did not regulate growth of either cell type. With fibroblastic cells this was evident from the finding that restriction of available dish surface did not affect the final cell number. With epithelial cells a dish surface restriction was the main factor stopping growth, but even here the effect was not mediated by cell contacts; epithelial cells stopped growth long after the cells started to touch each other. Furthermore, epithelial cells proliferating at the wound edge do not become free from each other (Dulbecco, 1971).

Stoker (1973) has shown that multiplication of the fibroblastic 3T3 cells is best explained by local variation in the fluid microenvironment of the cells; in Stoker's experiments, based on the use of a miniature pump to produce a local increase in medium velocity, cessation of cell growth in dense cultures was evidently caused by a diffusion boundary layer close to the cell surface. This diffusion barrier, originally suggested by Rubin and Rein (1967), would operate either by limiting the uptake of critical nutrients or growth factors from the medium or, alternatively, by preventing the escape of inhibitory molecules released by the cells. It may be noted that owing to the diffusion barrier, soluble inhibitory molecules, such as chalones, may be involved in the density-dependent inhibition, even if such factors are not detected in the whole culture medium.

In the light of the new evidence, it seems clear that the density-dependent inhibition is closely related to surface properties of the cells, but intimate cell-to-cell contacts are not critical in this phenomenon. Besides the diffusion boundary layer, other mechanisms may also be involved in the expression of the inhibition. For instance, crowding in itself may simply alter the cell form and lead to a reduced surface area, thus making it insufficient to permit the uptake of necessary nutrients or growth factors (Zetterberg and Auer, 1970) or, alternatively, insufficient to release inhibitory substances from the cells. Basically, therefore, density-dependent inhibition is not a unique expression of growth control which is difficult to explain in terms of the chalone concept (see also Garcia-Giralt et al., 1970a; Houck et al., 1972, 1973a); this conclusion is not invalidated by the obvious possibility that in some cell types or assay conditions other factors may become growth limiting much before the critical chalone concentration is reached.

Loss of density-dependent inhibition in transformed cells may even be easier to explain in terms of chalone concept than by any other mechanism. In particular, it is difficult to accept the common assumption (see, e.g., Stoker, 1973) that transformed cell variants break through density-dependent inhibition because they have acquired a lowered requirement for serum or other nutritional components. In the opinion of the present author, lowered requirement for nutrients is not likely to be an important universal property of malignant cells; it is more probable that malignant cells *in vitro* keep the mitotic engine running simply because they fail to switch it off. This assumption is, in fact, supported by experimental evidence which suggests that malignant cells are less responsive to inhibitory factors, possibly because of their deficient capability to retain or bind these substances (Bullough and Laurence, 1968a, 1968c; Rytömaa and Kiviniemi, 1968c, 1968d; Houck and Irasquin, 1973).

IX. Chalones and Cancer

It is quite clear that the chalone concept contains more than an element of truth, and that it offers tremendous *potential* for the control of a wide variety of diseases involving cell proliferation. However, I will not deal with the various possible applications of different putative chalones in clinical medicine, not even with the experimentally well supported potential of using the lymphocyte chalone(s) for immunosuppression (see Kieger *et al.*, 1972; Garcia-Giralt *et al.*, 1973; Houck *et al.*, 1973c; Chung and Hufnagel, 1973); several possible applications may be found in the recent book by Houck and Daugherty (1974). Instead, I will concentrate on the most controversial aspect of chalone research, the possibility of using these substances in the chemotherapy of cancer.

A. What Is Cancer?

There is no doubt that cancer cells differ from their normal counterparts; usually the difference is so conspicuous that it is readily detected under the microscope, sometimes even by an inexperienced eye. This is the very basis of histological and cytological diagnosis of cancer.

If malignant cells commonly display grossly altered cell morphology, it should not be surprising that cancer investigators, often working at a much higher level of sophistication than that involved in classical histology, have been able to discover a vast number of differences between cancer cells and their normal counterparts. What is surprising, however, is the common tendency to hope that any new difference discovered would be universal and, therefore, would hold the key to the solution of the cancer problem.

Even a superficial survey of the gigantic cancer literature reveals numerous aberrant properties of tumor cells. Besides altered cell morphology, these include changes in cell membrane (electric charge, lectin agglutinability, chemical composition, fluidity); loss of density-dependent inhibition; decreased cellular adhesiveness; alterations in cell metabolism (high rate of glycolysis, inability to synthesize L-asparagin, increased production or release of several enzymes); appearance of fetal antigens; presence of reverse transcriptase; chromosomal abnormalities (Philadelphia chromosome, increased susceptibility to breakage and rearrangement); altered genetic code or its expression (inherited, spontaneous; induced by chemicals, radiation, or viruses); alterations in regulatory signals (cAMP and cGMP); malfunction of immune system (surveillance, blocking factors, defective macrophages); presence of tumor-associated antigens; involvement of viruses (DNA and RNA viruses; oncogenes, proviruses, protoviruses).

This list of cancer cell properties is, of course, complex, incoherent, and incomplete; so are also the views of investigators in any subdiscipline of cancer research. At present no one knows how the aberrant properties of cancer cells are related; it is likely that they are not related at all. In any case, *none* of the aberrant properties known so far is specific to all cancer cells.

Yet, cancer cells display one property, not mentioned above, which is characteristic of the disease: the cells do not obey the normal rules of growth control.

In terms of population kinetics this means that the rate of cell production exceeds the rate of cell loss. The positive imbalance may have many possible causes of which pathologically increased cell proliferation is perhaps the least probable; it is more likely that tumor cells fail to mature, function, age, and die effectively as do their normal counterparts. In terms of an analogy, the unsocial behavior of tumor cells, perhaps arising from communication difficulties, is based on a meaningless expression of independence, i.e., tumor cells tend to behave like *unicellular* organisms.

B. Role of Chalones

Even if unsupported by direct experimental evidence, it is possible that cancer may result from some damage to the cells leading to an insufficient functioning of cell communication apparatus. *If* chalones are involved in carcinogenesis, then the damage must have affected one or more mechanisms that prevent the cells from receiving a signal or debilitate their capacity to respond to it adequately.

These ideas are, of course, speculative and, at this moment, it may not be wise to carry them any further. However, some fragmentary experimental evidence, relevant to the problem, is perhaps worth mentioning. Thus, it has been observed that in some transplanted animal tumors the chalone content is lower than in the corresponding normal cells (Bullough and Laurence, 1968a, 1968c; Rytömaa and Kiviniemi, 1968c,d), but the chalone content of the whole body is significantly increased (Rytömaa and Kiviniemi, 1967, 1968c,d; Bullough and Laurence, 1968a,c; Bullough and Deol, 1971a; Vilpo *et al.*, 1973; Ferris *et al.*, 1973a; Kariniemi and Rytömaa, 1976). The most obvious explanation for this seemingly paradoxical situation is a decreased ability of the tumor cells to retain or bind the chalone that they produce in excess (owing to the large number of tumor cells in the body).

Rather than discussing the possible role, if any, of chalones in carcinogenesis, the potential of using chalones in cancer therapy will be considered in detail. This is an intriguing subject (see Iversen, 1970, 1973a), and theoretical considerations cannot be avoided in the discussion.

It seems to be a popular misconception that cancer cells proliferate at a fast rate; in reality, however, cancer cells often proliferate more slowly than their normal counterparts (see, e.g., Baserga, 1965). As far as known, cancer cells seem to be less responsive to the chalone than the corresponding normal cells (Rytömaa and Kiviniemi, 1968c,d, 1969a; Houck and Irasquin, 1973). All this seems to mitigate against the possibility of using chalones, inhibitors of cell proliferation, in the treatment of cancer; however, available experimental evidence and closer "theoretical" analysis do not support this conclusion.

One essential requirement for cancer chemotherapy by chalones is that cancer cells are responsive to the inhibitors; this is usually the case as demonstrated by numerous observations made on different malignant cell lines, including a few spontaneous human tumors (Rytömaa and Kiviniemi, 1967, 1968c,d, 1969a, 1970; Bullough and Laurence, 1968a,b, 1970b; Jones et al., 1970; Bichel, 1970, 1971, 1972, 1973; Bullough and Deol, 1971a; Elgjo and Hennings, 1971b; Houck et al., 1971; Houck and Irasquin, 1973; Dewey, 1973; Cooper and Smith, 1973; Vilpo et al., 1973; Ferris et al., 1973a). It may be of some interest to note that if malignant cells were to deviate a little from the essential characteristics defining chalones, i.e., if chalone action were not strictly tissue specific regarding cancer cells, then the prospects of using chalones in cancer treatment would perhaps be even better. For instance, it might be possible to inhibit tumor cells by some chalone whose specific target in the body is of secondary importance to the well-being of the organism. Iversen's (1969) equivocal results on HeLa cells (see Section II,B) may be explicable in these terms.

It is self-evident that responsiveness of malignant cells to the inhibitory action of chalones is a necessary, but not sufficient, prerequisite for curing cancer with excess chalone. Chalones are, by definition, noncytotoxic substances, and therefore they cannot destroy tumors. However, the optimistic hopes for cures, arising from experimental evidence in animal models (see later), are based on the idea that chalone is used as an adjunct to the normal defense mechanisms of the body; thus the idea is merely an extension of the well known fact that bacteriostatic antibiotics can be used to cure infectious diseases. It must be realized that cancer cells live and grow in adverse conditions, including the common inadequacy of blood supply (see Bullough and Deol, 1971b), and that these cells commonly induce an immune reaction (see Mathé, 1969; Weiss, 1971). Because of the hostile environment, the death rate of tumor cells is indeed high and may be as much as 99% of the rate at which new cells are being produced by cell divisions (see Steel, 1967; Refsum and Berdal, 1967; Iversen, 1967; Cooper, 1973; Vilpo and Rytömaa, 1973). It is thus clear that, by artificially raising the chalone content, a situation may be achieved in which cell death exceeds cell proliferation; if this situation can be maintained for long enough, all tumor cells would, of course, disappear from the body.

Animal experiments have shown that, at least in rat chloroleukemia, permanent cures can be obtained by treatment with extracts containing the granulocyte chalone (Rytömaa and Kiviniemi, 1969a, 1970). Essentially similar results have also been obtained by Mohr et al. (1968), who treated mouse and hamster melanomata with pig skin and melanoma extracts; later, however, the same research team reported that the cures were caused not by the melanocyte chalone, but by *Clostridium* spores contaminating the test preparations (Mohr et al., 1972a,b).

The new evidence presented by Mohr and associates is not fully convincing to the present author. First, Mohr et al. (1968) reported in their original article that "spores of anaerobic bacteria which might lead to tumor regression as reported by Möse, were excluded as causative agents morphologically and microbiologically." Second, pure spore suspensions produced a rapid tumor lysis, but the animals were never entirely cured (Mohr et al., 1972b), although this sometimes happened when the crude tissue extracts were used (Mohr et al., 1968); it appears a little strange that the results cannot be reproduced with the purified causative agent. It may also be noted that when hamsters bearing an amelanotic melanoma were treated with a potent pig skin preparation, incorporation of ^{3}H-labeled thymidine into the tumor tissue was inhibited in comparison to that of control animals (Mohr et al., 1972a); however, when similar animals were treated with *Clostridium* spores, incorporation of ^{131}I-labeled iododeoxyuridine into DNA of the melanoma tumors was *increased* by a factor of 2 (Volm et al., 1974).

In spite of these controversial findings—and of the fact that (at least) a small-molecular-weight substance (MW $\leqslant$ 2000) in melanoma extracts has been directly shown to inhibit the growth of melanoma cells *in vitro* (Dewey, 1973)—it must be admitted that regression of melanoma tumors induced by melanocyte chalone has not been demonstrated. There is no *direct* proof that the chloroma cures induced by crude leukocyte extracts (Rytömaa and Kiviniemi, 1969a, 1970) were caused by the granulocyte chalone either. Nevertheless, it is clear that, in the case of chloroleukemia, cell lysis was at least not caused by *Clostridium* spores (the extracts used were dialyzates); it is also clear that massive death of chloroleukemia cells is "innate" to the tumor (Vilpo and Rytömaa, 1973); i.e., there is no need to provoke cell death by any material originating outside the animal. In fact, studies on the kinetics of chloroleukemia cells grown in diffusion chambers have indicated that the variable degree of success with chalone treatments (Rytömaa and Kiviniemi, 1969a, 1970) is based on the variable cell death of the leukemic cells from one individual to another (Vilpo and Rytömaa, 1973). Thus there *is* a distinct difference between the results obtained with melanoma and chloroma, respectively: in the case of melanoma, the results varied from one preparation to another, whereas in the case of chloroma the results varied from one animal to another.

In spite of the experimental results obtained with animal models and with tissue cultures, it has been argued, notably by Iversen (1970, 1973a), that chalone cannot be expected to destroy a tumor, that transplanted and "spontaneous" human tumors are not identical, and that the chalone treatment would stop the proliferation of normal cells long before it stops the proliferation of malignant cells. As far as is known, all these points are true but they do not disprove the possible, as yet not established, value of chalones in cancer treatment: (1) positive results are expected only on the assumption that a fair chance is given to the immunological defense mechanism to get rid of the tumor cells; (2) "spontaneous" human tumors may actually be more antigenic than transplanted tumors that have survived numerous passages in alien hosts; (3) chalone treatment does not suppress the immune reaction of the host (lymphocyte chalone evidently excluded), and hence it is possible to apply immunotherapy as an adjunct to chalone therapy; (4) the possibly slow proliferation rate in some "spontaneous" human tumors as compared to transplanted animal tumors is not important per se, because the primary aim is to reach a negative imbalance; (5) the higher sensitivity of normal cells to chalone action need not be fatal, because the normal tissue may fully recover after the cessation of the chalone treatment (e.g., the pluripotential hematopoietic stem cells automatically recruit the granulocytic system) and because many normal tissues can be destroyed without killing the host.

There is also another potential application of chalones to cancer treatment, which has been proposed in slightly different forms by Schütt and Langen (1972) and by Houck (1973). According to Schütt and Langen, chalones could be used to protect bone marrow cells by blocking them in the G_1 phase while treating cancer (originating from another cell line) by cytostatic agents. Houck, in turn, has suggested that tumor cells and the corresponding normal cells could first be arrested in the G_1 phase and then, by reducing the chalone dose, the less sensitive tumor cells be allowed to escape from the chalone control and to proceed to the S phase in a synchronized fashion; at this stage the malignant cell population would be "sensitized" to chemotherapy while normal cells, still blocked in the G_1 phase, would not be vulnerable.

One more potential application of chalone to cancer therapy has been suggested by Mathé (Mathé *et al.*, 1972), based on the immunosuppressive action of the lymphocyte chalone (thymic chalone). In this application, already tried in practice in a case of unresponsive leukemia, the main aim is to prevent graft-vs-host reaction in bone marrow transplantation by incubating the cells *in vitro* in the presence of the lymphocyte chalone (see, however, Section VI,B).

X. Conclusions

In the past 10 years evidence has accumulated indicating that cell proliferation is controlled by means of negative feedback, i.e., with the aid of endogenous hormonelike mitotic inhibitors which regulate cell division within each population in a cell-line specific manner. This new group of species nonspecific substances is now commonly known as chalones.

Experimental data indicating the existence and action of most chalones reported in the literature are often scarce, equivocal, and sometimes even of low scientific quality; in fact, all published work on chalones, if taken one by one, may be inadequate in one respect or the other. The most critical aspects of the chalone concept have been the inconclusive experimental demonstration of absolute specificity of action, and the fact that no one has been able to isolate any of these substances in a chemically pure form. Consequently, it has been difficult to develop the chalone concept experimentally, and, therefore, speculation has flourished. Much of the speculation advanced by the leading scientists in the chalone field, notably by Bullough, could be—and has been—negated by the lack of hard facts; in the opinion of the present author, however, this speculation is usually based on sound biological reasoning.

In spite of the many weaknesses in the published research on chalones, the combined evidence makes it clear that the existence and specificity of action of at least some chalones, especially those of the epidermis and the hemic cell lines, have been demonstrated beyond reasonable doubt. Only a few chalones have been extensively purified; full chemical characterization of these substances seems to be beset with enormous difficulties. It has been claimed that with increasing purification good biological activity remains, but the active substance has been reduced to a quantity that cannot be detected chemically even with methods working at the 10^{-12} mole level; the reason is either that some chalones are biologically extremely active or, possibly, that the investigators are seeking the wrong type of chemical substance.

The chemical nature of chalones is not merely of academic interest; the prospects for clinical applications are exciting in a wide variety of diseases involving uncontrolled or unwanted cell proliferation. However, it seems to be virtually impossible to isolate chalones in great enough quantities for more than a few preliminary clinical trials; if the results from such trials are promising—and there is reason to believe that they will be—one should try to synthesize individual chalones. Thus, for the time being, energetic research on chalones is justified; the concept contains more than an element of truth, and it offers a tremendous potential for the control of some diseases involving much suffering.

Acknowledgments

The author's original work reported in this article was supported by grants from the Sigrid Jusélius Foundation, Helsinki, The Finnish Cancer Society, Helsinki, and Weddel Pharmaceuticals Ltd., London.

References

Abercrombie, M., and Heaysman, J.E.M. (1954). *Exp. Cell Res.* 6, 293

Angeletti, R.H., Angeletti, P.U., and Levi-Montalcini, R. (1973). *In* "Humoral Control of Growth and Differentiation" (J. LoBue and A.S. Gordon, eds.), Vol. I, p. 229. Academic Press, New York.
Argyris, T.S. (1972). *Amer. Zool.* **12**, 137.
Baden, H.P., and Sviolka, S. (1968). *Exp. Cell Res.* **50**, 644.
Baker, H.S. (1935). *Lancet* **229**, 583.
Balázs, A., Fazekas, I, Bukulya, B., Blazsek, I., and Rappay, G. (1972). *Mech. Aging Develop.* **1**, 175.
Balls, M., and Billett, F.S., eds. (1973). "The Cell Cycle in Development and Differentiation." Cambridge Univ. Press, London and New York.
Bard, J. (1973). *Nat. Cancer Inst. Monogr.* **38**, 217.
Baserga, R. (1965). *Cancer Res.* **25**, 581.
Bateman, A.E. (1974). *Cell Tissue Kinet.* **7**, 451.
Benestad, H.B. (1974). See *Brit. J. Cancer* **29**, 84, 1974.
Benestad, H.B., Rytömaa, T., and Kiviniemi, K. (1973). *Cell Tissue Kinet.* **6**, 147.
Bertalanffy, L. von (1960). *In* "Fundamental Aspects of Normal and Malignant Growth" (W.W. Novinski, ed.), p. 137. Elsevier, Amsterdam.
Bichel, P. (1970). *Eur. J. Cancer* **6**, 291.
Bichel, P. (1971). *Nature (London)* **231**, 449.
Bichel, P. (1972). *Eur. J. Cancer* **8**, 167.
Bichel, P. (1973). *Nat. Cancer Inst. Monogr.* **38**, 197.
Bizzozero, G. (1894). *Brit. Med. J.* **1**, 728.
Boggs, D.R. (1967). *Semin. Hematol.* **4**, 359.
Brit. J. Cancer (1974). **29**, 84.
Brønstad, G.O., Elgjo, K., and Øye, I. (1971). *Nature (London), New Biol.* **233**, 78.
Brugal, G. (1973). *Cell Tissue Kinet.* **6**, 519.
Bullough, W.S. (1962). *Biol. Rev.* **37**, 307.
Bullough, W.S. (1963). *Nature (London)* **199**, 859.
Bullough, W.S. (1965). *Cancer Res.* **25**, 1683.
Bullough, W.S. (1967). "The Evolution of Differentiation." Academic Press, New York.
Bullough, W.S. (1969). *In* "Repair and Regeneration" (J.E. Dunphy and W. Van Winkle, eds.), p. 35. McGraw-Hill, New York.
Bullough, W.S. (1971a). *Agents Actions* **2**, 1.
Bullough, W.S. (1971b). *Nature (London)* **229**, 608.
Bullough, W.S. (1972). *Brit. J. Dermatol.* **87**, 187, 347.
Bullough, W.S. (1973a). *Nat. Cancer Inst. Monogr.* **38**, 5.
Bullough, W.S. (1973b). *Nat. Cancer Inst. Monogr.* **38**, 99.
Bullough, W.S. (1973c). *In* "Humoral Control of Growth and Differentiation" (J. LoBue and A.S. Gordon, eds.), p. 3. Academic Press, New York.
Bullough, W.S., and Deol, J.U.R. (1971a). *Symp. Soc. Exp. Biol.* **25**, 255.
Bullough, W.S., and Deol, J.U.R. (1971b). *Eur. J. Cancer* **7**, 425.
Bullough, W.S., and Deol, J.U.R. (1972). *Brit. J. Dermatol.* **86**, 586.
Bullough, W.S., and Laurence, E.B. (1960). *Proc. Roy. Soc., Ser. B* **151**, 517.
Bullough, W.S., and Laurence, E.B. (1961). *Proc. Roy. Soc., Ser. B* **154**, 540.
Bullough, W.S., and Laurence, E.B. (1964). *Exp. Cell Res.* **33**, 176.
Bullough, W.S., and Laurence, E.B. (1966a). *In* "Advances in Biology of Skin" (W. Montagna and R.L. Dobson, eds.), p. 1. Pergamon, Oxford.
Bullough, W.S., and Laurence, E.B. (1966b). *Exp. Cell Res.* **43**, 343.
Bullough, W.S., and Laurence, E.B. (1968a). *Eur. J. Cancer* **4**, 587.
Bullough, W.S., and Laurence, E.B. (1968b). *Eur. J. Cancer* **4**, 607.
Bullough, W.S., and Laurence, E.B. (1968c). *Nature (London)* **220**, 134.
Bullough, W.S., and Laurence, E.B. (1968d). *Nature (London)* **220**, 137.

Bullough, W.S., and Laurence, E.B. (1968e). *Cell Tissue Kinet.* **1**, 5.
Bullough, W.S., and Laurence, E.B. (1970a). *Cell Tissue Kinet.* **3**, 291.
Bullough, W.S., and Laurence, E.B. (1970b). *Eur. J. Cancer* **6**, 525.
Bullough, W.S., and Rytömaa, T. (1965). *Nature (London)* **205**, 573.
Bullough, W.S., Laurence, E.B., Iversen, O.H., and Elgjo, K. (1967). *Nature (London)* **214**, 578.
Burger, M.M. (1971). *Curr. Topics Cell. Regulation* **3**, 135.
Byron, J.W. (1971). *Nature (London)* **234**, 39.
Byron, J.W. (1973). *Nature (London), New Biol.* **241**, 152.
Carrel, A. (1925). *Ann. Surg.* **82**, 1.
Cercek, L., Cercek, B., and Ockey, C.H. (1973). *Biophysik* **10**, 187.
Cercek, L., Cercek, B., and Garrett, J.V. (1974). *In* "Proceedings of the 8th Leukocyte Culture Conference," Uppsala, p. 553. Academic Press, New York.
Chopra, D.P., and Simnett, J.D. (1969). *Exp. Cell Res.* **58**, 319.
Chopra, D.P., and Simnett, J.D. (1970). *Nature (London)* **225**, 657.
Chopra, D.P., and Simnett, J.D. (1971). *J. Embryol. Exp. Morphol.* **25**, 321.
Chopra, D.P., Ruey, J.Y.V., and Flaxman, B.A. (1972). *J. Invest. Dermatol.* **59**, 207.
Chung, A.C., and Hufnagel, A. (1973). *Nat. Cancer Inst. Monogr.* **38**, 131.
Clermont, Y., and Mauger, A. (1974). *Cell Tissue Kinet.* **7**, 165.
Cohen, S. (1965). *Develop. Biol.* **12**, 394.
Cone, C.D., Jr. (1971). *J. Theor. Biol.* **30**, 151, 183.
Cooper, E.H. (1973). *Cell Tissue Kinet.* **6**, 87.
Cooper, P.R., and Smith, H. (1973). *Nature (London)* **241**, 457.
Cowdry, E.V. (1950). "A Textbook of Histology." Kimpton, London.
Craddock, C.G. (1972). *In* "Hematology" (W.J. Williams, E. Beutler, A.J. Erslev, and R.W. Rundles, eds.), pp. 593, 607. McGraw-Hill, New York.
Cross, J.P., and Barer, R. (1972). *J. Anat.* **111**, 336.
Culliton, B.J. (1974). *Science* **184**, 1268.
Curtis, H.J. (1973). *Science* **141**, 686.
Dayan, A.D. (1971). *Brain* **94**, 31.
Dewey, D.L. (1973). *Nat. Cancer Inst. Monogr.* **38**, 213.
Donahue, D.M., Reiff, R.H., Hanson, M.L., Betson, Y., and Finch, C.A. (1958). *J. Clin. Invest.* **37**, 1571.
Dörmer, P., and Brinkmann, W. (1970). *In* "*In Vitro* Procedures with Radioisotopes in Medicine," p. 59. Int. At. Energy Agency, Vienna.
Dulbecco, R. (1970). *Nature (London)* **227**, 802.
Dulbecco, R. (1971). *In* "Ciba Foundation Symposium on Growth Control in Cell Cultures" (G.E.W. Wolstenholme and J. Knight, eds.), p. 203. Churchill, Edinburgh.
Dulbecco, R., and Elkington, J. (1973). *Nature (London)* **246**, 197.
Elgjo, K. (1972). *J. Invest. Dermatol.* **59**, 81.
Elgjo, K. (1973). *Nat. Cancer Inst. Monogr.* **38**, 71.
Elgjo, K., and Edgehill, W. (1973). *Virchows Arch. B* **13**, 14.
Elgjo, K., and Hennings, H. (1971a). *Virchows Arch. B* **7**, 1.
Elgjo, K., and Hennings, H. (1971b). *Virchows Arch. B* **7**, 342.
Elgjo, K.. Laerum, O.D., and Edgehill, W. (1972). *Virchows Arch. B* **10**, 229.
Epifanova, O. (1971). *In* "The Cell Cycle and Cancer" (R. Baserga, ed.), p. 145. Dekker, New York.
Fell, H.B. (1973). *Nat. Cancer Inst. Monogr.* **38**, 77.
Ferris, P., LoBue, J., and Gordon, A.S. (1973a). *In* "Humoral Control of Growth and Differentiation" (J. LoBue and A.S. Gordon, eds.), Vol. I, p. 213. Academic Press, New York.
Ferris, P., Molomut, N., and LoBue, J. (1973b) *In* "Humoral Control of Growth and

Differentiation" (J. LoBue and A.S. Gordon, eds.), Vol. I, p. 361. Academic Press, New York.
Finegold, M.J. (1965). *Proc. Soc. Exp. Biol. Med.* **119**, 96.
Fischer, A., and Parker, R.C. (1929). *Brit. J. Exp. Pathol.* **10**, 312.
Frankfurt, O.S. (1971). *Exp. Cell Res.* **64**, 140.
Franks, L.M. (1974). *Gerontologia* **20**, 51.
Franks, L.M., Wilson, P.D., and Whelan, R.D. (1974). *Gerontologia* **20**, 21.
Galjaard, H., Meer-Fieggen, W., and Giesen, J. (1972). *Exp Cell Res.* **73**, 197.
Garcia-Giralt, E. (1973). *Nat. Cancer Inst. Monogr.* **38**, 123.
Garcia-Giralt, E., and Macieira-Coelho, A. (1974). *In* "Proccedings of the 8th Leukocyte Culture Conference," Uppsala, p. 457. Academic Press, New York.
Garcia-Giralt, E., Berumen, L., and Macieira-Coelho, A. (1970a). *J. Nat. Cancer Inst.* **45**, 649.
Garcia-Giralt, E., Lasalvia, E., Florentin, I., and Mathé, G. (1970b). *Eur. J. Clin. Biol. Res.* **15**, 1012.
Garcia-Giralt, E., Rella, W., Morales, V.H., Diaz-Rubio, E., and Richaud, F. (1973). *Nat. Cancer Inst. Monogr.* **38**, 125.
Garry, R., and Hall, R. (1970). *Lancet* ii, 693.
Glinos, A. (1960). *Ann. N.Y. Acad. Sci.* **90**, 592.
Gordon, A.S., Handler, E.S., Siegel, C.D., Dornfest, B.S., and LoBue, J. (1964). *Ann. N.Y. Acad. Sci.* **113**, 766.
Gordon, A.S., Zanjani, E.D., Gidari, A.S., and Kuna, R.A. (1973). *In* "Humoral Control of Growth and Differentiation" (J. LoBue and A.S. Gordon, eds.), Vol. I, p. 25. Academic Press, New York.
Gospodarowicz, D. (1974). *Nature (London)* **240**, 123.
Goss, R.J. (1967). *In* "Control of Cellular Growth in Adult Organisms" (H. Teir and T. Rytömaa, eds.), p. 3. Academic Press, New York.
Hall, R.G. (1969). *Exp. Cell Res.* **58**, 429.
Heidrich, M.L., and Ryan, W.R. (1970). *Cancer Res.* **30**, 376.
Hennings, H., Iversen, O.H., and Elgjo, K. (1969). *Virchows Arch., B* **4**, 45.
Hinderer, H., Volm, M., and Wayss, K. (1970). *Exp. cell Res.* **59**, 464.
Holley, R.W., and Kiernan, J.A. (1968). *Proc. Nat. Acad. Sci. U.S.* **60**, 300.
Hondius Boldingh, W., and Laurence, E.B. (1968). *Eur. J. Biochem.* **5**, 191.
Houck, J.C. (1973). *Nat. Cancer Inst. Monogr.* **38**, 1.
Houck, J.C., and Cheng, R.F. (1973). *J. Cell Physiol.* **81**, 257.
Houck, J.C., and Daugherty, W.F., Jr. (1974). "Chalones: A Tissue-Specific Approach to Mitotic Control." Medcom, New York.
Houck, J.C., and Hennings, H. (1973). *FEBS Lett.* **32**, 1.
Houck, J.C., and Irasquin, H. (1973). *Nat. Cancer Inst. Monogr.* **38**, 117.
Houck, J.C., Irasquin, H., and Leikin, S. (1971). *Science* **173**, 1139.
Houck, J.C., Weil, R.L., and Sharma, V.K. (1972). *Nature (London), New Biol.* **240**, 210.
Houck, J.C., Sharma, V.K., and Cheng, R.F. (1973a). *Nature (London), New Biol.* **246**, 111.
Houck, J.C., Cheng, R.F., and Sharma, V.K. (1973b). *Nat. Cancer Inst. Monogr.* **38**, 161.
Houck, J.C., Attallah, A.M., and Lilly, J.R. (1973c). *Nature (London)* **245**, 148.
Hovi, T., and Vaheri, A. (1973). *Nature (London), New Biol.* **245**, 175.
Int. Comm. Radiol. Protection (ICRP) (1975). Publ. 23. Pergamon, Oxford.
Iversen, O.H. (1967). *Eur. J. Cancer* **3**, 389.
Iversen, O.H. (1968). *Nature (London)* **219**, 75.
Iversen, O.H. (1969). *In* "Ciba Foundation Symposium on Homeostatic Regulators" (G.E.W. Wolstenholme and J. Knight, eds.), p. 29. Churchill, London.
Iversen, O.H. (1970). *Cancer Res.* **30**, 1481.

Iversen, O.H. (1973a). *Nat. Cancer Inst. Monogr.* **38**, 225.
Iversen, O.H. (1973b). *Acta Pathol. Microbiol. Scand., Sect. A, Suppl.* **236**, 71.
Iversen, O.H., and Bjernes, R. (1963). *Acta Pathol. Microbiol. Scand., Suppl.* **165**, 1.
Iversen, O.H., and Elgjo, K. (1967). *In* "Control of Cellular Growth in Adult Organisms" (H. Teir and T. Rytömaa, eds.), p. 83. Academic Press, New York.
Iversen, O.H., Aandahl, E., and Elgjo, K. (1965). *Acta Pathol. Mocrobiol. Scand.* **64**, 506.
Iversen, O.H., Bhangoo, K.S., and Hansen, K. (1974). *Virchows Arch., B* **16**, 157.
Johnson, H.A. (1969). *Amer. J. Pathol.* **57**, 1.
Jones, J., Paraskova-Tchernozemska, E., and Moorhead, J.F. (1970). *Lancet* i, 654.
Jones, H.W., Jr., McKusick, V.A., Harper, P.S., and Wuu, K.-D. (1971). *Obstet. Gynecol.* **38**, 945.
Kariniemi, A.-L., and Rytömaa, T. (1976). *Brit. J. Dermatol.* **94** (in press).
Kieger, N. (1971). *Eur. J. Clin Biol. Res.* **16**, 566.
Kieger, N. (1974). *Image Roche* **58**, 2
Kieger, N., Florentin, N., and Mathé, G. (1972). *Transplantation* **14**, 448.
Kieger, N., Florentin, N., and Mathé, G. (1973). *Nat. Cancer Inst. Monogr.* **38**, 135.
Kirsch, Ch., Bentegeat, J., and Boisseau, M. (1972). *Bord. Med.* **5**, 11.
Kivilaakso, E. (1970). *Acta Physiol. Scand.* **80**, 436.
Kivilaakso, E., and Rytömaa, T. (1970). *Cell Tissue Kinet.* **3**, 385.
Kivilaakso, E., and Rytömaa, T. (1971). *Cell Tissue Kinet.* **4**, 1.
Kohn, A., and Fuchs, P. (1970). *Curr. Top. Microbiol. Immunol.* **52**, 94.
Kruse, P.F., Jr., Whittle, W., and Miedema, E. (1969). *J. Cell Biol.* **42**, 113.
Laerum, O.D., and Maurer, H.R. (1973). *Virchows Arch., B* **14**, 293.
Lajtha, L.G. (1963). *J. Cell Comp. Physiol.* **62**, 143.
Lajtha, L.G. (1973a). *Nat. Cancer Inst. Monogr.* **38**, 111.
Lajtha, L.G. (1973b). *Nat. Cancer Inst. Monogr.* **38**, 157.
Lasalvia, E., Garcia-Giralt, E., and Macieira-Coelho, A. (1970). *Eur. J. Clin. Biol. Res.* **15**, 789.
Laurence, E.B. (1973a). *Nat. Cancer Inst. Monogr.* **38**, 37.
Laurence, E.G. (1973b). *Nat. Cancer Inst. Monogr.* **38**, 61.
Laurence, E.B., and Randers Hansen, E. (1971). *Virchows Arch., B* **9**, 271.
Laurence, E.B., and Randers Hansen, E. (1972). *Virchows Arch., B* **11**, 34.
Laurence, E.B., Randers Hansen, E., Christophers, E., and Rytömaa, T. (1972). *Eur. J. Clin. Biol. Res.* **17**, 133.
Lee, R., and Hanson, W. (1947). "Protomorphology." Lee Found. Nutrit. Res., Milwaukee.
Lenfant, M., Kren-Proschek, L., and Verly, W.G. (1973). *Can. J. Biochem.* **51**, 654.
Lindeman, R. (1971). *Brit. J. Haematol.* **21**, 623.
Lord, B.I., Cercek, L., Cercek, B., Shah, G.P., Dexter, T.M., and Lajtha, L.G. (1974). *Brit. J. Cancer* **29**, 168.
MacManus, J.P., and Whitfield, J.F. (1969). *Exp. Cell Res.* **58**, 188.
Marks, F. (1971). *Hoppe-Seyler's Z. Physiol Chem.* **352**, 1273.
Marks, F. (1972). *Brit. J. Dermatol.* **86**, 543.
Marks, F. (1973). *Nat. Cancer Inst. Monogr.* **38**, 79.
Marks, F., and Grimm, W. (1972). *Nature (London), New Biol.* **140**, 178.
Marks, F., and Rebien, W. (1972). *Naturwissenschaften* **59**, 41.
Marrs, J., and Vorhees, J.J. (1971). *J. Invest. Dermatol.* **56**, 353.
Mathé, G. (1969). *Brit. Med. J.* iv, 7
Mathé, G. (1972). *Eur. J. Clin. Biol. Res.* **17**, 548.
Mathé, G., Garcia-Giralt, E., Kieger, N., Florentin, I., Halle-Pamenko, O., and Martyre, M.C. (1972). *Exp. Haematol.* **22**, 53.
Maurer, H.R., and Laerum, O.D. (1973). *Synopses Papers, Int. Symp. Chalone Control Mechanisms, Lane End* p. 14.

Mendelsohn, M.L. (1960). *Science* **132**, 1496.
Menkin, V. (1957). *Cancer Res.* **17**, 963.
Mercer, E.H. (1962). *Brit. Med. Bull.* **18**, 187.
Messier, B., and Leblond, C.P. (1960). *Amer. J. Anat.* **106**, 247.
Metcalf, D. (1971). *Advan. Cancer Res.* **14**, 181.
Metcalf, D. (1973). In "Humoral Control of Growth and Differentiation" (J. LoBue and A.S. Gordon, eds.), Vol. I, p. 91. Academic Press, New York.
Metcalf, D., and Moore, M.A.S. (1971). "Haemopoietic Cells." North-Holland Publ., Amsterdam.
Moberg, C., Olofsson, T., and Olsson, I. (1974). *Scand. J. Haematol.* **12**, 381.
Mohr, U., Althoff, J., Kinzel, V. Süss, R., and Volm, M. (1968). *Nature (London)* **220**, 138.
Mohr, U., Hondius Boldingh, W., and Althoff, J. (1972a). *Cancer Res.* **32**, 1117.
Mohr, U., Hondius Boldingh, W., Emminger, A., and Behagel, H.A. (1972b). *Cancer Res.* **32**, 1122.
Moorhead, J.F., Paraskova-Tchernozemska, E., Pirrie, A.J., and Hayes, C. (1969). *Nature (London)* **224**, 1207.
Moreau, D., and Bullough, W.S. (1973). *New Sci.* 4 October, 28.
Nelson-Rees, W.A., Flandermeyer, R.R., and Hawthorne, P.K. (1974). *Science* **184**, 1096.
Odell, T.T., Jr. (1973). In "Humoral Control of Growth and Differentiation" (J. LoBue and A.S. Gordon, eds.), Vol. I, p. 119. Academic Press, New York.
Osgood, E.E. (1957). *J. Nat. Cancer Inst.* **18**, 155.
Osgood, E.E. (1959). In "The Kinetics of Cellular Proliferation" (F. Stohlman, Jr., ed.), p. 282. Grune & Stratton, New York.
Otsuka, H., and Együd, L.G. (1968). *Currents Mod. Biol.* **2**, 106.
Paran, M., Ichikawa, Y., and Sachs, L. (1969). *Proc. Nat. Acad. Sci. U.S.* **62**, 81.
Paukovits, W.R. (1971). *Cell Tissue Kinet.* **4**, 539.
Paukovits, W.R. (1973a). In "Leukämien und maligne Lymphome" (A. Stacher, ed.), p. 62. Urban & Schwarzenberg, München.
Paukovits, W.R. (1973b). *Blut* **27**, 217.
Paukovits, W.R. (1973c). *Nat. Cancer Inst. Monogr.* **38**, 147.
Paukovits, W.R. (1974). See *Brit. J. Cancer* **29**, 84.
Philpott, G.W. (1971). *Gastroenterology* **61**, 25.
Pickart, L., and Thaler, M.M. (1973). *Nature (London), New Biol.* **243**, 85.
Pohjanpelto, P., and Raina, A. (1972). *Nature (London), New Biol.* **235**, 247.
Pontén, J. (1971). "Spontaneous and Virus-Induced Transformation in Cell Culture." Springer-Verlag, Berlin and New York.
Powell, J.A., Duell, E.A., and Vorhees, J.J. (1971). *Arch. Dermatol.* **104**, 359.
Randers Hansen, E. (1967). *Odontol. Tidsk.* **75**, 480.
Refsum, S.B., and Berdal, P. (1967). *Eur. J. Cancer* **3**, 235.
Ribbert, H. (1895). *Virchows Arch. Pathol. Anat. Physiol.* **141**, 153.
Riley, P.A. (1969). *Nature (London)* **223**, 1382.
Riley, P.A. (1972). In "Cell Differentiation" (R. Harris, P. Allin, and D. Viza, eds.), p. 288. Munksgaard, Copenhagen.
Robertson, T.B. (1923). "Chemical Basis of Growth and Senescence." Lippincott, Philadelphia.
Rose, S.M. (1957). *Biol. Rev.* **32**, 351.
Rose, S.M. (1958). *J. Nat. Cancer Inst.* **20**, 653.
Rothberg, S., and Arp, B.C. (1973). *Nat. Cancer Inst. Monogr.* **38**, 93.
Rubin, H., and Rein, A. (1967). In "Growth Regulating Substances for Animal Cells in Culture" (V. Defendi and M.G.P. Stoker, eds.), Wistar Inst. Symp. Monogr. 7, p. 51. Wistar Inst. Press, Philadelphia, Pennsylvania.

Rytömaa, T. (1969). *In Vitro* **4**, 47.
Rytömaa, T. (1970). *Ann. Clin. Res.* **2**, 94.
Rytömaa, T. (1973a). *Brit. J. Haematol.* **24**, 141.
Rytömaa, T. (1973b). In "The Cell Cycle in Development and Differentiation" (M. Balls and F.S. Billett, eds.), p. 457. Cambridge Univ. Press, London and New York.
Rytömaa, T. (1973c). *Nat. Cancer Inst. Monogr.* **38**, 143.
Rytömaa, T., and Kiviniemi, K. (1964). In "Proceedings of the XIV Scandinavian Congress of Pathology and Microbiology," p. 169. Universitetsforlaget, Oslo.
Rytömaa, T., and Kiviniemi, K. (1967). In "Control of Cellular Growth in Adult Organisms" (H. Teir and T. Rytömaa, eds.). p. 106. Academic Press, New York.
Rytömaa, T., and Kiviniemi, K. (1968a). *Cell Tissue Kinet.* **1**, 329.
Rytömaa, T., and Kiviniemi, K. (1968b). *Cell Tissue Kinet.* **1**, 341.
Rytömaa, T., and Kiviniemi, K. (1968c). *Eur. J. Cancer* **4**, 595.
Rytömaa, T., and Kiviniemi, K. (1968d). *Nature (London)* **220**, 136.
Rytömaa, T., and Kiviniemi, K. (1969a). *Nature (London)* **222**, 995.
Rytömaa, T., and Kiviniemi, K. (1969b). *Cell Tissue Kinet.* **2**, 263.
Rytömaa, T., and Kiviniemi, K. (1970). *Eur. J. Cancer* **6**, 401.
Rytömaa, T., and Kiviniemi, K. (1975). *In Vitro* **11**, 1.
Saetren, H. (1956). *Exp. Cell Res.* **11**, 229.
Saetren, H. (1970). *Acta Pathol. Microbiol. Scand., Sect. A* **78**, 55.
Savage, C.R., and Cohen, S. (1972). *J. Biol. Chem.* **247**, 7609.
Scaife, J.F. (1970). *Experientia* **26**, 1071.
Schäfer, E.A. (1916). "The Endocrine Organs." Longmans, London.
Schultz, E.F., Lapin, D.M., and LoBue, J. (1973). In "Humoral Control of Growth and Differentiation" (J. LoBue and A.S. Gordon, eds.), Vol. I, p. 51. Academic Press, New York.
Schütt, M., and Langen, P. (1972). *Studia Biophys.* **31/32**, 211.
Shadduck, R.K. (1971). *Blood* **38**, 820.
Sheldrake, A.R. (1974). *Nature (London)* **250**, 381.
Simms, H.S., and Stillman, N.P. (1937). *J. Gen. Physiol.* **20**, 621.
Simnett, J.D., and Chopra, D.P. (1969). *Nature (London)* **222**, 1189.
Simnett, J.D., and Fisher, J.M. (1973). *Nat. Cancer Inst. Monogr.* **38**, 29.
Simnett, J.D., Fisher, J.M., and Heppleston, A.G. (1969). *Nature (London)* **223**, 944.
Simpson, G.E.C., and Finckh, E.S. (1963). *J. Pathol. Bacteriol.* **86**, 361.
Smeby, W. (1974). Ph.D. Thesis, Inst. Physics, University of Oslo.
Smith, J.A., and Martin, L. (1973). *Proc. Nat. Acad. Sci. U.S.* **70**, 1263.
Spielhoff, R. (1971). *Proc. Soc. Exp. Biol. Med.* **138**, 43.
Steel, G.G. (1967). *Eur. J. Cancer* **3**, 381.
Stich, H.F., and Florian, M.L. (1958). *Can. J. Biochem. Physiol.* **36**, 855.
Stoker, M.G.P. (1973). *Nature (London)* **246**, 200.
Stoker, M.G.P., and Rubin, H. (1967). *Nature (London)* **215**, 171.
Stone, L.S., and Vultee, J.H. (1949). *Anat. Rec.* **103**, 144.
Szent-Györgyi, A. (1966). *Biochem. J.* **98**, 641.
Szent-Györgyi, A. (1968). "Bioelectronics." Academic Press, New York.
Tardent, P. (1955). *Rev. Suisse Zool.* **62**, 289.
Teir, H. (1951). *Soc. Sci. Fenn., Commentat. Biol.* **13**, 1.
Teir, H. (1952). *Acta Pathol. Microbiol. Scand.* **30**, 158.
Tisman, G., and Herbert, V. (1973). *In Vitro* **9**, 86.
Todaro, G.J., Lazar, G.K., and Green, H. (1965). *J. Cell Comp. Physiol.* **66**, 325.
Tsanev, R., and Sendov, B. (1966). *J. Theoret. Biol.* **12**, 327.
Tyler, A. (1946). *Growth, Suppl.* **7**.

Vaheri, A., Ruoslahti, E., and Nordling, S. (1972). *Nature (London), New Biol.* **238**, 211.
Verly, W.G. (1973). *Nat. Cancer Inst. Monogr.* **38**, 175.
Verly, W.G., Deschamps, Y., Pushpathadam, J., and Desrosiers, M. (1971). *Can. J. Biochem.* **49**, 1376.
Vilpo, J.A., and Rytömaa, T. (1973). *Cell Tissue Kinet.* **6**, 489.
Vilpo, J.A., Kiviniemi, K., and Rytömaa, T. (1973). *Eur. J. Cancer* **9**, 515.
Voaden, M.J. (1968). *Exp Eye Res.* **7**, 313.
Voaden, M.J., and Leeson, S.J. (1970). *Exp. Eye Res.* **9**, 57, 67.
Volm, M., and Wayss, K. (1971). *Naturwissenschaften* **58**, 458.
Volm, M., Wayss, K., and Hinderer, H. (1969). *Naturwissenschaften* **56**, 566.
Volm, M., Mattern, J., and Wayss, K. (1972). *Exp. Pathol.* **7**, 84.
Volm, M., Gericke, D., Schuhmacher, J., and Wayss, K. (1974). *Naturwissenschaften* **61**, 458.
Vorhees, J.J., Duell, E.A., Bass, L.J., and Harrell, E.R. (1973). *Nat. Cancer Inst. Monogr.* **38**, 47.
Wayss, K., Mattern, J., and Volm, M. (1973). *Naturwissenschaften* **60**, 354.
Weiss, D.W., ed. (1971). "Immunological Parameters of Host-Tumor Relationships." Academic Press, New York.
Weiss, P. (1952). *Science* **115**, 487.
Weiss, P. (1955). *In* "Biological Specificity and Growth" (E.G. Butler, ed.), p. 195. Princeton Univ. Press, Princeton, New Jersey.
Weiss, P., and Kavanau, J.L. (1957). *J. Gen. Physiol.* **41**, 1.
Wheldon, T.E., Gray, W.M., Kirk, J., and Orr, J.S. (1970). *Nature (London)* **226**, 547.
Whitfield, J.F., McManus, J.P., and Gillan, D.J. (1973). *J. Cell Physiol.* **81**, 241.
Zetterberg, L., and Auer, G. (1970). *Exp. Cell Res.* **62**, 262.

Note Added in Proof

It has recently been shown that granulocyte chalone is indeed biologically active against myeloid leukemia in man: it was observed in the first clinical tests in 7 patients that i.v. injection of partially purified chalone inhibits leukemic growth and that this inhibition is followed by actual regression of the leukemia (Rytömaa, Vilpo, Levanto and Jones: *Scand. J. Haematol. 1976* [in press]).

Relation of Vascular Proliferation to Tumor Growth[1]

JUDAH FOLKMAN and RAMZI COTRAN[2]

Department of Surgery, Children's Hospital Medical Center, Department of Pathology, Peter Bent Brigham Hospital, and Harvard Medical School, Boston, Massachusetts

I.	Endothelial Turnover and Capillary Regeneration	208
	A. Introduction	208
	B. Normal Endothelial Turnover	208
	C. Endothelial Proliferation	210
	D. Studies of Endothelial Cell Turnover *in Vitro*	211
II.	Biology of Tumor Angiogenesis	214
	A. General Background	214
	B. Tumor Growth in the Isolated Perfused Organ	215
	C. Tumor Angiogenesis in the Dorsal Air Sac of the Rat	216
	D. Tumor Growth and Neovascularization in the Rabbit Eye	218
	E. Tumor Angiogenesis on the Chorioallantoic Membrane	220
	F. Vascularization of Transplanted Tissues, Normal and Neoplastic	222
	G. Effect of Irradiation on the Capacity of Tumor to Induce Angiogenesis	224
	H. Soft Agar Suspension Culture	225
III.	Tumor Angiogenesis Factor	228
	A. Purification	228
	B. Bioassay	230
IV.	Discussion	230
	A. The Avascular and Vascular Phases of Tumor Growth	230
	B. Specificity of Tumor Angiogenesis	233
	C. Inhibition of Angiogenesis	238
	References	245

---

[1] This work was supported by Grants Nos. CA-14019 from the National Cancer Institute, DT-2A from the American Cancer Society, and HL08251 from the National Heart and Lung Institute.

[2] Recipient of a Career Development Award from the National Heart and Lung Institute.

I. Endothelial Turnover and Capillary Regeneration

A. INTRODUCTION

Proliferation of vascular endothelial cells plays a key role in a variety of important biological processes. These include wound healing, the formation of inflammatory granulation tissue, the organization of thrombi, the healing of large vessel defects, the repopulation of endothelium in grafts, the development of collateral vessels, and the growth of tumors. Yet despite extensive research on cell proliferation in various organs and types of normal and malignant tissue, there has been comparatively little work on the kinetics of endothelial cell turnover and the mechanisms responsible for endothelial proliferation.

Our interest in endothelial proliferation arose from experiments on the biology of tumor neovascularization, (angiogenesis) and was further stimulated by the isolation of an extract derived from tumor cells that can induce new blood vessel formation *in vivo* (Folkman *et al.*, 1971). Here we shall briefly review what is presently known about normal endothelial cell replication in general, and then summarize the studies on tumor angiogenesis carried out in our laboratories over the past 5 years.

We are indebted to our colleagues, much of whose work is included here: Drs. Robert Auerbach, Dianna Ausprunk, Henry Brem, Tito Cavallo, Michael Gimbrone, Christian Haudenschild, Michael Klagsbrun, David Knighton, and Milton Sholley. The review will not deal with the morphology of regenerating vessels since several light and electron microscopic studies have been published and have been reviewed recently (Cliff, 1963; Schoefl, 1963; Schoefl and Majno, 1964; Cavallo *et al.*, 1973).

B. NORMAL ENDOTHELIAL TURNOVER

It is now well established that normal adult vascular endothelium represents a slow renewal population of cells (Tannock and Hayashi, 1972; see review in Cavallo *et al.*, 1972). Mitoses are rarely encountered in normal adult endothelium, and a number of autoradiographic studies with ^{3}H-labeled thymidine have in general confirmed this view. It is to be emphasized, however, that there is considerable variability in the normal rate of endothelial labeling among different tissues. For example, using the same schedule of thymidine, Engerman *et al.* (1967) found the labeling index in the myocardium to be 0.13%, while it was only 0.01% in the retina. Most published thymidine-^{3}H labeling indices for *capillary* endothelium have been less than 1%, and most often in the vicinity of 0.1%. Some of the higher figures appearing in the literature (e.g., Crane and Dutta, 1964) almost certainly are due to difficulty in clearly identifying capillary endothelial cells in paraffin sections, since they can often be confused with pericytes or adventitial cells. For this reason, in quantitative studies, we do autoradiography on 1 μm-thick plastic sections in which labeled endothelial cells can be identified with relative ease.

In adult, nongrowing animals, capillaries in certain organs grow in response to physiological stimuli. For example, endothelial proliferation occurs in the endometrium during the menstrual cycle. We have induced endothelial mitosis in the endometrium and myometrium of rats injected with diethylstilbestrol (Widman and Cotran, 1975). Capillaries around hair follicles undergo cyclic changes during the hair growth cycle (Durward and Rudall, 1958). Autoradiographic studies using thymidine-^{3}H in the skin should take into account the normal increase in endothelial labeling around hair follicles during hair growth (Sholley and Cotran, 1976).

Endothelial turnover in the aorta has been studied with autoradiography of en face preparations of sheets of endothelium. These studies also indicate that a very small proportion of endothelial cells synthesize DNA under normal conditions (Fig. 1). Labeling appears to be greater in areas of bifurcations and branching (Wright, 1970) and in younger, growing animals (Sade et al., 1972).

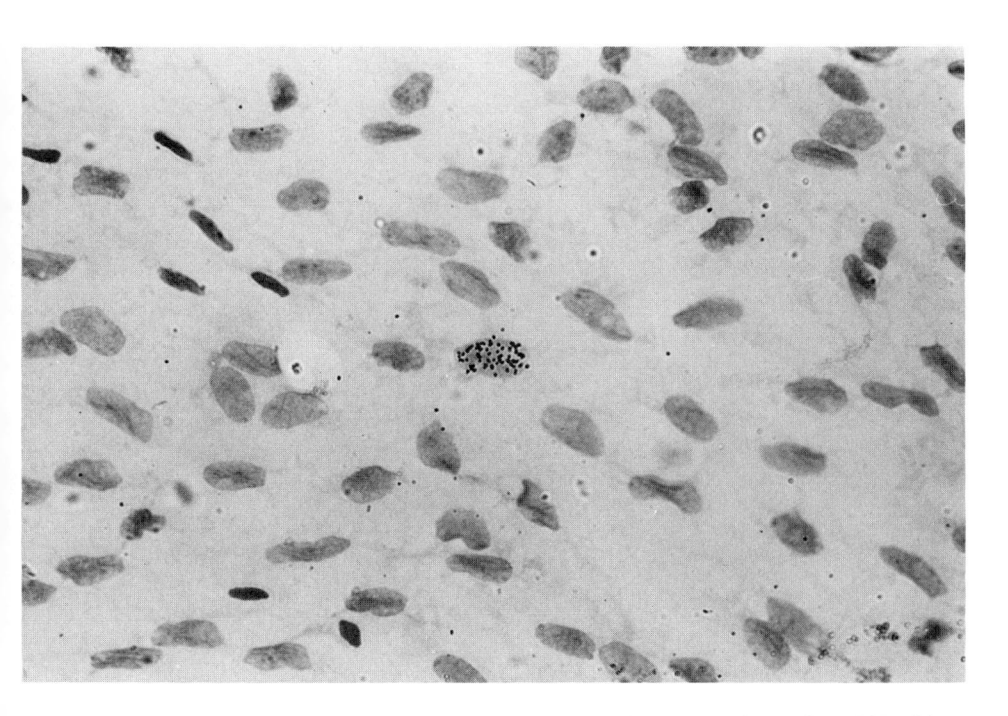

FIG. 1. En face preparation of aortic segment cultured for 6 hours in Medium 199 with 10% calf serum in the presence of ^{3}H-labeled thymidine. The oval endothelial cell nuclei can be differentiated from smooth muscle cells (upper left) when the latter are not removed by the stripping procedure. One labeled cell can be seen. × 400. From Sade et al. (1972) with permission of the publisher.

The most extensive study of endothelial labeling in the aorta is that reported by Schwartz and Benditt (1973). They mapped labeled endothelial nuclei in various regions of the rat aorta and found loci of heavy labeling not related to areas of bifurcation. Caplan and Schwartz (1973) further showed in normal pigs that foci of increased thymidine labeling in the aorta correlated with foci of increased permeability of the endothelium. This was demonstrated by aortic uptake of intravenously injected Evans blue. These authors concluded that the increased labeling reflects increased endothelial regeneration resulting from hemodynamically induced endothelial injury. This may be important in the early development of atheromatous plaques. Gaynor (1971) reported higher mitotic activity in the normal renal and pulmonary arteries than in the aorta of rabbits.

C. Endothelial Proliferation

While normal endothelium has a low mitotic index, a variety of pathologic stimuli can induce endothelial proliferation. In large vessels, such as the aorta, this endothelial proliferation serves to heal endothelial defects, while in the microcirculation it results, in addition, in the formation of new blood channels, so-called neovascularization.

The capacity of aortic and venous endothelial cells to undergo mitosis was initially shown by light microscopy of en face preparations of aortic endothelium after traumatic injury. The sequence of events resulting in reendothelialization of small endothelial defects was described in detail in the classic experiments of Poole *et al.* (1958). These studies have since been repeated with the use of more elegant techniques of traumatic injury to endothelium, such as ballooning (Baumgartner and Studer, 1966). Increased endothelial labeling, measured by autoradiography, has also been reported after traumatic, chemical, physical, and immunological injury to the aorta (Cavallo *et al.*, 1972). Increased labeling also follows feeding of cholesterol for 3 days (Florentin *et al.*, 1969), and is seen in the aorta of rabbits after a single injection of endotoxin (Gaynor, 1971). In these experiments, a common denominator appears to be injury leading to detachment of endothelial cells and regeneration of adjacent endothelium. Endothelial regeneration often can also be induced after injury in aortic segments *in vitro* (Sade *et al.*, 1972) (Fig. 2). Thus, it appears, the primary stimulus for endothelial proliferation in large vessels is some form of endothelial injury. Further, most observations suggest that endothelial regeneration ceases when the endothelial defect has been reconstituted.

The proliferation of capillaries in healing wounds has been studied extensively in such systems as the rabbit ear chamber, the hamster cheek pouch, the cornea, and the cremaster muscle. The light and electron microscopic sequence of events in the growth and formation of new blood vessels have been well described (Schoefl, 1963). In addition, a variety of necrotizing inflammatory stimuli, which cause tissue necrosis, induce the formation of granulation tissue. It has

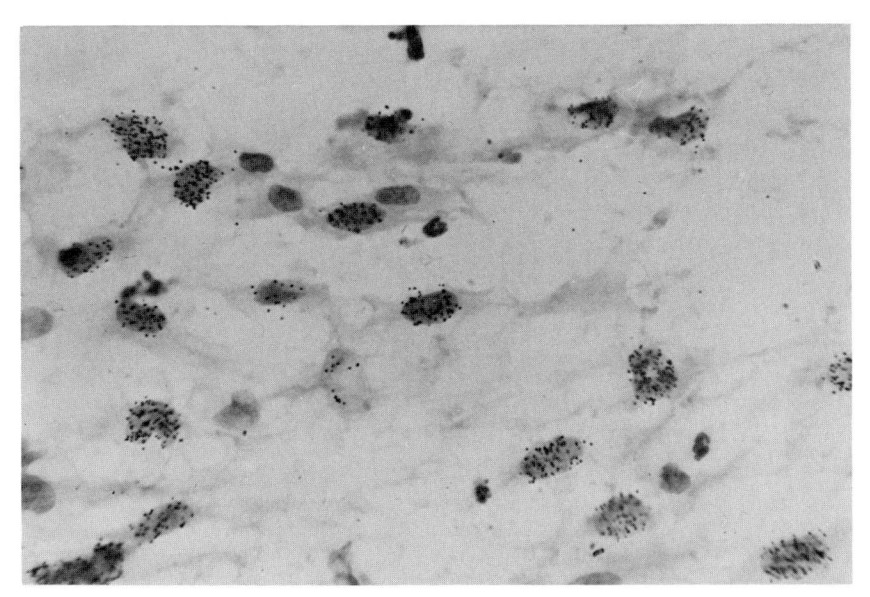

FIG. 2. En face preparation of endothelium adjacent to an area that was crushed *in vivo* 48 hours before the segment was removed and incubated with ^{3}H-labeled thymidine *in vitro*. × 350. From Sade *et al*. (1972) with permission of the publisher.

been assumed that the vascular proliferation which occurs under these circumstances is similar to that in healing wounds. Studies of the mechanisms of capillary proliferation, however, have been inconclusive. Release of a substance from mast cells, vasoactive mediators, local hypoxia or change in oxygen tension, accumulation of cell metabolites, tissue extracts, and other factors have been implicated as stimuli of vascular proliferation in wound healing (Florey, 1970; Remensnyder and Majno, 1968). This subject has been recently reviewed in some detail by Ryan (1973) and is considered briefly later in this review, in relation to the specificity of tumor angiogenesis.

D. STUDIES OF ENDOTHELIAL CELL TURNOVER *in Vitro*

In order to study the effects of possible neoplastic and nonneoplastic mediators of endothelial mitoses, we developed methods for culture of endothelium either in aortic segments, or, more recently, in pure monolayer cultures.

Over the past 25 years a number of investigators have attempted to grow endothelium in culture with little success; in most instances growth ceased after a few days. In the few successful attempts (e.g., Maruyama, 1963), it was not possible clearly to identify the cultured cells as endothelium.

In our first attempts, 3–5-mm circular segments of rat aorta (which had been dissected aseptically) were cultured in Medium 199 and 10% calf serum (Sade *et al.*, 1972). By this method it was possible to maintain endothelium in a viable state for at least 48 hours. Ultrastructural studies showed that approximately 70% of the endothelial layer was intact at that time. By making autoradiographs of Häutchen preparations of endothelium after exposure to ^{3}H-labeled thymidine, we found that the labeling index in control untraumatized segments varied according to the age of the animal. In 6-month-old breeders after a 6-hour exposure to ^{3}H-labeled thymidine, the labeling index was 0.01–0.1% (Fig. 3). It was possible to induce increases in endothelial labeling *in vitro* by traumatizing the segment, e.g., with the pinch of a clamp, which resulted in a zone of labeled cells immediately adjacent to the pinched area. It was also noted that smooth muscle cells showed increased labeling in culture after traumatic injury.

More recently, we have used cultures of human umbilical vein endothelium to study *in vitro* kinetics (Jaffe *et al.*, 1973; Gimbrone *et al.*, 1973a, b, c, 1974a). Because the culture work is being reviewed separately by Gimbrone, it will be summarized here only briefly.

Human vascular endothelial cells are obtained by perfusion of term umbilical cord veins with collagenase (Gimbrone *et al.*, 1974a). After 10 minutes of incubation with the enzyme, the cells are centrifuged and cultured in Falcon plastic dishes in Medium 199 containing 20% fetal calf serum. Small clumps of endothelial cells stick to the substrate, and after a lapse of about 24 hours begin to spread, coalesce, and multiply. By 6 or 7 days, a confluent monolayer of polygonal epithelioid cells results. The cells can be shown by electron microscopy to possess the Weibel–Palade granules that are characteristic of native umbilical vein endothelium. In some cultures these Weibel–Palade bodies are maintained for up to 19 passages (Haudenschild *et al.*, 1975a). By exposure of cultures at various intervals to ^{3}H-labeled thymidine, we calculated labeling indices of up to 50% in the growing phase of the culture, before confluence.

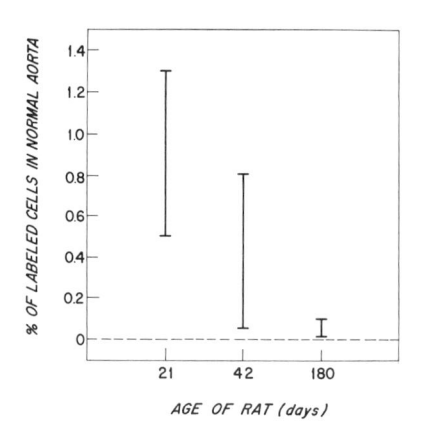

FIG. 3. Labeling index (thymidine-^{3}H) of aortic endothelium decreases with increasing age of rats.

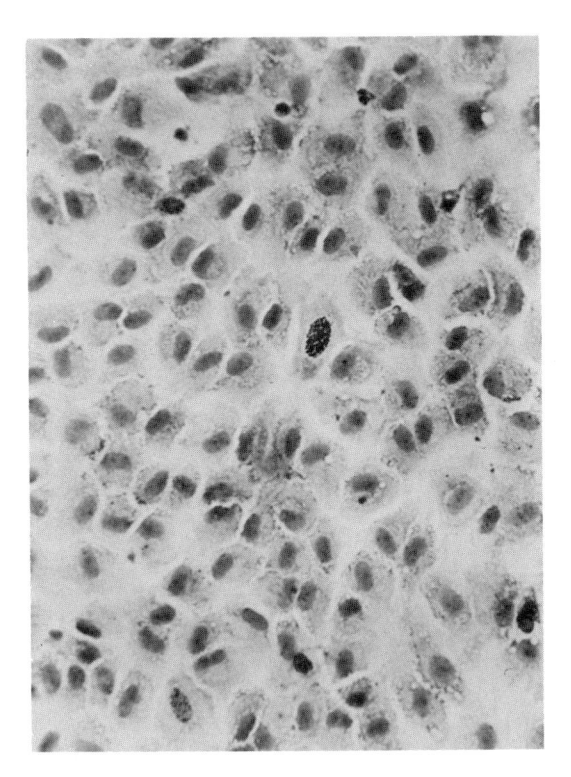

RELATION OF VASCULAR PROLIFERATION TO TUMOR GROWTH 213

FIG. 4. Autoradiograph from the central region of a confluent primary endothelial culture after exposure to ^{3}H-labeled thymidine. There are two lightly labeled cells and one heavily labeled cell. × 200. From Gimbrone et al. (1974a) with permission of the publisher.

Three days postconfluence, however, the labeling index in all experiments was consistently below 4% (Fig. 4). When the culture was wounded by a scratch, a wave of increased labeling at the periphery of the wound occurred and within 24–48 hours the wound had been reconstituted. Human endothelial cells from umbilical cord veins resembled large vessel endothelium in the native state in these respects: they exhibited density-dependent inhibition of cell division, and were stimulated to divide by denudation. Thus far, it has not been possible to induce increased labeling in such endothelial cells in culture with angiogenesis factor derived from tumor cells. In fact, it has not been possible to stimulate endothelial mitosis with a number of substances that seem to be active in other cell lines, such as fibroblasts. In recent studies Haudenschild et al. (1975b) have shown that, unlike a 3T3 fibroblast or primary human skin fibroblast, endothelial cells *do not* respond to addition of serum after a short period of serum deprivation. In this respect, therefore, endothelial cells seem to be under a stringent mechanism of control of cell growth.

II. Biology of Tumor Angiogenesis

A. GENERAL BACKGROUND

For more than 100 years, morphologists have noted the increased number of blood vessels associated with solid tumors. Virchow, in 1863, commented on the size and abnormal number of capillaries in the tumor mass. Goldman (1907) carried out some of the earliest anatomical studies of human and animal tumor vessels. He concluded that host vessels in the tumor bed undergo proliferation and "chaotic" growth. Succeeding papers were limited to studies of anatomical and postmortem material until the 1930s, when tumor vessels were first studied *in vivo*. Hasegawe (1934) applied the new technique of contrast medium radiography to tumors in live rabbits. Newly formed capillary sprouts were observed to grow toward the tumor and to establish a tortuous circulation within its advancing borders. This line of investigation has continued with the use of advanced techniques, such as microcineangiography and injection of radio-opaque cast material (Lien and Ackerman, 1974). Another technique, the transparent ear chamber, was first used by Clark and Clark (1932) to study growing capillaries in wounds. This chamber was soon adopted by a number of workers to study the earliest onset of vascular growth in transplanted tumors. Algire and Chalkley (1945) were the first to appreciate that growing malignancies could continuously elicit new capillary growth from the host. They suggested that this might be an underlying factor responsible for autonomous growth of these tumors. Wood (1958) carried out detailed studies of tumor angiogenesis by using these chambers. With high-powered time-lapse movies of rabbit ear chambers, he showed that new capillary sprouts began to grow as early as 18 hours after a metastatic focus of tumor cells appeared in the extravascular space. Warren and Shubik (1966) used the transparent chamber in the hamster cheek pouch to study the structure of tumor vessels.

Thus, until the 1960s, the literature of tumor angiogenesis was mainly descriptive, not mechanistic. These studies are briefly summarized in reviews by Urbach (1961), Day (1964), and Ryan (1973).

Not until 1967 was there an experiment suggesting a mechanism for tumor angiogenesis. Greenblatt and Shubik (1968) implanted tumors in a Millipore chamber in the hamster cheek pouch. The tumor was capable of inducing new vessels on the opposite side of the Millipore filter. Since the pore size of the filter was 0.45 μm, cells could not traverse it. It was, therefore, assumed that some diffusible material crossed through the filter and induced the neovascularization. Ehrmann and Knoth (1968) and Gitterman and Luell (1969) later confirmed this phenomenon with tumor-filled Millipore chambers placed on the chorioallantoic membrane.

Our own interest in tumor angiogenesis arose from an entirely different line of investigation, begun in 1960. We were studying the behavior of transplanted tumors (Folkman *et al.*, 1963, 1966; Folkman, 1970; Folkman and Gimbrone, 1971) in isolated perfused organs. Initially, it was assumed that tumors implanted into isolated perfused organs would become vascularized as they grew, because the organs themselves contained a vascular network. All our tumor implants failed to vascularize and stopped growing at small diameters of less than 2 mm. Further studies in the isolated perfused organ were redirected to explore the relationship between the tumor and the host vessels.

B. Tumor Growth in the Isolated Perfused Organ

In these experiments a single lobe of thyroid gland was removed from a dog or rabbit under sterile conditions. The superior thyroid artery was cannulated, and the organ was placed in a glass chamber. The arterial circulation was perfused with a pulsatile pump, and the perfusate was passed through a silicone rubber oxygenator. A variety of perfusates were used. These included culture medium, hemoglobin solutions, and autologous plasma, both platelet rich and platelet poor (Gimbrone *et al.*, 1969).

Perfusions lasted up to 1 week. The B-16 mouse melanoma from C57 black mice was implanted in the organ. The implants, 1 mm or less, were observed daily, and histological sections were made at the conclusion of the perfusion. In general, the outer third of the gland remained viable during this time while the central portion became necrotic. Although the majority of vessels were patent, vascular endothelium always degenerated. In more than 100 perfusions studied over a period of four years, endothelial regeneration and capillary proliferation were never observed. Tumor implants remained viable and often grew to 2 mm in diameter although there was always a large area of central necrosis. The tumor implants tended to grow in three-dimensional, spheroidal configurations rather than spreading out as a monolayer of cells. When the implants failed to grow beyond 1.5–2 mm, our first thought was that the area of central necrosis was in some way toxic to the peripheral cell layer. However, when the tumors were removed from these isolated organs and transplanted back to the host animals, large tumors grew that killed the host. When histological sections of the *in vitro* implants were compared to the *in vivo* implants, there was a striking difference. The *in vitro* implants were avascular whereas the *in vivo* implants were large and well vascularized.

These experiments suggested that the absence of angiogenesis, or the prevention of vascularization of a solid tumor, would in some way limit its growth to a small population of small diameter. Why tumor growth should be limited in this way was completely unclear at that time; also very little was known about the mechanism of tumor neovascularization. Furthermore, we did not know why the vascular endothelium of the isolated perfused organ would not regenerate or proliferate. This artifact of isolated perfusion provided our first insight that tumor angiogenesis might be a control point in tumor growth. However, the inability of the vessels to grow in the isolated perfused organ prohibited this method from being useful in further investigations.

C. Tumor Angiogenesis in the Dorsal Air Sac of the Rat

The major problem was to develop a system in which tumor could be separated from the vascular bed, or in which tumor extracts could be tested. The rat dorsal air sac technique originally used by Selye (1953) to study inflammation was modified. When air is injected subcutaneously the skin is lifted up from an area of white fascia which is only sparsely vascularized. When Millipore chambers containing Walker tumor cells were implanted into the air sacs, a vascular response was observed beneath the filter, but was not seen with nonmalignant tissues (see Section IV, B, 1). The vascular response, which was apparent 48 hours after tumor implantation, consisted of vasodilatation and an increase in the number of visible vascular channels. Endothelial mitoses were seen histologically, and labeled endothelial cells were present in autoradiographs after local injection of ^{3}H-labeled thymidine. Soluble, cell-free fractions were extracted from cytoplasm and nuclei of Walker tumor cells. These extracts were administered to a local zone in the subcutaneous air sac (see Section III, A for preparation of extract). This was accomplished by an intermittent infusion system, with a silicone tube implanted into the air sac (Folkman et al., 1970, 1971). A similar vascular response occurred. This study first showed that a soluble extract from tumor cells could produce a vascular reaction, part of which was endothelial proliferation, as demonstrated by autoradiography and histologically. A limited number of control tissues studied did not produce neovascularization. Furthermore, inflammation was not a major component of the vascular response.

The rat air sac was used in two additional studies by Cavallo et al. (1972) to document these findings more precisely. In the first, Walker ascites tumor cells and an extract derived from such cells (tumor angiogenesis factor, TAF) were injected into the fascial floor of the dorsal air sac. At intervals thereafter, ^{3}H-labeled thymidine was injected into the air sac and the tissues were examined by autoradiography and electron microscopy. Autoradiographs showed thymidine-^{3}H labeling in endothelial cells of small vessels, 1–3 mm from the site of the implantation, as early as 6–8 hours after exposure to live tumor cells. DNA synthesis by endothelium subsequently increased, and within 48 hours new blood vessel formation was detected. The presence of labeled endothelial nuclei (Fig. 5), endothelial mitosis, and regenerating endothelium was confirmed by electron microscopy. TAF also induced neovascularization and endothelial cell DNA synthesis after 48 hours. A similar response was not evoked in saline controls. Formic acid, which elicited an intense inflammatory response, was

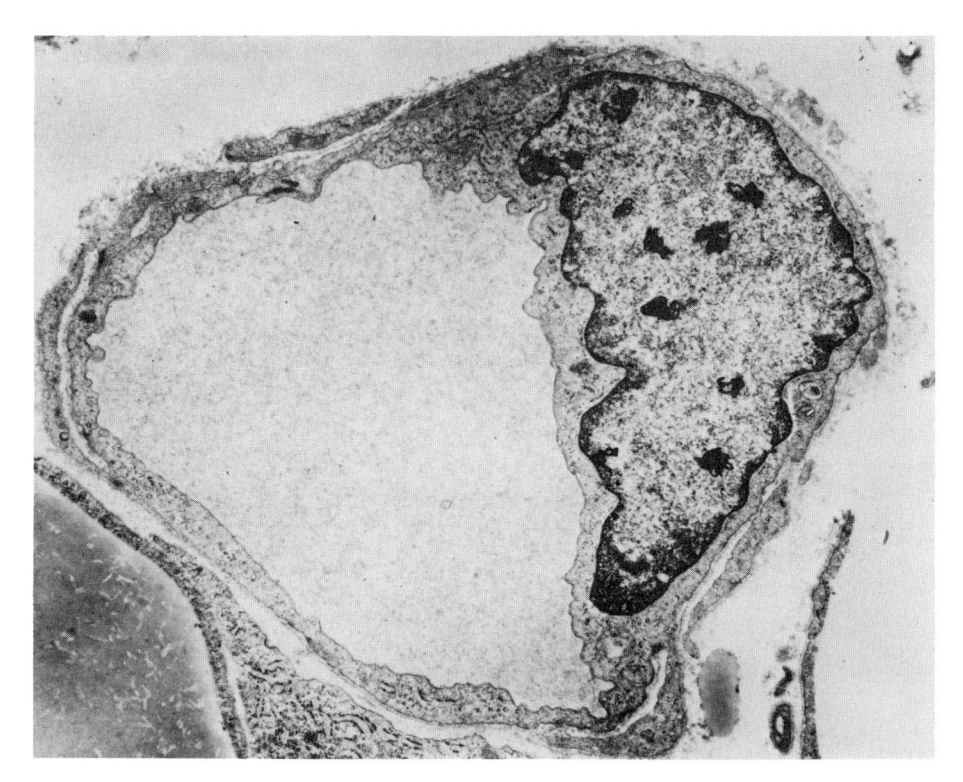

FIG. 5. Electron microscopic autoradiograph of a capillary 50 hours after injection of 1.0 × 10⁶ Walker tumor cells and 2 hours after injection of ³H-labeled thymidine into dorsal air sac of rat. The endothelial cell nucleus is labeled. × 8700. From Cavallo *et al.* (1972) with permission of the publisher.

associated with less endothelial labeling and neovascularization at the times studied.

Further ultrastructural autoradiographic studies were carried out with the same model (Cavallo *et al.*, 1973). It was apparent that by 48 hours there was ultrastructural evidence of regenerating endothelium, including marked increase in ribosomes and endoplasmic reticulum, scarce or absent pinocytotic vesicles, and discontinuous basement membrane. Labeled endothelial cells were seen along newly formed sprouts as well as in parent vessels. Furthermore, pericytes were also shown to synthesize DNA.

These studies were important in that they provided more precise evidence for: (1) endothelial proliferation and new capillary sprouts in response to tumor cells or tumor extract (TAF), (2) response at distances of up to 3 mm from the nearest tumor cell, (3) early onset of endothelial DNA synthesis. These studies also documented in a better way that the observed neovascularization was not accompanied by significant inflammation.

The limitations of the dorsal air sac method are that vascular growth cannot be quantitated, and tumor implants are so quickly vascularized that it is not possible to observe the behavior of tumor in the prolonged avascular state.

D. Tumor Growth and Neovascularization in the Rabbit Eye

The relationships of tumor growth and neovascularization have been demonstrated most clearly in experiments in the rabbit eye. Studies were carried out in both the cornea and the anterior chamber.

1. Cornea

Fragments of Brown-Pearce and V2 carcinomas, homologous to the rabbit, were implanted into the avascular corneal stroma of rabbits at distances from the limbus of 1–6 mm (Gimbrone et al., 1974b). The tumor implants were usually 1 mm in size. Tumor growth and neovascular response of limbal vessels were studied by (a) slit-lamp stereomicroscopy, (b) histologic examination, (c) colloidal carbon injections, and (d) autoradiography after exposure to ^{3}H-labeled thymidine. Centrally placed tumors, i.e., 5–6 mm from the limbus, spread as

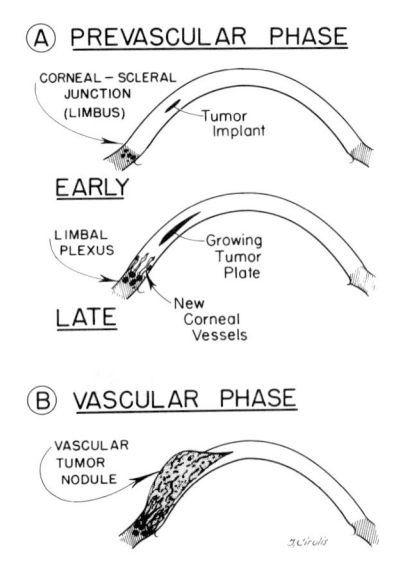

FIG. 6. Intracorneal implants of Brown-Pearce tumor during avascular phase before penetration by new capillaries and during vascular phase, after penetration by new capillaries. From Gimbrone et al. (1974b) with permission of the publisher.

thin plates toward the limbus. When the tumor edge reached within 2.5 ± 0.5 mm of the limbus, new vessels began to grow from the limbal plexus toward the tumor. When new capillaries penetrated the tumor, it grew rapidly into a large exophytic mass (Fig. 6). Mouse tumors, immunologically incompatible with the rabbit, grew in a similar fashion prior to vascularization and elicited new vessels in a similar way. After vascularization, immunologically incompatible tumors regressed. Intracorneal polyacrylamide gel implants containing tumor extracts (TAF) also elicited corneal neovascularization. This study, by prolonging the avascular phase of tumor growth, emphasized the importance of considering solid tumor growth in two stages: avascular and vascular. It provided further evidence that cytoplasmic contact between tumor cell and responding vascular bed was not essential for tumor-induced angiogenesis. The effective range for the humoral TAF in the cornea appeared to be up to 3.0 mm. This approximated the findings in the rat dorsal air sac experiments. Finally, the relative absence of inflammation of the cornea during tumor angiogenesis was striking. The cornea model was also used to study the ability of cartilage implants to inhibit capillary proliferation (Brem and Folkman, 1975) (see Section IV, C).

2. *Anterior Chamber*

Tumors were suspended in the aqueous humor of the anterior chamber. These tumors were placed at various distances from the iris vessels, and compared with tumors implanted directly on the iris and with those implanted in the cornea (Gimbrone *et al.*, 1973d). Autoradiographic and stereomicroscopic studies were made as before, but in addition, the entire microvascular tree of the iris was outlined with colloidal carbon and studied in glycerol-cleared, flat-embedded preparations. Iris neovascularization was induced even by remote intraocular tumor implants at distances up to 6 mm. Again, there was little or no evidence of inflammation associated with iris neovascularization.

In a parallel study (Gimbrone *et al.*, 1972), tumor implants placed in the anterior chamber remote from the iris, were observed for periods up to 6 weeks during which they did not become vascularized. Although these tumors failed to grow beyond 1 mm^3, they contained a population of viable and mitotically active tumor cells. When implanted on the iris, these tumors became vascularized (Fig. 7) and grew rapidly, often reaching a volume 16,000 times their original size after a period of 2 weeks (Fig. 8). This experiment introduced the concept of tumor dormancy brought about by prevention of neovascularization. The term dormancy was not meant to indicate a single resting cell, but was used in the sense of "population dormancy." In a crowded population of tumor cells, growing in a three-dimensional configuration and not penetrated by new capillaries, there is an outer proliferating compartment balanced by dying cells in a central necrotic compartment. This explains why expansion of the tumor mass stops.

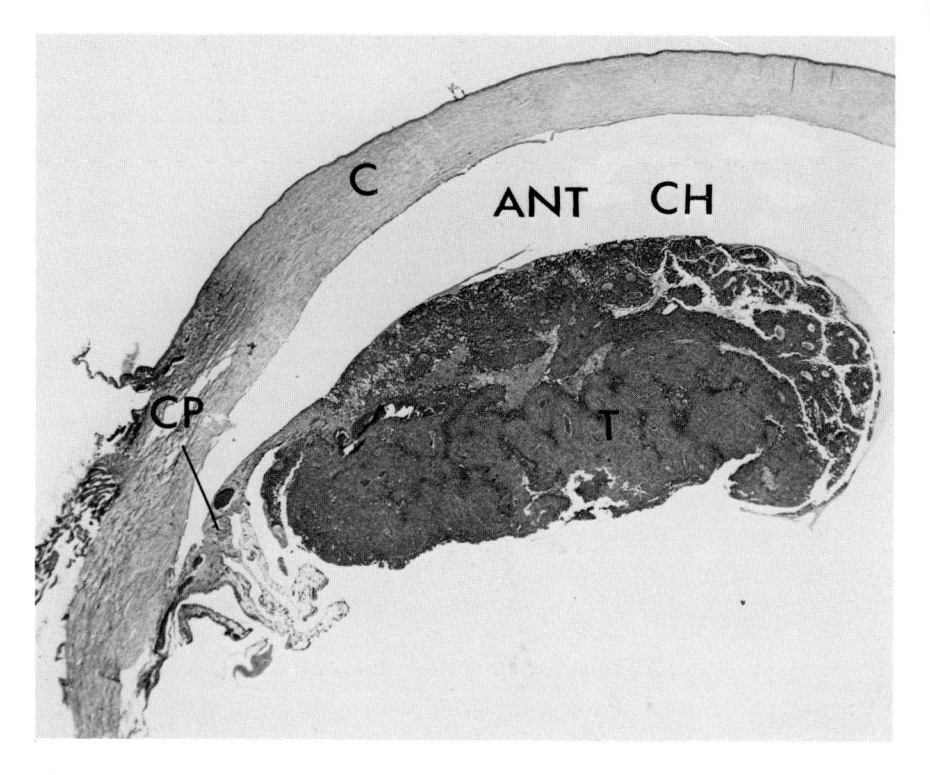

FIG. 7. Light micrograph of a large vascularized tumor 8 days after implantation on the iris. The tumor (T) has completely replaced the iris proper and invaded the ciliary body. ANT CH, anterior chamber; C, cornea; CP, ciliary process. Stained with hemotoxylin and eosin. × 15. From Gimbrone et al. (1972) with permission of the publisher.

E. Tumor Angiogenesis on the Chorioallantoic Membrane

Further studies required a system that would permit assay and quantitation of tumor angiogenesis. This was not practical in the cornea, the anterior chamber or the subcutaneous rat back. Therefore, the chorioallantoic membrane (CAM) was selected. However, before CAM could be used as an assay for tumor angiogenesis, it was necessary to know the normal growth pattern of the vessels of this membrane throughout the development of the chick. Accordingly, the maturation of vascular endothelial cells in the CAM from 8 to 18 days after fertilization was investigated by light and electron microscopy and by autoradiography (Ausprunk et al., 1974). From this study, we determined that prior to day 11 of incubation, endothelial cells have the morphological characteristics of immature and relatively undifferentiated cells. During this time, they exhibit a high labeling index with thymidine-^{3}H of approximately 23% (Fig. 9). At 11 days,

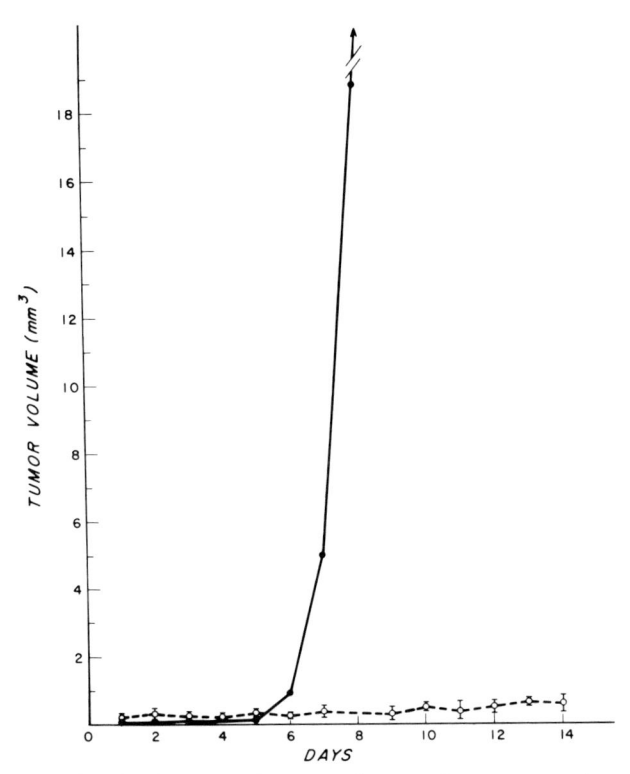

FIG. 8. A typical iris implant growth curve of Brown-Pearce tumor (●———●) and the mean daily volumes of 10 avascular anterior chamber implants (○– – –○) are plotted on a linear scale for comparison. Positive fluorescein test on day 6 indicates time of vascularization of iris tumor. Final volume on day 14 = 394 mm^3 ~ 16,000 × initial volume. From Gimbrone et al. (1972) with permission of the publisher.

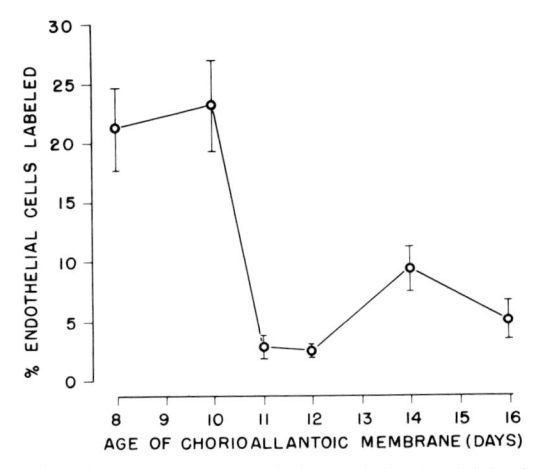

FIG. 9. Thymidine labeling index of endothelial cells in the chick chorioallantoic membrane as a function of age of the embryo. Vertical brackets represent standard deviation. From Ausprunk et al. (1974) with permission of the publisher.

the labeling index decreases to 2.8%, and subsequently the cells begin to acquire the structural characteristics of matured, differentiated endothelium. These data suggest that during the period of high endothelial cell mitosis (i.e., before day 11), the capillary network of the growing CAM is expanding by an overall proliferation of endothelial cells and existing capillaries, rather than by formation of new capillary sprouts.

With this information in hand, we proceeded to implant 1-mm fragments of fresh Walker 256 carcinoma into the embryo each day of incubation from day 3 to day 16. On days 3, 4, and 5, implants were made among the yolk sac vessels using a method described by Auerbach *et al.* (1974). From day 5 to day 16, tumor implants were made on the (CAM) (Knighton *et al.*, 1974). The size of the tumors was measured daily, and the onset of vascularization of each tumor was determined *in vivo* with a stereoscope and confirmed with histological sections. From these studies, the following points were made:

1. Proliferation of chick capillaries occurred in the neighborhood of the tumor graft by 24 hours after implantation, but capillary sprouts did not penetrate the tumor graft until approximately 72 hours. The 72-hour delay prior to the onset of vascularization was the same, regardless of whether the tumor was implanted on day 3 or at some later date in incubation.

2, During the avascular period, tumor diameter did not exceed 1 mm. Small tumor implants of 0.5 mm or less grew to 1 mm and stopped expanding. Larger tumor implants of 2 or 3 mm shrank until they reached the 1-mm diameter. During the first 24 hours after penetration by capillaries, there was rapid tumor growth, in some cases at an exponential rate.

3. The time of onset of vascularization was independent of the immune status of the chick embryo. The chick embryo does not become immunocompetent until day 12–14 of incubation. However, tumor angiogenesis evolved at the same rate both before and after the appearance of immunocompetence.

4. Although the neovascularization induced by either tumor or TAF could be seen on histological sections as early as day 6 on the CAM, neovascularization was not grossly observable with the stereomicroscope until after day 10 or 11. The gross detection of neovascularization required a pattern of vessels that converged on the implant or the TAF fraction. This was difficult to see before day 10, possibly because all of the other CAM vessels themselves were in a state of growth. These experiments suggested that the 10-day egg was optimum for use as an assay for tumor angiogenesis factor.

F. Vascularization of Transplanted Tissue, Normal and Neoplastic

In a third study (Ausprunk *et al.*, 1975), the behavior of tumor grafts on the CAM was compared to grafts of normal adult and embryonic tissues. Adult and embryonic tissue from rats were grafted to the CAM of the chick embryo. A rat tumor, the Walker carcinoma, was also grafted to the CAM. The grafts were all 1 mm or less and were examined daily by stereomicrosopy *in vivo* and by colloidal carbon injections to determine the precise onset of graft circulation, by histological sections, and thymidine-^{3}H-labeled autoradiographs. In tumor tissue, preexisting blood vessels within the tumor graft disintegrated by 24 hours after implantation. Revascularization did not occur until after at least 3 days, and only by penetration of proliferating *host* vessels into the tumor tissue. There was marked neovascularization of host vessels in the neighborhood of the tumor graft. By contrast, in the embryonic graft, preexisting vessels did not disintegrate. They reattached by anastomosis to the host vessels within 1–2 days, but with minimal or almost no neovascularization on the part of the host vessels. The embryonic tissue did not stimulate capillary proliferation in the host. In adult tissues, the preexisting graft vessels disintegrated although this took longer than in tumor vessels, i.e., 9 days. Also, adult tissues did not stimulate capillary proliferation in the host. There was *no* reattachment of their circulation with the host.

These studies suggest that only tumor grafts are capable of stimulating formation of new blood vessels in the host and thus acquiring a blood supply. In sharp distinction, revascularization of normal tissue grafts, when it does occur, is predominantly the result of fusion of preexisting vessels with the host circulation (Fig. 10).

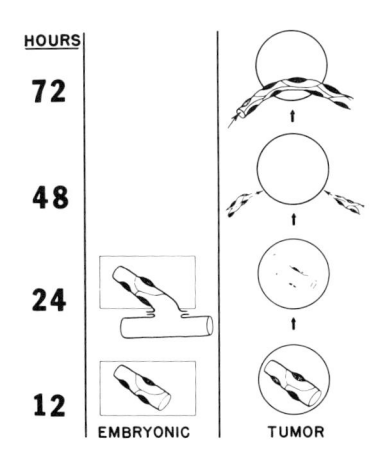

FIG. 10. Diagram to show that free grafts of embryonic tissue retain their own vessels. These vessels anastomose with host vessels by 24 hours after the graft is implanted on the chorioallantoic membrane. By contrast, the vessels in a tumor graft disintegrate by 24–48 hours. The tumor remains avascular until newly generated host vessels penetrate the graft at approximately 72 hours. From Ausprunk *et al.* (1975) with permission of the publisher.

TABLE I

IRRADIATED TUMOR GRAFT: ABILITY TO INDUCE
ANGIOGENESIS ON CHORIOALLANTOIC MEMBRANE

Tissue	No irradiation	2000 R	4000 R
Walker sarcoma	9/10[a]	14/19	7/8
Mouse teratoma	8/11	5/6	6/6
Mouse melanoma	5/6	4/5	5/5
V2 carcinoma	7/7	7/8	
Mouse placenta	0/7	0/7	
Mouse muscle	0/4	0/2	

[a]Number positive/total.

G. Effect of Irradiation on the Capacity of Tumors to Induce Angiogenesis

In a further study, Auerbach et al. (1975) used the CAM to study the effect of irradiated tumor grafts. Grafts of V2 carcinoma, Walker carcinoma, mouse melanoma and teratoma were irradiated with 2000 R or 4000 R just prior to implantation on the CAM (Table I). These grafts did not grow, and incubation with ^{3}H-labeled thymidine revealed no DNA synthesis. However, the tumor cells remained viable as demonstrated histologically. More important, the irradiated tumor grafts did induce capillary proliferation at the rate elicited by nonirradiated tumors, as demonstrated by light microscopy and histology. Control tissues, such as muscle and placenta from both mouse and rabbit, did not induce angiogenesis either before or after irradiation. Similar results were obtained when irradiated grafts were implanted in the cornea (Table II). These experiments demonstrate that the capacity of tumor grafts to induce angiogenesis is

TABLE II

IRRADIATED TUMOR GRAFT:
ABILITY TO INDUCE ANGIOGENESIS IN CORNEA

Tissue	No irradiation	4000 R
V2 carcinoma	10/10[a]	14/16
Muscle (rabbit)	0/4	0/4
Placenta (13-day mouse)	0/3	0/4

[a]Number positive/total.

not inhibited by 4000 R, even though this dose may be sufficient to stop mitosis. This is important evidence that angiogenesis capacity (or synthesis of TAF) operates independently of the mitotic rate.

H. SOFT AGAR SUSPENSION CULTURE

Although tumor dormancy was first observed in the anterior chamber, its mechanism could not be studied there. Therefore, an *in vitro* experiment was designed to simulate the conditions of the anterior chamber in order to understand just why the avascular tumor stops growing at such a tiny diameter.

B-16 mouse melanoma, V-79 Chinese hamster lung cells, and L-5178 Y murine leukemia cells were plated in soft agar (Folkman and Hochberg, 1973; Folkman *et al.*, 1974). After 6–7 days of incubation, spheroidal colonies of 0.1 mm were visible. Each spheroidal colony was transferred with a wide-bore pipette to a new flask containing 10 ml of fresh soft agar every 2–3 days, i.e., before there was time for pH change. The diameter of each spheroid was measured every 2–3 days by projecting its image on a white table top at 20 power magnification. Ten thousand transfers of spheroids to new medium were made over a period of one year. All spheroids first enlarged exponentially for a few days and then continued on a linear growth curve for 5–23 weeks before reaching a diameter beyond which there was no further expansion. This was termed the dormant phase. For murine leukemic cells, the mean diameter of the dormant phase was 3.8 mm ± 0.5 at approximately 24 days. For V-79 cells, the dormant diameter was 4.0 mm ± 0.8 mm at 175 days. Spheroids of B-16 melanoma cells stopped growing at 2.4 mm ± 0.4 mm at approximately 100 days.

After the dormant diameter was reached, these spheroids remained viable for 3–5 months, or as long as they were frequently transferred to new medium. Cells in the periphery of the spheroid incorporated ^{3}H-labeled thymidine while cells in the center died. This is a form of population dormancy in which the proliferating cells near the surface of the spheroid just balance those dying cells deep in the center of the spheroid. We have proposed as a possible mechanism that dormancy begins when the volume of cells has reached a point where their aggregate surface area is insufficient to allow absorption of nutrients and escape of catabolites. By contrast, the same cells grown in a flat configuration are not restricted since there is always sufficient surface area for the aggregate population to absorb nutrients and release catabolites.

In both experiments, unlimited fresh medium and space are provided; geometry becomes the critical variable. Growth in three dimensions is self-regulating; growth in two dimensions is not. The mechanism of dormancy of avascular tumors *in vivo* may be similar to what goes on in the dormant spheroid in soft agar. The onset of penetration by new vessels would enlarge the effective surface area of a three-dimensional population of cells.

TABLE III
TUMOR ANGIOGENESIS FACTOR (TAF) ACTIVITY IN TISSUE CULTURED CELLS AS MEASURED BY A VASCULAR RESPONSE ON THE CHORIOALLANTOIC MEMBRANE

Part A

Cells with TAF activity	Species	Number of eggs assayed	Strongly positive	Weakly positive[a]	Negative	Minimum number of cells needed for a positive vascular response
SVT2 (BALB/c 3T3 transformed by SV40	Mouse	42	24	16	2	$2-4 \times 10^6$
BALB/c 3T3	Mouse	14	7	5	2	$2-4 \times 10^6$
B-16 melanoma	Mouse	10	5	3	2	$2-4 \times 10^6$
Walker 256 carcinoma	Rat	13	8	2	3	$4-6 \times 10^6$
W138 embryonic lung	Human	9	2	5	2	$4-6 \times 10^6$
SVW126 (W126) embryonic lung transformed by SV40	Human	20	9	7	4	$4-6 \times 10^6$
Glioblastoma (brain)	Human	5	5	0	0	$0.5-1 \times 10^6$
Meningioma (brain)	Human	10	6	2	2	$1-2 \times 10^5$

Part B

Cells with no detectable TAF activity

Cells with no detectable TAF activity	Species	Number of eggs assayed	Number of eggs with following vascular response			Highest number of cells tested yielding a negative vascular response[b]
			Strongly positive	Weakly positive[a]	Negative	
BALB/c primary embryo	Mouse	14	0	1	13	$0.6-1 \times 10^7$
Skin fibroblasts (passage 11)	Human	12	0	3	9	$1-2 \times 10^7$

[a] These responses are characterized by a smaller number of vessels directed toward the test samples than is the case with strong responses. However, they differ significantly from blank filter controls.
[b] This does not imply that larger numbers of cells gave positive response but rather that larger numbers of cells were not tested.

III. Tumor Angiogenesis Factor

A. Purification

The capacity of neoplastic tissue to stimulate capillary proliferation appears to be mediated by a material (TAF) secreted from tumor cells. TAF is capable of diffusing through tissues and acting upon host vessels lying 2–5 mm from the tumor edge (Cavallo et al., 1972; Gimbrone et al., 1973d). When the tumor cell is disrupted, both the cytoplasm and nuclear pellets will stimulate angiogenesis. In our original attempts at purification, tumor cells from the solid or ascites phase were disrupted and the cytoplasmic and nuclear components were worked up separately. When the cytoplasmic components were separated by gel filtration on Sephadex G-100, a fraction with potent angiogenesis activity was found in the range of 10^5 daltons (Folkman et al., 1971). In parallel studies of the nuclear component, angiogenesis activity was associated with chromatin, but not with the DNA separated from the chromatin (Tuan et al., 1973). Further fractionation of the chromatin revealed TAF activity in the pool of nonhistone proteins. No activity was found in the cytoplasm or nucleus of normal liver cells disrupted in a similar manner.

Recently, TAF has been extracted without cell disruption from a variety of tumor lines grown in tissue culture (Folkman and Klagsbrun, 1975). Cells are grown in large roller bottles and when nearly confluent, the medium is discarded. Ringer's solution is added for 3 hours, then dialyzed against distilled water and lyophilized. The cells can be fed with fresh medium and used repeatedly every few days. The lyophilyzate contains serum proteins which had previously been absorbed by the cells, as well as newly synthesized proteins, as determined by feeding the cells with radiolabeled precursors. This material contains angiogenesis activity and is used as the crude preparation for further purification by Sephadex chromatography and ion-exchange separation. Purification is still in progress at this writing; no characterization has been carried out. Approximately 1–3 μg of protein containing TAF activity are released from 1 × 10^7 cells when roller bottles are used, and slightly higher yields are obtained from flat monolayer cultures. TAF activity has been found in cultures of mouse tumors (BALB/c SVT2) and B-16 melanoma; in a meningioma, a glioblastoma, and SVW126. TAF activity has also been found in two established lines, the W138 human embryonic lung at passage 24, and the mouse BALB/c3T3 embryo cell line (Folkman and Klagsbrun, 1975). However, this particular mouse 3T3 line produces tumors when implanted into the chick embryo (Table IIIA).

No TAF activity has been recovered from primary cultures of nonneoplastic cells such as BALB/c primary embryo cells or human skin fibroblast (Table IIIB).

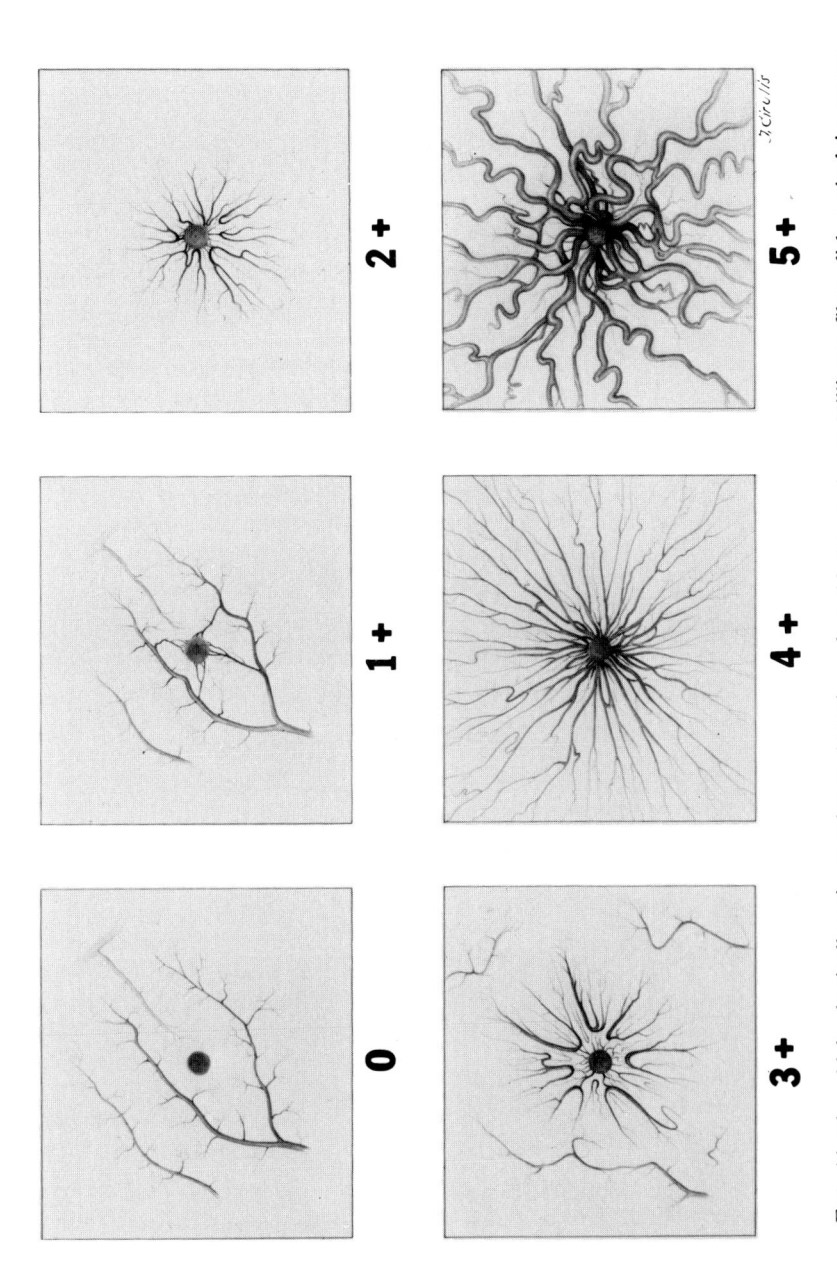

FIG. 11. The chick chorioallantoic membrane (CAM) at days 13–15. A 1-mm Millipore filter disk soaked in tumor angiogenesis factor is placed over a tiny needle hole in the CAM. New vascular loops, consisting of capillaries and venules, converge on the disk of the fraction is active. The density of these new vessels is assigned a grade of 0 to 5+.

B. Bioassy

In our original studies, test fractions were injected intermittently over 48 hours into the subcutaneous dorsal air sac of the rat through an implanted silicone rubber tube. The animals were then anesthetized and the fascia examined for intensity of neovascularization. This method is no longer used because it is cumbersome and requires up to 500 μg of total protein containing TAF activity.

Presently, the CAM of the chick embryo and the cornea of the rabbit eye are used to assay test fractions. A shell window is made in the 9- or 10-day chick embryo to expose the CAM. Protein fractions containing TAF are soaked into a 1-mm piece of Millipore filter, or implanted as a lyophilized crystal next to the filter. The CAM is examined under a low-power stereoscope at 48–72 hours, and the vascular reaction of new capillaries and venules converging on the Millipore filter are graded on a scale of 1 to 5 according to their intensity (Fig. 11). Very active fractions may be read as early as 48 hours, while weak fractions may be given a low score even after 4 days. Approximately 10^6 tumor cells in culture will release enough TAF activity after one wash with Ringer's solution to give a 2+ reaction on the CAM in 48 hours.

When the rabbit cornea is used for assay, 1-mm pieces of tissue are implanted into a corneal pocket 1.5 × 2.0 mm, and 2.0 mm or less from the limbal edge (Gimbrone et al., 1974b). TAF fractions are tested by adding lyophilized crystals to the pocket or dispersing concentrated fluid fractions in the pocket, either alone or in acrylamide gel which has been prepared under sterile conditions and thoroughly washed. Positive fractions stimulate new vessels to grow from the limbal edge toward the pocket. The rate of growth and the density of vessels can be used to determine activity.

We emphasize that these assays are essentially nonquantitative and are subject to biological variations. There is currently no *in vitro* assay for TAF. The type of endothelial cells from human umbilical veins that can be cultivated *in vitro* (Gimbrone et al., 1974a) are not stimulated by TAF fractions. Until an *in vitro* assay can be developed, purification will progress slowly.

IV. Discussion

A. The Avascular and Vascular Phases of Tumor Growth

The cells of solid tumors, in contrast to those of leukemia, live most of their life outside the blood stream or bone marrow. Solid tumor cells grow in densely packed populations, usually a three-dimensional configuration approximating a spheroid or ellipsoid. A surface tension, which is proportional to the mean curvature of the tumor surface, is assumed to maintain the colony as a compact mass (Greenspan, 1974) within the interstitial fluid of the host tissues. This aggregate of cells survives by exchanging nutrients and catabolites through simple diffusion with the surrounding environment. Only a small population can be maintained in this way. Population increase requires proliferation of new capillaries from the host, and these vessels must *penetrate* the small tumor nodule. Thus, neovascularization separates the development of any solid tumor into two stages: (1) the avascular stage and (2) the vascular stage (Folkman, 1974a).

1. *The Avascular Stage*

The avascular phase denotes the early aggregation of cells in a small tumor nodule, whether arising from a single cell, a metastatic implant, or a transplanted tumor. The maximum size of this population is on the order of 1 million cells, or a spheroid of about 1–2 mm diameter. When this maximum population is reached, only cells in the periphery (approximately 0.15 mm thick) are proliferating. As a new cell forms in the outer mitotic layer, it must push aside neighboring tumor cells. The forces of displacement are transmitted with attenuation (Greenspan, 1974) cell to cell, throughout the crowded population. Central necrosis begins as the nodule approaches 1 mm in diameter. In the experimental animal this stage is usually microscopic. It is also brief, lasting about 2–3 days for most tumor cells implanted subcutaneously in the mouse. However, in some special situations, the avascular phase is easily observed. Tumors implanted into the CAM of the chick embryo remain avascular for about 72 hours (Knighton *et al.*, 1974). The transparent chamber in the rabbit ear (Algire and Chalkley, 1945), or in the hamster cheek pouch (Greenblatt and Shubik, 1968), or in the rat skin (Yamaura and Sato, 1973) also provide a good view of the avascular phase. When silicone rubber casts are made of the blood supply of experimental liver tumors in rabbits, it can be shown that tumors up to 1 mm in diameter remain avascular (Lien and Ackerman, 1974). Capillaries do not penetrate the tumor surface. Beyond that size tumors are vascularized. In some situations the duration of the avascular phase can be prolonged. Tumors implanted (cells or grafts) in the anterior chamber of the rabbit eye, will persist for weeks in the avascular phase (Gimbrone *et al.*, 1972). When tumors are implanted in the corneal stroma the time to vascularization is directly proportional to the distance between the tumor and the limbus. Implants in the central cornea (4–5 mm from the limbus) may remain unvascularized for up to 2 months (Gimbrone *et al.*, 1973d).

In some clinical situations the avascular phase of tumor growth is also visible. Carcinoma *in situ* can be diagnosed in the skin, in the eye (Folkman, 1974b), in the bladder, and in the uterine cervix. In the cervix (Suess *et al.*, 1973), neoplastic cell masses sit superficial to the basement membrane and may remain avascular for years without penetrating it. At some point the small tumor mass penetrates

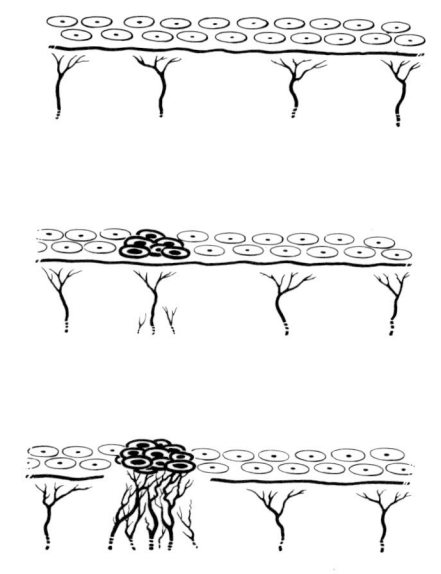

FIG. 12. A diagram of a theoretical progression of carcinoma of the uterine cervix *in situ*. This can be thought of as a model of other human carcinomas, which begin in an avascular compartment of epithelium separated from vessels by a basement membrane.

the basement membrane and becomes vascularized. Carcinoma of the cervix *in situ* can be thought of as a model of the avascular state of many other carcinomas (Fig. 12). There is a common pattern in the skin, gastrointestinal tract, pharynx, genitourinary tract, and respiratory tract in which the avascular epithelial compartment is separated from blood vessels by a basement membrane. Most carcinomas begin in this avascular compartment. In summary, the hallmark of the avascular stage of tumor development is limited growth with a minuscule population of 10^6 cells in a mass less than 2 mm in diameter. When vascularization is delayed or prevented, the avascular tumor enters a dormant state. This is a form of population dormancy or steady state in which proliferating cells in the outer portion of the nodule just balance those dying cells in the center. There is no further growth.

2. *The Vascular Phase*

Once new capillaries have penetrated the avascular spheroid, rapid growth begins. In some tumors exponential growth starts with vascularization. In the rabbit anterior chamber, a Brown–Pearce tumor implanted near iris vessels will be penetrated by new capillaries in 5–6 days (Gimbrone *et al.*, 1972). During the next 2 weeks, growth is so rapid that the tumor reaches a maximum size of up to 16,000 times it original volume. In the chick embryo, tumor implants on the CAM remain at a mean diameter of 0.93 ± 0.29 mm during the avascular phase.

These implants begin rapid growth 24 hours after vascularization and achieve a mean diameter of 8.0 ± 2.5 mm by 7 days. The area of central necrosis, so common in the avascular spheroid, disappears 2 days after vascularization (Ausprunk et al., 1975). The 1 cm^3 tumor contains capillaries throughout, and the tumor cells within it have a high mitotic index from the center to the periphery (Goldacre and Sylven, 1962). Central necrosis reappears as tumors exceed 1 cm^3 despite vascularization. This is primarily the result of high tissue pressure generated in the center of the expanding tumor, which compresses the deeper capillaries, stopping blood flow (Young et al., 1959). In very large tumors, capillary blood flow is present only in a thin rind at the periphery while the large central area is necrotic.

In summary, the hallmark of the vascular phase is rapid growth. It is also possible that vascularization is largely responsible for shedding of antigenic material into the circulation (Currie, 1973), release of metastases (Butler and Gullino, 1975), and malignant progression (Folkman, 1974a).

B. Specificity of Tumor Angiogenesis

1. Angiogenesis by Control Tissues and Extracts

The experiments summarized in the preceding sections show that malignant tumors, or an extract derived from such tumors, induce neovascularization. Further, this neovascularization plays an important role in the propensity of individual tumor nodules for uncontrolled growth. The question arises whether this capacity is unique to malignant tumors, or whether benign tumors, normal organs, or rapidly proliferating tissues can also induce neovascularization. We have not tested all tissues in all the bioassay systems used. In the rather crude assays used, it has not been possible to quantitate exact cell count, biochemical composition, or purity of the preparations used as controls in relation to tumor tissue. However, as seen in Table IV, the only other normal tissue that consistently caused appreciable angiogenesis in our hands was the salivary gland. Occasionally mouse embryonic kidney induced weak neovascularization. This was also true of bone. Sidky and Auerbach (1975) have shown that in some instances heterologous lymphoid tissue implants caused a vascular response interpreted as neovascularization. In some series of experiments tissues like pancreas and placenta occasionally produced apparent neovascularization, but further study indicated that the response was either caused by a necrotizing inflammatory reaction or was inconsistent. Of the tumors tested, the following consistently induced neovascularization: mouse mammary carcinoma, mouse plasmacytoma (MOPC and TEPC), mouse B-16 malanoma, mouse teratoma, SV3T3, Walker 256 sarcoma, Brown—Pearce tumor, and V2 carcinoma.

It has been suggested that angiogenesis may be a property of embryonic tissue. For this reason a detailed study of embryonic, adult, and tumor tissue was

TABLE IV
TESTING OF NORMAL TISSUES FOR ABILITY TO INDUCE ANGIOGENSIS

Tissue	Source	Test system	Result	Reference
Adipose tissue, white	Mouse, adult	Anterior chamber	−	Gimbrone and Gullino, unpublished
Adrenal	Mouse, adult	Anterior chamber	±	Gimbrone and Gullino, unpublished
Adrenal	Mouse, embryonic	CAM	−	Stacpoole and Folkman, unpublished
Bone, scapular	Rabbit, neonatal	Cornea	+	Brem and Folkman (1975)
Bone, scapular	Rabbit, neonatal	CAM	+	Brem and Folkman (unpublished)
CAM[a]	Chick embryo	CAM	−	Ausprunk et al. (1975)
Cartilage, scapular	Rabbit, adult	Cornea	−	Brem and Folkman (unpublished)
Cartilage, scapular	Rabbit, neonatal	Cornea	−	Brem and Folkman (1975)
Cartilage, scapular	Rabbit, neonatal	CAM	−	Brem and Folkman (1975)
Cartilage, scapular	Rabbit, neonatal (boiled)	Cornea	−	Brem and Folkman (1975)
Cartilage, rib	Human	CAM	−	Brem and Folkman, unpublished
Cornea	Rabbit, neonatal	Cornea	−	Brem, unpublished
Heart muscle	Rat, adult	CAM	−	Ausprunk et al. (1975)
Heart muscle	Rat, embryonic	CAM	−	Ausprunk et al. (1975)
Heart muscle	Chick embryo	CAM	−	Ausprunk et al. (1975)
Intestine	Mouse, embryonic	CAM	−	Stacpoole and Folkman, unpublished
Kidney	Mouse, adult	Anterior chamber	+	Gimbrone and Gullino, unpublished
Kidney	Mouse, adult	CAM	Weak +	Auerbach et al., unpublished
Kidney	Mouse, embryonic	CAM	Weak +	Auerbach et al., unpublished
Kidney	Rat, adult	CAM	−	Ausprunk et al. (1975)
Kidney	Rat, adult	Rat back	−	Folkman et al. (1971)
Kidney	Rat, embryonic	CAM	±	Ausprunk et al. (1975)
Limb bud	Mouse, embryonic	CAM	−	Stacpoole and Folkman, unpublished
Limb bud	Rat, embryonic	CAM	−	Ausprunk et al. (1975)

Tissue	Species/Age	Site	Result	Reference
Liver	Mouse, adult	Anterior chamber	—	Gimbrone and Gullino, unpublished
Liver	Mouse, embryonic	CAM	—	Stacpoole and Folkman, unpublished
Liver	Rabbit, fetal	Cornea	—	Brem, unpublished
Liver	Rat, adult	CAM	—	Ausprunk et al. (1975)
Liver	Rat, adult	Rat back	—	Folkman et al. (1971)
Liver	Rat, embryonic	CAM	—	Ausprunk et al. (1975)
Lung	Mouse, embryonic	CAM	—	Stacpoole and Folkman, unpublished
Lymph node	Mouse, adult	Anterior chamber	+	Gimbrone and Gullino, unpublished
Lymph node	Rabbit, adult (autologous)	Cornea	—	Auerbach, unpublished
Lymph node	Rabbit, adult (homologous)	Cornea	+	Auerbach, unpublished
Mast cells (5×10^5)	Rat, adult	CAM	—	Ausprunk et al., unpublished
Pancreas	Mouse, embryonic	CAM	—	Stacpoole and Folkman, unpublished
Paraspinous muscle	Rabbit, adult	Cornea	—	Auerbach et al. (1975)
Placenta	Mouse	CAM	—	Auerbach et al. (1975)
Placenta	Mouse	Cornea	—	Auerbach et al. (1975)
Placenta	Mouse	Anterior chamber	—	Gimbrone and Gullino, unpublished
Placenta	Human, 18 weeks	Rat back	—	Auerbach, unpublished
Placenta	Rabbit	CAM	—	Auerbach, unpublished
Salivary gland	Mouse, adult	CAM	+ + +	Folkman and Knighton, unpublished
Skeletal muscle	Rabbit, adult	CAM	—	Auerbach et al. (1975)
Skeletal muscle	Rabbit, adult	Cornea	—	Auerbach et al. (1975)
Skeletal muscle	Rat, adult	CAM	—	Ausprunk et al. (1975)
Skin	Mouse, embryonic	CAM	—	Stacpoole and Folkman, unpublished
Spleen	Mouse, embryonic	CAM	—	Stacpoole and Folkman, unpublished
Thyroid	Mouse, adult	Anterior chamber	+	Gimbrone and Gullino, unpublished
Thyroid	Rat, 4 months	CAM	—	Brem, unpublished
Trophoblasts	Human	Cornea	—	Stacpoole and Folkman, unpublished
Trophoblasts	Rabbit	Cornea	—	Brem and Arensman, unpublished

[a] CAM, chorioallantoic membrane.

performed in the CAM (Ausprunk *et al.*, 1975). The findings, summarized above (Section II, F), show that embryonic grafts become vascularized by anastomosis of host and graft vessels, not by induction of neovascularization in the host.

2. *The Relationship of Tumor Neovascularization to the Inflammatory Process*

Formation of new blood vessels is an important event in wound healing and in chronic inflammatory processes. It could be argued that tumors or tumor extracts induce new blood vessel formation by acting as inflammatory stimuli. For example, it is conceivable that products of necrotic tumor cells, or perhaps invading leukocytes, are released in the adjacent connective tissue, which then responds with an inflammatory reaction. This process could lead to the formation of new vessels. This argument against the specificity of tumor angiogenesis is important, even though the mechanism of neovascularition in wound healing is far from understood (Ryan, 1973). Alternatively, it is possible that a specific factor from tumor cells can induce angiogenesis by activating a mechanism, e.g., a chemical, or cellular mediator, which is shared with inflammatory neovascularization. While the issue cannot be settled, the following facts emerge from our experiments:

1. In experimental models in which either tumor or tumor extracts were used, histological sections of the responding site showed only mild cellular infiltrate. This was true in the corneal experiments, where early examination of the limbal vessels as well as the zone between the tumor and limbus showed very few neutrophils and monocytes. In the rat air sac model thymidine-^{3}H-labeled endothelial cells were seen in small vessels devoid of infiltrate. This was demonstrated by light and electron microscopy in vessels 1–3 mm from the site of injection of tumor (Cavallo *et al.*, 1972). It is interesting to note that Fauve *et al.* (1974), and more recently Bronza and Ward (1975), have reported anti-inflammatory and antichemotactic substances in tumors. This may account for the finding of only slight inflammation in our experiments.

2. The key mediator of neovascularization in inflammation may be related to a serum factor, and therefore to edema rather than cell infiltrate. Edema is easily visible by slit-lamp examination in the cornea, and it was absent prior to neovascularization induced by tumors. Electron microscopy of blood vessels as early as 6–24 hours after tumor implant, when thymidine-^{3}H-labeled cells were already present, showed no ultrastructural evidence of increased vascular permeability. At later intervals, when newly formed vessels were more leaky, our findings were consistent with the findings of Schoefl and Majno (1964).

3. In early experiments with the "rat back" model, it was shown that administration of formic acid as an "inflammatory" control for tumor extract resulted in little neovascularization and significantly less endothelial labeling. Despite the increased inflammation, endothelial labeling was decreased compared to animals implanted with tumor. More recently, we have initiated a series

of experiments to reexamine endothelial replication in acute inflammation, and to determine the possible contribution of inflammatory cells to endothelial regeneration.

Localized thermal injuries were induced in rat skin by applying heated copper disks for 20 seconds. The disks were heated to 54°C or 60°C by a circulating-water bath. Previous studies in this laboratory (Cotran and Majno, 1964; Cotran 1965, 1967; Cotran and Remensynder, 1968) have shown that the 54°C stimulus induces moderate injury, with a delayed-prolonged phase of increased vascular permeability. The 60°C lesion is overtly necrotizing and induces immediate and sustained vascular leakage. At various intervals thereafter, thymidine-^{3}H was injected and the labeling index was determined in autoradiographs of 1 μm plastic sections (Cavallo and Cotran, 1973; Sholley et al., 1974; Sholley and Cotran, 1975). With both stimuli, endothelial labeling began 24 hours after injury and reached a peak between 48 and 72 hours. Labeling at 54°C (7% labeling index at 72 hours) was less than at 60°C (11% at 72 hours). In order to determine whether leukocytic infiltration, which is prominent in the 60°C response, is necessary for the endothelial proliferation, rats were made severely leukopenic by total body irradiation of 800 rads accompanied by shielding of the site of thermal injury. At 2–5 days after irradiation, when the leukocyte count was 1–10% of normal, the animals were subjected to thermal injury, and they were studied 3 days later. The data indicate no statistical difference in the proportion of labeled endothelial cells between control and severely leukopenic animals. These experiments suggest that, in the skin, a significant amount of endothelial proliferation can occur in the absence of a prominent cellular inflammatory response.

4. When pieces of necrotic tumor, or tumor tissue killed by boiling, were implanted in the cornea, no neovascularization was induced.

5. Endothelial mitosis and capillary proliferation may be a feature of immunological reactions. Graham and Shannon (1972) noted endothelial mitosis in peroxidase-induced immunological arthritis in conjunction with lymphocytic emigration. We have recently shown that the so-called "activation" of endothelial cells previously observed in delayed hypersensitivity reactions is associated with endothelial proliferation (Polverini and Cotran, 1975). Sidky and Auerbach (1975) showed neovascularization in the graft-vs-host reaction and postulated that sensitized lymphocytes have angiogenic activity. Whether tumor angiogenesis is at all related to this phenomenon is at present unclear. It appears unlikely since angiogenesis occurs after injection of tumor cells in previously unsensitized animals or in immunoincompetent chick embryos and begins very early, within 24 hours of administration of tumor cells or extracts. Recent studies suggest that lymphocytes and macrophages, under certain conditions, induce both stimulatory and inhibitory effects on multiplication of other cells. For example, Calderon et al. (1975) have shown that activated macrophages in culture secrete two different substances: one causing inhibition of lymphocytes, fibroblasts, and

other cells, and the other stimulating lymphocytes *in vitro*. The possibility that these "multispecialty" cells may also be involved in endothelial proliferation deserves further study.

In summary, it appears that the ability of tumor cells to induce angiogenesis is not related to initiation of classical inflammatory or immune responses. Whether the final mechanism of action of tumor and inflammatory stimuli on endothelial replication is similar, remains open to question.

3. *Relationship of TAF to Other Tumor Factors*

Finally, it can be asked whether the factors that induce angiogenesis are related to other important factors produced by tumors, for example, those that result in fibroplasia, or spread of tumor through connective tissue. At present the purification procedures for tumor angiogenesis factor result in materials that are biochemically rather crude. With the present extract, we have observed thymidine-^{3}H labeling as well as mitosis not only in endothelial cells, but also in pericytes, adventitial cells, and, in some instances, fibroblasts. It is too early to tell whether further purification will separate such activities.

C. Inhibition of Angiogensis

In previous experiments, the avascular phase was prolonged by an experimental artifact. Tumors were implanted under special conditions so that a long time was required for capillaries to reach the tumor edge (as in the cornea). In the case of the anterior chamber, capillaries proliferated in the iris, but never reached the tumor.

A more recent study (Brem and Folkman, 1975), showed that a diffusible material from normal cartilage was capable of inhibiting the growth of new capillaries.

1. *Inhibition of Tumor Angiogenesis by a Diffusible Factor from Cartilage*

Human embryonic cartilage is known to be vascularized, but vessels disappear in the early neonatal period (Haraldsson, 1962; Blackwood, 1965). A possible explanation is that a factor inhibitory for capillary proliferation might be turned on during the maturation of neonatal cartilage. Eisenstein *et al.* (1973) have reported that cartilage placed on the CAM did not become vascularized. Recently, we have shown that tumor-induced vessels are inhibited by a diffusible factor from neonatal rabbit cartilage (Brem and Folkman, 1975; Brem *et al.*, 1975). Keuttner *et al.* (1975) have demonstrated that endothelial cells in culture are inhibited by a factor isolated from cartilage.

In our studies (Brem and Folkman, 1975), Walker carcinosarcoma or TAF obtained from the Walker tumor were implanted on chick CAM as sources of neovascularization. A 1-mm piece of neonatal cartilage from rabbit scapula was implanted 1–2 mm from the neovascularizing source. An avascular zone of 1–2 mm width developed around the cartilage (Fig. 13). A similar experiment was

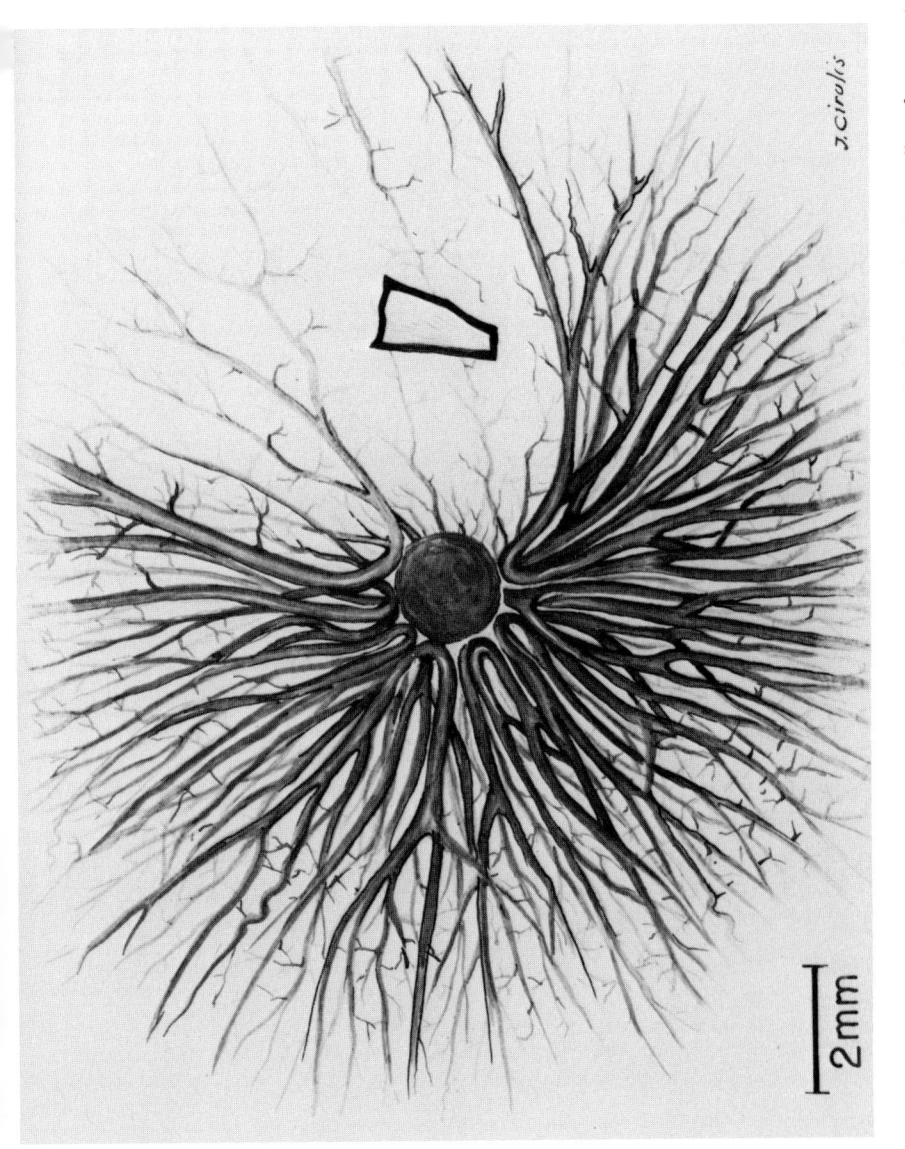

FIG. 13. Diagram of experiment in which tumor angiogenesis factor (TAF) granules (circle in center) and a cartilage fragment (on right side) were implanted on the chorioallantoic membrane. The neovascularization produced by TAF was inhibited in the zone surrounding the cartilage. From Brem and Folkman (1975) with permission of the publisher.

repeated in the rabbit cornea in order to quantitate the inhibitory effect of cartilage on vessel growth. Pieces of neonatal rabbit cartilage (1.0 × 1.5 mm) were implanted in a pocket made in the corneal stroma. V2 carcinoma (1.5 × 1.5 mm) was also implanted in the pocket according to the configuration in Fig. 14. Controls for the active cartilage included cartilage which was boiled, pieces

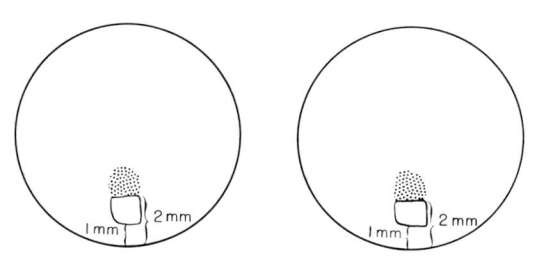

FIG. 14. Diagram of rabbit cornea. V2 carcinoma and neonatal rabbit cartilage (left) are implanted together in a corneal pocket. As a control for neonatal cartilage, boiled cartilage, or pieces of neonatal cornea are used (right).

of neonatal cornea of the same size as the cartilage implant, and fragments of neonatal bone.

Each cornea was examined every other day with a slit-lamp stereomicroscope. One hundred and forty corneas were studied. Measurements of the growth rate of new vessels were made with an accuracy of ± 0.1 mm. The results are summarized in Figs. 15 and 16. In every case, tumor grew slowly, as a thin intracorneal plate. It remained avascular until one edge grew within 2.5 ± 0.5 mm of the limbus. At that point, preexisting vessels in the limbus began to proliferate. New capillaries grew toward the tumor. When tumor was alone, or with cartilage inactivated by boiling, capillaries grew toward the tumor at 0.22 ± 0.12 mm/day during the first week. By the end of the first week, there were up to 30 new capillaries advancing toward the tumor. The rate increased to 0.48 ± 0.16 mm/day by the second week. Within 3 weeks after the onset of neovas-

FIG. 15. Representative corneas after implantation of tumor with active cartilage or with boiled cartilage. This diagram was drawn to scale by tracing color photographs of the actual specimens. The diameter of the cornea is 12 mm. When cartilage is implanted with tumor, the vessels are inhibited from reaching the tumor (A, B, C). With inactive cartilage, the vessels enter the tumor by day 15 and rapid tumor growth follows (E), leading to a large exophytic mass (F). A similar result (D, E, F) is obtained if the boiled cartilage is replaced by neonatal cornea or if tumor alone is implanted. From Brem and Folkman (1975) with permission of the publisher.

30 DAYS	C	F
20 DAYS	B	E
10 DAYS	A	D

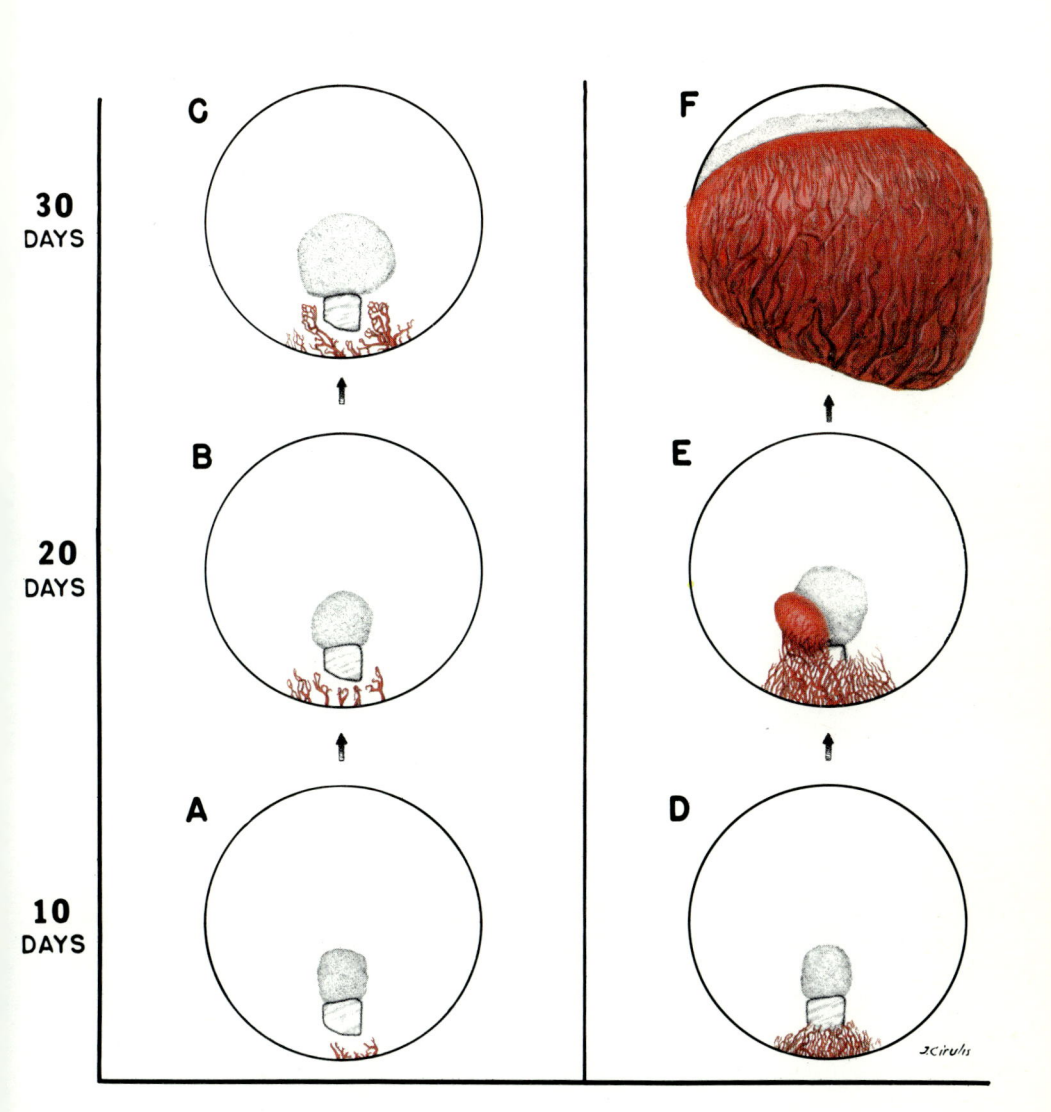

cularization, all the tumors were large, exophytic masses enveloping the eye (Fig. 15F). At this time the capillaries were growing at the rate of 0.6 ± 0.14 mm/day. None of these tumors regressed.

When the tumor was implanted with active neonatal cartilage, the time of onset of neovascularization was similar to that for corneas containing only tumor or tumor with inactive cartilage control. By the end of the first week, a major difference was observed: the density of vessel growth was less (Fig. 15A). Only approximately five new capillaries were advancing toward the tumor. By the second week, another major difference was observed: as the vessel tips grew close to the cartilage, the rate of vessel growth slowed. The average vessel growth rate was only 0.12 ± 0.16 mm/day (Figs. 15B, 16). In some corneas, the vessels

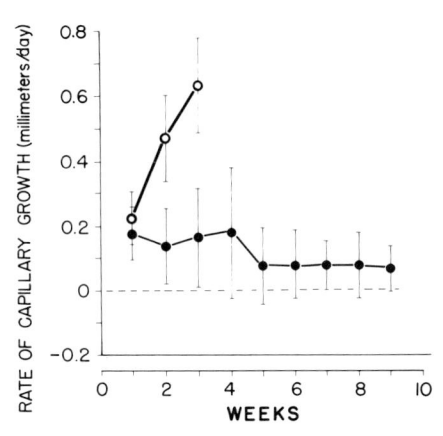

FIG. 16. Rate of capillary growth in rabbit corneas with (●) and without (○) cartilage. Note that some vessels exposed to cartilage actually regressed at the 4th to 10th week. From Brem and Folkman (1975) with permission of the publisher.

stopped advancing and regressed. In other corneas, vessels appeared to oscillate between brief periods of growth and regression, but without forward progress. Twenty-eight percent of these tumors had not vascularized by the end of 3 months, compared to vascularization times of 3 weeks for tumors implanted without cartilage or with inactivated carilage. The unvascularized tumors eventually underwent immunological rejection. No rejections had previously been seen with this tumor during the 4 years it had been carried in the cornea and intramuscularly in our laboratory.

The remaining tumors implanted intracorneally with cartilage eventually became vascularized. This vascularization occurred following the steady growth of the tumor plate in two dimensions within the corneal lamellae. Vessels were elicited at sites of the limbus remote from the cartilage. Once the tumor was

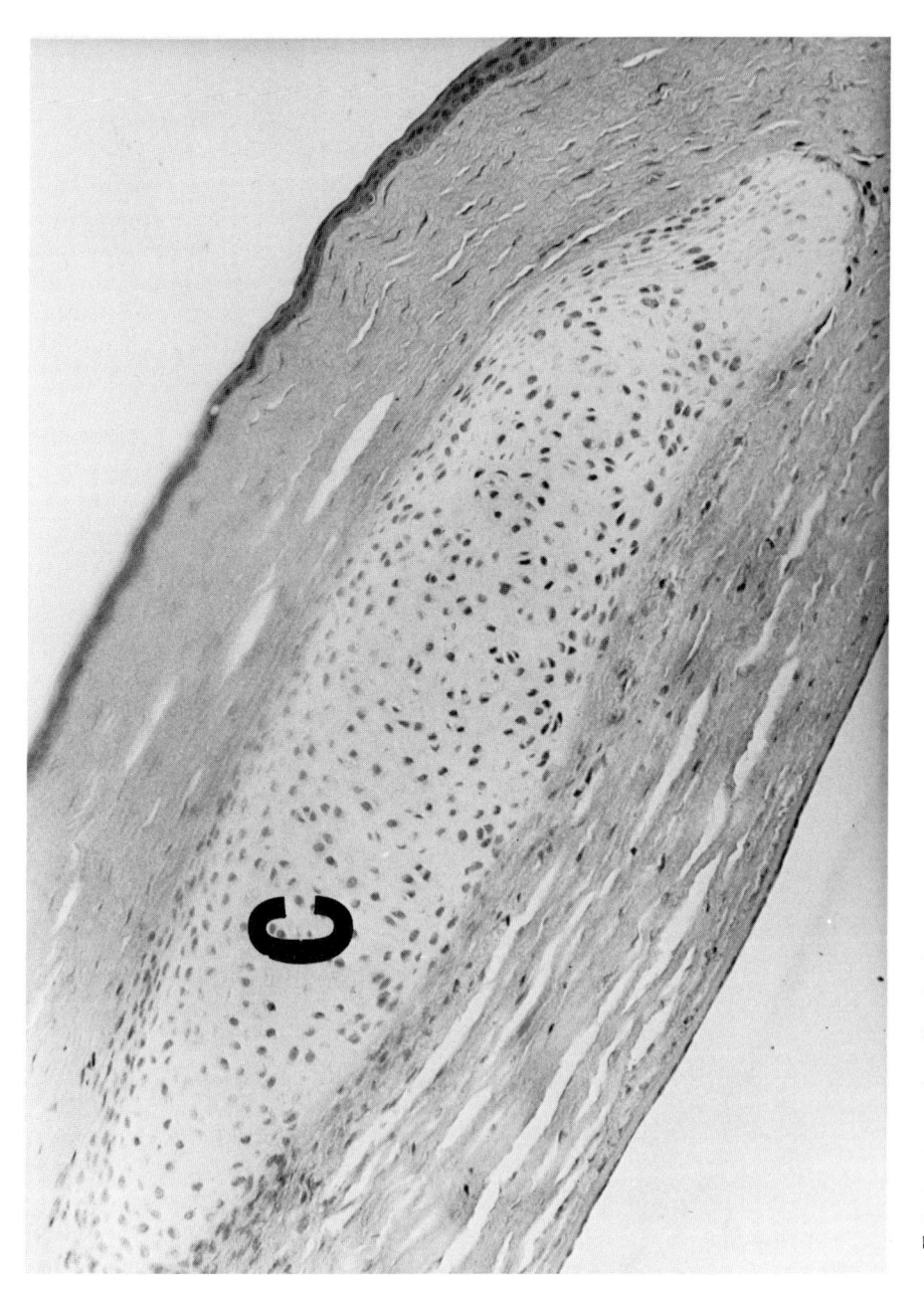

FIG. 17. Neonatal cartilage implant (C) in the rabbit cornea at 30 days. Cartilage is healthy, and there is no inflammatory reaction.

vascularized, rapid exponential growth ensued and the cartilage was completely covered by tumor.

In all corneas, the cartilage implant appeared healthy throughout, by histologic examination. It was not associated with any inflammatory reaction (Fig. 17).

These studies indicate that a diffusible material released from neonatal cartilage inhibits capillary proliferation induced by tumor. The inhibitory effect operates over short distances of up to 2.0 mm and displays a gradient from cartilage source to limbal edge of the cornea. The highest concentration of the inhibitor seems to be closest to the cartilage, because capillary tips slow their growth as they approach the cartilage. The inhibitor is effective even in the face of a rising concentration of TAF stimulator which meets the advancing vessels, because the tumor is implanted just beyond the cartilage. The cartilage inhibitor does not appear to neutralize TAF. If this were the case, lesser amounts of TAF should arrive at the limbus. The *onset* of capillary proliferation in the presence of active cartilage should be delayed. In fact, there was no significant difference between the first appearance of vessels in the corneas containing active cartilage and those containing no cartilage or boiled cartilage. Cartilage appears to produce inhibitor continuously, because the inhibitory effect upon capillary growth lasted through the longest observation period of 4 months. At that time the cartilage appeared histologically viable.

This is the first time, to our knowledge, that a diffusible material from normal tissue has been shown to inhibit capillary proliferation induced by tumors. The material is not inflammatory in the cornea. When this inhibitory factor is further purified and characterized, it may prove useful as a means of maintaining tumor dormancy (Folkman, 1971, 1972).

REFERENCES

Ackerman, N.B. (1974). *Surgery* 75, 589.
Algire, G.H., and Chalkley, H.W. (1945). *J. Nat. Cancer Inst.* 6, 73.
Auerbach, R., Kubai, L., Knighton, D.R., and Folkman, J. (1974). *Develop. Biol.* 41, 391.
Auerbach, R., Arensman, R., Kubai, L., and Folkman, J. (1975). *Int. J. Cancer* 15, 241.
Ausprunk, D.H., Knighton, D.R., and Folkman, J. (1974). *Develop. Biol.* 38, 237.
Ausprunk, D.H., Knighton, D.R., and Folkman, J. (1975). *Amer. J. Pathol.* 79, 597.
Baumgartner, H.R., and Studer, A. (1966). *Pathol. Microbiol.* 29, 393.
Blackwood, H.J.J. (1965). *J. Anat.* 99, 551.
Brem, H., and Folkman, J. (1975). *J. Exp. Med.* 141, 427.
Brem, H., Arensman, R., and Folkman, J. (1975). In "Extracellular Matrix Influences on Gene Expression" (H. Slavkin and R.C. Greulich, eds.), pp. 767–772. Academic Press, New York.
Bronza, J., and Ward, P.A. (1975). *Federation Proc.* 34, 842.
Butler, T., and Gullino, P. (1975). *Cancer Res.* 35, 512.
Calderon J., Kiely, J.M., and Unanue, E. (1975). *Federation Proc.* 34, 959.
Caplan, B.A., and Schwartz, C.J. (1973). *Atherosclerosis* 17, 401.

Cavallo, T., and Cotran, R.S. (1973). *Federation Proc.* **32**, 823.
Cavallo, T., Sade, R., Folkman, J., and Cotran, R.S. (1972). *J. Cell Biol.* **54**, 408.
Cavallo, T., Sade, R., Folkman, J., and Cotran, R.S. (1973). *Amer. J. Pathol.* **70**, 345.
Clark, E.R., and Clark, E.L. (1932). *Amer. J. Anat.* **49**, 441.
Cliff, W.J. (1963). *Phil. Trans. Roy Soc. London, Ser. B* **246**, 305.
Cotran, R.S. (1965). *Amer. J. Pathol.* **46**, 589.
Cotran, R.S. (1967). *Exp. Mol. Pathol.* **6**, 143.
Cotran, R.S., and Majno, G. (1964). *Amer. J. Pathol.* **45**, 261.
Cotran, R.S., and Remensnyder, J.P. (1968). *Ann. N.Y. Acad. Sci.* **150**, 495.
Crane, W.A.J., and Dutta, L.P. (1964). *J. Pathol. Bacteriol.* **88**, 291.
Currie, G. (1973). *Brit. J. Cancer* **28**, 153.
Day, E.D. (1964). In "Progress in Experimental Tumor Research" (F. Homburger, ed.), pp. 58–84. Hafner, New York.
Durward, A., and Rudall, K.M. (1958). In "The Biology of Hair Growth" (W. Montagna and R.A. Ellis, eds.), pp. 189–218. Academic Press, New York.
Ehrmann, R.L., and Knoth, M. (1968). *J. Nat. Cancer Inst.* **41**, 1329.
Eisenstein, R., Sorgente, N., Soble, L.W., Miller, A., and Kuettner, K.E. (1973). *Amer. J. Pathol.* **73**, 765.
Engerman, R.L., Pfaffenbach, D., and Davis, M.D. (1967). *Lab. Invest.* **17**, 738.
Fauve, R.M., Hevin, B., Jacob, H., Gaillard, J.A., and Jacob, F. (1974). *Proc. Nat. Acad. Sci. U.S.* **71**, 4052.
Florentin, R.A., Nam, S.C., Lee, K.T., Lee, K.J., and Thomas, W.A. (1969). *Arch. Pathol.* **88**, 463.
Florey, H. (ed.) (1970). "General Pathology," 4th ed. Lloyd-Luke, London.
Folkman, J. (1970). In "Carcinoma of the Colon and Antecedent Epithelium" (W.J. Burdette, ed.), Chapter 6. Thomas, Springfield, Illinois.
Folkman, J. (1971). *New Engl. J. Med.* **285**, 1182.
Folkman, J. (1972). *Ann. Surg.* **175**, 409.
Folkman, J. (1974a). *Advan. Cancer Res.* **19**, 331–358.
Folkman, J. (1974b). *Cancer Res.* **34**, 2109.
Folkman, J. (1975). *Ann. Int. Med.* **82**, 96.
Folkman, J., and Gimbrone, M. (1971). In "Karolinska Symposia on Research Methods in Reproductive Endocrinology," 4th Symp.: Perfusion Techniques (E. Diczfalusy, ed.). Karolinska Institutet, Stockholm.
Folkman, J., and Hochberg, M. (1973). *J. Exp. Med.* **138**, 745.
Folkman, J., and Klagsbrun, M. (1975). In "Symposium on Fundamental Aspects of Neoplasia" (A. Gottlieb, ed.), pp. 401–412. Springer-Verlag, Berlin and New York.
Folkman, J., Long, D.C., and Becker, F.F. (1963). *Cancer* **16**, 453.
Folkman, J., Cole, P., and Zimmerman, S. (1966). *Ann. Surg.* **164**, 491.
Folkman, J., Merler, E., Abernathy, C., and Williams, G. (1970). *J. Clin. Invest.* **49**, 30a.
Folkman, J., Merler, E., Abernathy, C., and Williams, G. (1971). *J. Exp. Med.* **133**, 275.
Folkman, J., Hochberg, M., and Knighton, D. (1974). "Control of Proliferation in Animal Cells" (B. Clarkson and R. Baserga, (eds.), Cold Spring Harbor Conf. Cell Proliferation Vol. I, pp. 833–842.
Gaynor, E. (1971). *Lab. Invest.* **24**, 318.
Gimbrone, M.A. (1975). In "Progress in Hemostasis and Thrombosis" (T. Spaet, ed.), Vol. III. Grune & Stratton, New York. In press.
Gimbrone, M.A., and Gullino, P.M. (1974). *Fed. Proc.* **33**, 596.
Gimbrone, M.A., Aster, R.H., Cotran, R.S., Corkery, J., Jandl, J., and Folkman, J. (1969). *Nature (London)* **222**, 33.

Gimbrone, M.A., Leapman, S., Cotran, R.S., and Folkman, J. (1972). *J. Exp. Med.* **136**, 261.
Gimbrone, M.A., Cotran, R.S., and Folkman, J. (1973a). *Ser. Haematol.* **4**, 453.
Gimbrone, M.A., Cotran, R.S., Haudenschild, C., and Folkman, J. (1973b). *J. Cell Biol.* **59**, 109a.
Gimbrone, M.A., Cotran, R.S., and Folkman, J. (1973c). *Microvasc. Res.* **6**, 249.
Gimbrone, M.A., Leapman, S., Cotran, R.S., and Folkman, J. (1973d). *J. Nat. Cancer Inst.* **50**, 219.
Gimbrone, M.A., Cotran, R.S., and Folkman, J. (1974a). *J. Cell Biol.* **60**, 673.
Gimbrone, M.A., Cotran, R.S., and Folkman, J. (1974b). *J. Nat. Cancer Inst.* **52**, 413.
Gitterman, C.A., and Luell, S. (1969). *Proc. Amer. Ass. Cancer Res.* **10**, 29.
Goldacre, R.J., and Sylven, B. (1962). *Brit. J. Cancer* **16**, 306.
Goldman, E. (1907). *Lancet* **2**, 1236.
Graham, R.C., and Shannon, S.L. (1972). *Amer. J. Pathol.* **69**, 7.
Greenblatt, M., and Shubik, P. (1968). *J. Nat. Cancer Inst.* **41**, 111.
Greenspan, H.P. (1974). *Growth* **38** (1), 81.
Haraldsson, S. (1962). *Acta Anat.* **48**, 156.
Hasegawe, K. (1934). *Gann* **28**, 32.
Haudenschild, C.C., Cotran, R.S., Gimbrone, M.A., and Folkman, J. (1975a). *J. Ultrastruc. Res.* **50**, 22.
Haudenschild, C.C., Zahniser, D., and Klagsbrun, M. (1975b). *J. Cell Biol.* In press.
Jaffe, E.A., Nachman, R.L., Becker, C.G., and Minick, R.C. (1973). *J. Clin. Invest.* **52**, 2745.
Knighton, D., Ausprunk, D., Tapper, D., and Folkman, J. (1974). Unpublished data.
Kuettner, K.E., Pita, J.C., Howell, D.S., Sorgente, N., Eisenstein, R. (1975). *In* "Extracellular Matrix Influences on Gene Expression" (H. Slavkin, ed.), pp. 435–440. Academic Press, New York.
Maruyama, Y. (1963). *Z. Zellforsch. Mikrosk. Anat.* **60**, 69.
Polverini, P., and Cotran, R.S. (1975). *J. Dental Res.* In press.
Poole, J.C.F., Sanders, A.G., and Florey, H.W. (1958). *J. Pathol. Bacteriol.* **75**, 133.
Remensnyder, J., and Majno, G. (1968). *Amer. J. Pathol.* **52**, 301.
Ryan, T.J. (1973). *In* "The Physiology and Pathophysiology of the Skin" (A. Jarret, ed.), pp. 779–805. Academic Press, New York.
Sade, R.M., Folkman, J., and Cotran, R.S. (1972). *Exp. Cell. Res.* **74**, 297.
Schoefl, G.I. (1963). *Virchows Arch. Pathol. Anat. Physiol.* **337**, 97.
Schoefl, G.I., and Majno, G. (1964). *In* "Advances in Biology of Skin" (W. Montagna and R.A. Ellis, eds.), pp. 173–193. Pergamon, N.Y.
Schwartz, S., and Benditt, E. (1973). *Lab. Invest.* **28**, 699.
Selye, H., (1953). *J. Amer. Med. Ass.* **152**, 1207.
Sholley, M.M., and Cotran, R.S. (1976). Unpublished.
Sholley, M.M., Cavallo, T., and Cotran, R.S. (1974). *Anat. Record* **178**, 462.
Sidky, Y.A., and Auerbach, R. (1975). *Fed. Proc.* **34**, 1040.
Süss, R., Kinzel, V., and Scribner, J.D., eds. (1973). *In* "Cancer Experiments and Concepts," p. 70. Springer-Verlag, Berlin and New York.
Tannock, I.F., and Hayashi, S. (1972). *Cancer Res.* **32**, 77.
Tuan, D., Smith, S., Folkman, J., and Merler, E. (1973). *Biochemistry* **12**, 3159.
Urbach, F. (1961). *In* "Advances in Biology of the Skin" (W. Montagna and R.A. Ellis, eds.), pp. 123–149. Pergamon, N.Y.
Virchow, R. (1863). "Die Krankhaften Geschwülste." Hirschwald, Berlin.
Warren, B.A., and Shubik, P (1966). *Lab. Invest.* **15**, 464.

Widman, J., and Cotran, R.S. (1975). Unpublished.
Wood, S. (1958). *Arch. Pathol.* **66**, 550.
Wright, H.P. (1970). *Thromb. Diath. Haemorrh. Suppl.* **40**, 79.
Yamagami, I. (1970). *Jap. J. Ophthalmol.* **14**, 41.
Yamaura, H., and Sato, H. (1973). *In* "Chemotherapy of Cancer Dissemination and Metastasis" (S. Garattini and G. Franchi, eds.), pp. 149–175. Raven Press, New York.
Young, J.S., Lumsden, C.E., and Stalker, A.L. (1950). *J. Pathol. Bacteriol.* **62**, 313.

Biochemical, Functional, and Structural Aspects of Phagocytosis

ANTHONY J. SBARRA, RATNAM J. SELVARAJ, BENOY B. PAUL, PAULA K. F. POSKITT, JAN M. ZGLICZYNSKI, GEORGE W. MITCHELL, JR., and FARID LOUIS

Department of Medical Research and Laboratories and Department of Pathology, St. Margaret's Hospital, and Department of Obstetrics and Gynecology, Tufts University School of Medicine, Boston, Massachusetts

I.	Introduction	249
II.	Production and Maturation	250
	A. Polymorphonuclear Leukocytes	250
	B. Monocytes and Macrophages	252
III.	Chemotaxis	252
IV.	Recognition Factors	253
V.	Morphological Events during Phagocytosis	254
VI.	Biochemical and Antimicrobial Activities of Different Cells	255
	A. Polymorphonuclear Leukocytes	255
	B. Macrophages	259
	C. Bactericidal and Associated Metabolic Activities of Mouse Spleen Cells	260
	D. Relationships between Metabolic and Bactericidal Activities	263
VII.	Alterations and Decreased Resistance to Infections	263
	A. Altered Chemotaxis	264
	B. Altered Recognition Activity	264
	C. Altered Biochemical and Microbicidal Activity	265
	References	269

I. Introduction

It was in Messina, Italy, in 1882 that Elie Metchnikoff the zoologist became a pathologist. Metchnikoff loved Messina, with its rich marine fauna and beautiful scenery. The view of the sea and the calm outline of the Calabrian coast across the straits were a delight to him. It was here that he entered a new arena in which all his later activity was to be exerted. It all began one quiet afternoon when, while observing through his microscope life in the mobile cells of a transparent starfish larva, a thought suddenly occurred to him. Could similar cells serve in the defense of the organisms against intruders? After some thought and a walk along the seashore, he reasoned that if a splinter is introduced into the body of a starfish larva, free of blood vessels and of a nervous system, it should soon be surrounded by mobile cells, as is observed in man with a splinter in his finger. Quickly he obtained a few rose thorns and introduced them under the skin of the starfish larva. These experiments formed the basis of the phagocytic theory to which he completely devoted the next 25 years of his life. During this time the theory was developed and defended, heatedly at times, in numerous publications and congresses. The importance of phagocytosis as a defense mechanism against infectious disease has not been seriously questioned since.

Surprisingly, however, the mechanisms by which phagocytes engulf and destroy microbes are not completely known. Even more surprising is our relative ignorance regarding marrow production and storage of phagocytes, delivery to the blood, margination and immigration, and actual contact with the microbes. Information relative to all the above areas is essential in order to fully comprehend phagocytosis. Within the last decade or so significant information has appeared regarding the interactions of the phagocyte with the microbe and antimicrobial activity. Since these activities are of major importance and have been and are of interest in our laboratory, we will focus in this chapter on the recent developments and current understanding in this area. We will discuss the structure and the biochemical activities of the cell as they relate to antimicrobial activities in the polymorphonuclear leukocyte, the monocyte and macrophage, and the lymphocyte. Also, alterations in biochemical and antimicrobial activities will be shown to correlate with decreased resistance to infectious disease.

We realize that we are discussing only a part of the phagocytic process. Information relative to other aspects of phagocytosis (i.e., chemotaxis, recognition factors) is emerging, and one can confidently predict that significant advances in these critical areas will be forthcoming.

II. Production and Maturation

A. POLYMORPHONUCLEAR LEUKOCYTES

In general, agreement has been reached on the overall granulocyte maturation process. Six developmental stages are recognized in smears of bone marrow stained with Wright's stain. The most immature precursor cell of the granulocytes is the myeloblast, recognized by its large oval nucleus and strongly basophilic cytoplasm, free of granules. With the appearance of metachromatic azurophilic granules staining red-to-purple, the cell becomes a progranulocyte. As specific granules emerge, it becomes a myelocyte. This can be of the eosinophilic, basophilic, or heterophilic variety in a given cell.

When a distinct indentation of the nucleus occurs and the cell size is reduced, the cell is designated a metamyelocyte. When the nuclear indentation becomes marked, the cell is termed a "band" cell. It becomes a mature granulocyte when nuclear segmentation into distinct lobes occurs. Under ordinary circumstances the total maturation process takes approximately 96 hours. The cell undergoes 4 to 5 mitotic divisions. These occur only during the first three stages.

As it is well known that polymorphonuclear leukocyte (PMN) granules are intimately related to the antimicrobial activities of the cell, a brief discussion of their origin, nature, and distribution would be in order. Two distinct types of granules can be distinguished: azurophilic and specific. Both are produced by the Golgi complex, but at different stages of maturation and from different faces of the Golgi complex. Azurophilic granules are formed only during the progranulocyte stage and originate from the proximal or concave face of the Golgi complex. They are larger and more dense than the specific granules. The latter arise from the distal or convex face of the Golgi complex and are formed during the myelocyte stage. Progranulocytes contain only azurophilic granules. In mature PMN, relatively few azurophils are noted. Most of the granules present are of the specific type. The inversion of the azurophilic granule to specific granule ratio occurs during the myelocyte stage. Additional information relative to the development of these granules can be obtained by consulting papers of Bainton and Farquhar (1966, 1968).

The possibility that the two different granular types might have different compositions has been explored. Briefly, the azurophils contain approximately 90% of the cell's myeloperoxidase (MPO) activity. On the other hand, the specific granules are essentially devoid of MPO; however, they contain essentially all the lactoferrin and 50% of the lysozyme. Lactoferrin and MPO, as measured immunochemically, appear to be the most reliable markers for specific and azurophilic granules (Spitznagel et al., 1974). In addition to MPO, the azurophilic granules also contain acid phosphatase, arylsulfatase, β-glucuronidase, esterase, and 5'-nucleotidase. The finding of these lysosomal enzymes in the azurophilic granules suggests that this granule is a primary lysosome. Alkaline phosphatase was originally thought to originate in the specific granules. However, some recent work in Spitznagel's laboratory has challenged this. Perhaps the enzyme is located on the membranous surfaces of granules and its associations with specific granules is different from that of lactoferrin and lysozyme. Moreover, Spitznagel has recently suggested that azurophilic granules can be further resolved during velocity centrifugation into two subclasses. This is a new finding, not noted in earlier biochemical and morphological studies, and obviously will require further study (Spitznagel et al., 1974).

B. Monocytes and Macrophages

The origin of curculating monocytes is now established. Monocytes originate from precursor cells in the bone marrow and eventually migrate into the tissues to become macrophages. The life cycle of monocytes consists of maturation in the bone marrow for a 1—3-day period; they circulate for a 24- to 36-hour period in the blood and then migrate in the tissues, where they function as macrophages. Monocytes contain azurophilic granules, and also lysosomal enzymes, including peroxidase. It seems likely that the azurophilic granules of monocytes are primary lysosomes comparable to the azurophils of the PMN leukocytes (Nichols et al., 1971).

A monocytic origin has been established for macrophages residing in the serous cavities (e.g., peritoneal) and in many other sites, such as the liver, lung, and connective tissue of the skin. Considerable attention has been and is being focused on the alveolar macrophage. Certainly, the methodology advanced by Myrvik permitting us to obtain relatively pure preparations of pulmonary mononuclear cells, mainly alveolar macrophages by pulmonary lavage in experimental animals and man has been the impetus. The alveolar macrophage is characterized by phagocytic and migratory properties. It has a large nucleus, smooth and rough endoplasmic reticulum, numerous mitochondria and vacuolar structures representing varying stages of lysosome and phagosome interactions (Gee, 1970).

Recently, van Furth has advanced the concept that the mononuclear phagocytes of the bone marrow, peripheral blood and tissues are closely related with respect to morphology, origin, and function. As a result, he has grouped them together in the "mononuclear phagocyte system" (van Furth and Thompson, 1971). The relationship of these cells is schematically outlined below.

Bone marrow	Peripheral blood	Tissue
Promonocyte	Monocyte	Peritoneal macrophage, alveolar macrophage, Kupffer cells, skin macrophage

III. Chemotaxis

The term chemotaxis refers to the directional motion of a cell along a concentration gradient. There is some agreement that chemotaxis is a major mechanism by which phagocytic cells are induced to move to the site of infection. Two different, major methodologies have been developed for the study of movement of cells toward a site: The "skin window" technique of Rebuck and Crowley (1955) and the chemotaxis chambers of Boyden (1962).

The making of a "skin window" has been adequately described by Rebuck and Crowley. In normal adults, 2–4 hours after abrasion, the cells observed are almost exclusively neutrophils. By 8 hours approximately 50% of the adherent cells are mononuclear, and at 24 hours mononuclear cells predominate.

In vitro chemotactic studies have generally utilized a chamber described by Boyden (1962). The chamber contains two adjacent compartments separated by a Millipore filter with pores sufficiently large to permit leukocytes to pass. By placing a leukocytic suspension in one compartment and a test substance in the other, one may measure the number of leukocytes migrating through the filter. This provides a measure of the chemotactic activity and the nature of the test substance. It does not provide any information relative to mechanisms of the motile response by the phagocytes.

Release of chemotactic factors has been shown to occur when microorganisms interact with host tissue. Certain microorganisms liberate substances that are able to attract phagocytes (e.g., endotoxin). The principal mechanism by which bacteria produce chemotactic factors, however, is by activating serum complement. For example, antibody can react with the microbial surface, and the resulting antigen–antibody complex activates the hemolytic complement components C1, C4, and C2. This complex can in turn attack C3 and C5 to yield C3a and C5a. Both of these are low-molecular-weight peptides with chemotactic activity (Sorkin et al., 1970). In the absence of specific antibody, microorganisms can generate C5a from C5 and C3a from C3 in serum by activating the alternative complement pathway or the properdin system (Sandberg et al., 1972). Also, nonspecific bacterial or damaged tissue proteases can attack directly C3 and C5, thus producing C3a and C5a. Chemotactic activity can also be generated by other serum reactions. Hageman factor activation can lead to the formation of kallikrein and plasminogen activator, and both these substances have chemotactic activity (Kaplan et al., 1972, 1973). Furthermore, ingestion of particulate material by PMN may cause them to release a factor that can attract other neutrophils in the absence of serum (Zigmond and Hirsch, 1973). Finally, lymphocytes, in response to antigens, may elaborate lymphokines, which have chemotactic activity for monocytes (David, 1966).

It is apparent from the above that the generation of soluble chemotactic factors can be demonstrated in vitro. The possible significance of this in vivo, however, has yet to be determined.

IV. Recognition Factors

In general, in order for a phagocyte to ingest microbes, it must first recognize them. Phagocytosis of pathogens is often facilitated by serum factors called opsonins. In some, as yet unknown, way the bacterial surface is modified so that it becomes more easily ingested by the phagocytes. A number of opsonic factors have been described in serum. Activated C3 and IgG are apparently the most important and best characterized opsonins of serum.

Interestingly, opsonization of particles by complement proteins has been noted only with the active fragment of C3. Other C3 fragments may bind to particles and be immunologically detectable, but the particle is not opsonized or ingested. Of the immunoglobulins, only IgG_1 and IgG_3 molecules with intact F_c and F_{ab} regions opsonize.

These specificities suggest that ingestion of opsonized particles involves receptor molecules on the phagocyte surface. Considerable work on the receptor problem is currently underway. However, before major contributions will occur, our knowledge regarding the nature and composition of the phagocytic membrane and the chemical and physical nature of the microbial surface will need to be increased.

V. Morphological Events during Phagocytosis

During phagocytosis leukocytic cytoplasmic granules release their contents into the phagocytic vacuoles containing ingested microorganisms. As pointed out above, two general granular types have been described, specific and azurophilic granules. Both are bound by membranes. The azurophilic granules contain approximately 90% of the MPO activity. Since MPO has been shown to be a critical reactant in the antimicrobial activity of the cell, the fate of the azurophilic granule during phagocytosis is of interest. During phagocytosis the granules appear to move forcibly into proximity to the phagosome. They subsequently fuse with the phagosomal vacuole and disappear. This phenomenon has been referred to as degranulation and is considered a mechanism whereby MPO and other enzymes are released to the microbial site without dilution into the cytoplasm. Degranulation and ingestion seem to be triggered by a similar, if not the same, mechanism. The primary and secondary granules of granulocytes degranulate at somewhat different rates during phagocytosis. The secondary granules appear to fuse with the phagosome before the primary granules (Stossel, 1974).

The release of lysosomal enzymes outside of the cell has also been reported. This extracellular release can result from the leakage of granule contents out of incompletely sequestered phagosomes, from disruptions of the cell or possibly by active secretion after exposure of the cell to different agents (Henson, 1971).

Microtubules and microfilaments appear to be involved in the mechanism of degranulation. Apparently, microfilaments closely apposed to cell membranes break away and allow the granules to fuse with the phagosome. The phagosome is bound by plasma membrane. An alteration in degranulation can be expected to result in altered bactericidal activity.

A distinct abnormality in degranulation has been noted in monocytes and neutrophils collected from patients with the Chediak–Higashi syndrome. The phagocytes in this disorder have giant primary granules that fail to fuse with the phagosome. This results in a functional MPO deficiency and a deficient bactericidal effect. Delayed degranulation has been occasionally observed in neutrophils of patients with chronic granulomatous disease. This certainly can contribute to impaired killing activity noted in these cells.

VI. Biochemical and Antimicrobial Activities of Different Cells

Within the past decade an enormous amount of effort has been directed at identifying the specific biochemical reactions responsible for the antimicrobial activity of phagocytes. Without doubt, the impetus for these concentrated efforts has been the elucidation of the dramatic metabolic changes which occur when phagocytic cells are challenged with particulate material. In this section we shall highlight those metabolic events that are enhanced in the PMN during phagocytosis and shall correlate the stimulated activities with antimicrobial activity of the cell. A possible mechanism of action of a particle-activated antimicrobial system will also be presented. Attention will be focused on the PMN, as the bulk of the information available relates to this cell type. To show that the phagocytic and antimicrobial activities of the PMN are not unique to this cell type, two other cell types will be discussed, namely, the rabbit alveolar macrophage and the mouse spleen lymphocyte. It is known that the alveolar macrophage is a phagocytic cell and is capable of being metabolically stimulated when challenged with particulate material. The degree of stimulation is lower in these cells than in the PMN; however, the stimulated activities appear to be similarly related to antimicrobial function. The mouse spleen lymphocytes will also be discussed. Conventional phagocytosis of particles by these cells is not demonstrable by either light or electron microscopy. However, particle challenge elicits metabolic enhancement similar to that found in particle-stimulated, conventional phagocytes. Interestingly, the splenic lymphocytes exhibit bactericidal activity by mechanisms that are similar in many aspects to those of the PMN.

A. Polymorphonuclear Leukocytes

1. *Metabolic Activities*

Phagocytosis and intracellular killing of microorganisms seem to be two separate and distinct physiological functions of PMN. Engulfment of bacteria and other particulate material is an endergonic process dependent upon energy derived from glycolysis (Sbarra and Karnovsky, 1959). Postengulfment metabolic activity of phagocytes is mainly oxidative in nature and has been related to intracellular antimicrobial activity (Selvaraj and Sbarra, 1966). Evidence for these statements is provided by the observations that particle engulfment by PMN is inhibited by the glycolytic antagonists iodoacetic acid (IAA) and sodium fluoride, but not by inhibitors of oxidative metabolism, such as antimycin A, and that bactericidal activity by these cells is markedly reduced under anaerobic conditions (Selvaraj and Sbarra, 1966; McRipley and Sbarra, 1967b). Oxygen consumption, the flow of glucose through the HMS and certain oxidative activities, namely, NADPH oxidase (Rossi et al., 1972; Paul et al., 1972), NADH oxidase (Cagan and Karnovsky, 1964), glutathione (GSSG) reductase (Reed, 1969; Strauss et al., 1969), and MPO (Paul et al., 1970a) are all significantly increased during phagocytosis by PMN. Production of H_2O_2, an end product of NADPH and NADH oxidation (Roberts and Quastel, 1964), as well as D- and L-amino acid oxidases (Cline and Lehrer, 1969; Skarnes, 1970) is also increased in PMN stimulated by phagocytosis. The anti-inflammatory drug phenylbutazone inhibits the HMS at the level of glucose-6-phosphate dehydrogenase (G6PDH) and 6-phosphogluconate dehydrogenase (6PGDH) and also inhibits H_2O_2 production in phagocytizing PMN. This compound also inhibits the killing of phagocytized bacteria by these cells (Strauss et al., 1968; Kvarstein and Stormorken, 1971). The increased production of H_2O_2 by phagocytizing leukocytes is most interesting. This substance has long been known to be a potent antimicrobial agent. However, the amount of H_2O_2 produced by PMN neutrophils during phagocytosis by itself does not appear to be sufficient for the observed bactericidal activity by these cells. If, however, one reacts sublethal concentrations of H_2O_2 and peroxidase with a halide, either I^-, Cl^-, or Br^-, at acid pH, significant bactericidal activity is obtained (Klebanoff, 1968; McRipley and Sbarra, 1967b).

2. Peroxidase Activity

This H_2O_2–peroxidase–halide antimicrobial system is now generally accepted as at least one mechanism by which phagocytes can kill some engulfed microorganisms. The system has been found in human peripheral blood PMNs, guinea pig exudate PMNs (Paul et al., 1970b; Jacobs et al., 1970; Strauss et al., 1971), and recently in mouse spleen cells (Strauss et al., 1972a,b), guinea pig bone marrow cells (Paul et al., 1973a), and rabbit alveolar macrophages (Paul et al., 1973b). The spectrum of organisms affected by this system includes gram-negative and gram-positive bacteria (McRipley and Sbarra, 1967a,b), fungi and yeasts (Lehrer, 1969), viruses (Belding et al., 1970), and mycoplasma (Jacobs et al., 1972).

The MPO of neutrophils appears unique in that it is capable of catalyzing the decarboxylation and deamination of amino acids in the presence of H_2O_2 and Cl^- (Zgliczynski et al., 1968; Jacobs et al., 1970). Subsequently, it was shown that this MPO–H_2O_2–Cl^- system can chlorinate amino acids, with resulting formation of chloramines of amino acids. Formation of chloramines most likely occurs through the MPO-catalyzed oxidation of Cl^- by H_2O_2 to yield an active species, possibly Cl^+. The decomposition of α-amino acid chloramines results in the formation of NH_3, CO_2, Cl^-, and corresponding aldehydes (Zgliczynski et al., 1971). The conditions required for chlorination of amino acids appear to be similar to those required for the antimicrobial activity of the $MPO-H_2O_2-Cl^-$ system. The correlation between amino acid chlorination and antimicrobial activity is supported by findings that taurine inhibits both decarboxylation (Zgliczynski et al., 1968) and bactericidal ability of the MPO system (Jacobs et al., 1970). The questions arises whether all the necessary requirements for chlorination and bactericidal activity of the $MPO-H_2O_2-Cl^-$ system are present in PMN. The available evidence indicates that phagocytizing PMN do possess all the required factors for the optimal activity of this system. The absolute requirement for H_2O_2 is satisfactorily covered by enhanced H_2O_2 production during phagocytosis (Paul and Sbarra, 1968). The pH inside phagocytic vacuole is slightly acidic (Mandell, 1970), and this has been considered to be important for chlorination and killing of bacteria. Some question has been raised as to the extent of the pH drop in human cells. Since the $MPO-H_2O_2$-halide system has been shown to function optimally at a pH of approximately 5.0, the possibility that this level of acidity is not reached would cast considerable doubt on the physiological function of the system. However, recent observations from our laboratory have revealed that the $MPO-H_2O_2-Cl^-$ system can function efficiently at a neutral pH. This can occur providing sufficiently low concentrations of H_2O_2 and high concentrations of Cl^- ions are present. The affinity between H_2O_2 and MPO decreases when the concentration of H^+ ion increases (Zgliczynski et al., 1976). This finding indicates that the MPO system can be made to function in chlorination reactions essentially independent of pH. For example, either by using lower concentrations of H_2O_2 at neutral pH or by using higher concentrations of H_2O_2 at lower pH, an efficient velocity of the reaction can be obtained.

The physiological importance of the chlorination reaction was recently emphasized by the observation that human leukocytes incubated with bacteria (*Staphylococcus epidermidis*), autologous serum, and $Na^{36}Cl$ incorporate radioactivity into the insoluble fraction of the cells. The incorporation of ^{36}Cl occurs only in the presence of bacteria (Zgliczynski and Stelmaszynska, 1975). Iodination of bacteria has also been reported to occur when the halide employed is I^- (Klebanoff, 1967). However, iodination has been shown to occur independent of killing. Further, the concentration of I^- required *in vitro* for killing is generally not reached *in vivo*. The physiological significance of this iodination reaction in killing remains to be clarified.

3. *Chlorination and Decarboxylation: A Possible Mechanism of Action of $MPO-H_2O_2-Cl^-$ Antimicrobial System*

The precise mechanism responsible for the antimicrobial activity of $MPO-H_2O_2-Cl^-$ system is presently under study. However, it is likely that chlorination is the first important step in this system. $MPO-H_2O_2-Cl^-$ mixture needs intimate contact with bacteria to exert its bactericidal activity (Paul et al., 1970b). This was demonstrated by incubation of microorganisms with MPO–Cl⁻ and H_2O_2, but MPO and bacteria were separated by a dialysis membrane. Under these conditions no cidal activity was observd (Paul et al., 1970b). When MPO has the opportunity to bind to bacteria in phagosomes, direct chlorination may take place. Electron microscopic evidence has also been presented by Klebanoff (1970) to show that bacteria in phagosomes are coated by MPO. This chlorination of bacterial cell wall may give rise to structural changes sufficiently grave to result in killing. One possibility of this kind of action is being investigated. By labeling bacterial cell wall proteins with [1,7-^{14}C] diaminopimelic acid (DAP), we have noted directly that this antimicrobial system can attack carboxyl groups of protein-bound DAP. Furthermore, according, to the current concept of the structure of DAP-containing glycosaminopeptides in the cell wall, for every two DAP molecules only two of the four carboxyl groups are free: Of these two carboxyl groups, only one has a free α-amino group. So the maximal $^{14}CO_2$ production from DAP in the labeled bacteria should be (1) <25%, if only free α-amino carboxyl groups are attacked; (2) 25–50%, if all free carboxyl groups are attacked; and (3) >50%, if all the carboxyl groups, including those in peptide linkage are attacked. We have noted that under appropriate conditions, over 80% of the radioactivity can be recovered as $^{14}CO_2$ from DAP-labeled bacteria. These data suggest that a universal reaction in which peptide bonds are broken may occur rather than a specific reaction confined to DAP-containing proteins (Selvaraj et al., 1974).

Exactly how the MPO–H_2O_2–Cl⁻ system splits the peptide bonds for decarboxylation of amino acids is not yet certain. However, it has been demonstrated that MPO–H_2O_2–Cl⁻ and free amino acids interact to form amino acid chloramines (Stelmaszynska and Zgliczynski, 1974). The chloramines are unstable and, in the presence of water, spontaneously decompose to form aldehydes, CO_2, and NH_4Cl. It is likely, therefore, that MPO–H_2O_2–Cl⁻ similarly chlorinates peptide bonds with the formation of amino acid chloramines and, thus, results in peptide cleavage. It may be inferred that chlorination of microorganisms is a mechanism by which the antimicrobial effect of MPO–H_2O_2–Cl⁻ is exerted. The possible sequence of reactions is illustrated in Fig. 1.

Furthermore, it has been demonstrated that singlet oxygen can be formed by MPO–H_2O_2 in the presence of chloride ions (Allen et al., 1972). Being a potent oxidant, singlet oxygen could participate in oxidative cleavage of peptide bonds. Krinsky (1974) has recently shown that human PMN can kill a colorless mutant strain of *Sarcina lutea* much more readily than a carotenoid-containing strain. A similar protective effect has been reported in the organism during photodynamic inactivation, where it is attributable to the quenching of singlet excited oxygen by carotenoids. This recent finding is further support that singlet oxygen can act as a mediator of PMN bactericidal activity. In addition, it has been shown that the superoxide anion and superoxide dismutase may also have a role in the

$$2H_2O_2 \qquad 2Cl^- + 2H^+$$
$$\downarrow \text{MPO}$$

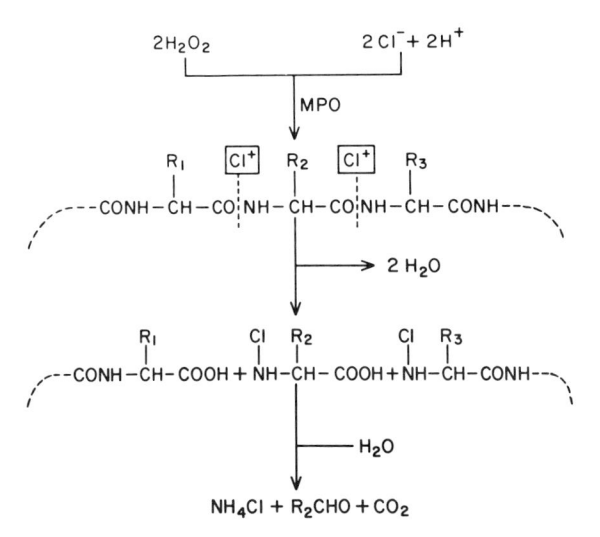

[Structure: ---CONH–CH(R₁)–CO·NH–CH(R₂)–CO·NH–CH(R₃)–CONH--- with Cl⁺ inserted between residues]

$$\longrightarrow 2H_2O$$

[---CONH–CH(R₁)–COOH + NH–CH(Cl)(R₂)–COOH + NH–CH(Cl)(R₃)–CONH---]

$$\longleftarrow H_2O$$

$$NH_4Cl + R_2CHO + CO_2$$

FIG. 1. Possible mechanism of chlorination and aldehyde formation by the myeloperoxidase (MPO)–H_2O_2–Cl^- antimicrobial system.

antimicrobial activity of PMN. The superoxide anion can result from the oxidation of NADPH by its oxidase. Also, it has been found that the reduction of cytochrome *c* by intact leukocytes is inhibited by superoxide dismutase. The above suggests that the superoxide anion is formed by the cell. Incubation of cells in the presence of latex particles increases its formation. Recently, it has been shown that superoxide dismutase and scavengers of superoxide anion and hydroxyl radicals influence microbicidal activity, possibly through their effect on H_2O_2 formation (Klebanoff, 1974).

B. Macrophages

The macrophage is an important cell in the expression of antimicrobial resistance against a wide variety of infections. The immediate source of exudative macrophages are the circulating monocytes. Although circulating monocytes are a minor constituent of blood, kinetic data indicate that removal of monocytes from the circulation runs at an elevated level during infection. Histochemical studies indicate that macrophages arrive in an unmodified form at sites of bacterial implantation. However, shortly after arrival they change to an activated form. They appear larger and show a markedly increased content of lysosomal enzymes. Further, these adaptive changes are accentuated in animals that are already hypersensitive to the infective agent.

The precise mechanism of macrophage activation is of interest and puzzling. For example, Simon and Sheagren (1972) have shown that macrophages which had been incubated with Bacillus Calmette-Guérin (BCG)-immune lymphocytes in the presence of BCG displayed a markedly enhanced listericidal activity. In parallel experiments, the same antigen-stimulated lymphocytes were shown to inhibit the migration of normal macropages. In spite of this, the exact molecular basis of the macrophage–lymphocyte interaction, and subsequent activation must await further study.

The ability of the rabbit alveolar macrophage to engulf and kill microorganisms is well accepted. The cell responds to particle challenge by enhanced metabolism, which is qualitatively similar to, but quantitatively less than, that seen in PMN (Ouchi et al., 1965). Since peroxidase activity was not found histochemically in this cell, the stimulated oxidative activities appeared to be of questionable significance. However, recent demonstrations that the alveolar macrophage has low but detectable peroxidase activity suggest that a similar correlation between biochemical and antimicrobial activity may occur with this cell type as with the PMN. Increased activities may be noted if the assay is performed under somewhat different assay conditions. For example, if the assay is carried out in the absence of sucrose, with increased H_2O_2 concentration, at 37°C and in the presence of cetyltrimethylammonium bromide, significant peroxidase activity is detectable. Admittedly, the enzyme activity is significantly less on a per cell basis than in the PMN. Nevertheless, it can participate in the antimicrobial activities of the cell. The peroxidase activity of this cell is similar to horseradish and lactoperoxidase in that the functional halide in the antimicrobial system is iodide, not chloride (Paul et al., 1973b).

The possibility that catalase is behaving as a peroxidase has not been completely ruled out. However, the bulk of catalase is present in the 20,000 g supernatant fraction, whereas the peroxidase and bactericidal activity reside principally in the 20,000 g pellet. It appears then that a peroxidase H_2O_2–halide system is present in the alveolar macrophage and potentially available as a killing mechanism.

C. Bactericidal and Associated Metabolic Activities of Mouse Spleen Cells

Spleen cells, predominantly lymphocytes by morphology, collected from non-leukemic AKR and CD-1 mice, are able to kill *Escherichia coli in vitro*. When these cells are incubated with particles such as heat-killed bacteria or polystyrene latex spheres, there is significant increase in glucose-1-^{14}C oxidation, a measure of hexose monophosphate shunt (HMS) activity, NADPH oxidation and formate ^{14}C oxidation (Strauss et al., 1972b). The latter is an indirect measurement of H_2O_2. These cells also contain peroxidase activity, which is increased in the presence of particles. The 20,000 g pellet fraction of mouse spleen cell homogenates contains a peroxidase–H_2O_2–Cl^- bactericidal system which is qualitatively similar to that found in PMN of other species. This enzyme has an absolute requirement for both H_2O_2 and chloride for bactericidal and amino acid decarboxylation activities. Like the MPO-mediated system, it functions optimally at pH 5.5. There is also a linear correlation between bactericidal activity and peroxidase-mediated amino acid decarboxylation. On a "per guaiacol unit" basis, however, splenoperoxidase (SPO) is not as potent as MPO for amino acid decarboxylation or bactericidal activity (Strauss et al., 1972a,b). The choride requirement of SPO is about 20 times greater than that of MPO for these activities when compared on the same basis of guaiacol units.

Whole-body X-irradiation of mice provides another means of differentiating the activity of SPO from that of MPO in the spleen. Spleen cell suspensions from irradiated animals contain a significantly greater percentage of PMN than those from nonirradiated controls. Irradiation also caused a marked decrease in the percentage of cells identified as lymphocytes in these preparations. The peroxidase activity of the 20,000 g pellet fraction from homogenates of these cells is similar to that of MPO with respect to bactericidal potency and amino acid decarboxylation activity per unit of guaiacol activity (Paul et al., 1970c).

In contrast to spleen cells from normal animals, spleen cells from leukemic AKR mice are unable to kill bacteria when tested under identical conditions. Metabolic studies of cells from leukemic animals indicate significant decreases in G6PDH, GSSG reductase, and peroxidase activities when compared to those of spleen cells from normal AKR mice. Formate-^{14}C oxidation by cells from leukemic animals is markedly increased. These results are derived from data based on the total cell population. If the data are calculated on the basis of the number of PMN present in the cell suspensions, there is no significant difference between cells from normal and leukemic mice with respect to GSSG reductase and G6PDH activities. The differences in formate oxidation and peroxidase activities are significant by either calculation. The increased H_2O_2 content as determined by formate oxidation is probably directly related to the decrease in peroxidase activity. The marked decrease in peroxidase activity, as determined either by guaiacol oxidation or amino acid decarboxylation is a likely reason for the lack of bactericidal activity by both intact spleen cells and 20,000 g pellet fractions thereof from leukemic mice (Strauss et al., 1974).

Further studies of the 20,000 g pellet fraction of spleen cell homogenates from leukemic animals indicate the presence of a factor inhibitory to some peroxidase-mediated functions of normal mouse spleen cells. This factor significantly inhibits peroxidase-mediated amino acid decarboxylation activity of normal spleen cell homogenate fractions and is both heat stable and nondialyzable. As might be expected, spleen cell homogenates from leukemic animals inhibit peroxidase–H_2O_2–Cl^- bactericidal activity of normal mouse spleen homogenate fractions without having a significant effect upon guaiacol oxidation. The factor is not present in the 20,000 g pellet fraction of spleen cell homogenates from normal mice, and its inhibitory action is a function of its concentration (Strauss et al., 1974).

The data obtained to this time indicate that the peroxidase–H_2O_2–Cl^- system plays an important role in the bactericidal function of mouse spleen cells. The presence of an inhibitory factor in the 20,000 g pellet fraction of spleen cells from leukemic animals has helped to clarify this role. It appears from these preliminary data that the inhibitory factor is a heat-stable macromolecule. Since it does not significantly alter guaiacol oxidation activity, it probably does not interfere with H_2O_2 or SPO per se. Its mechanism of action is more likely involved with the substrate of peroxidase-mediated decarboxylation and bactericidal activity.

This recently acquired information on the SPO–H_2O_2–Cl^- system in spleen cells from normal and leukemic mice may be significant. It could provide a useful tool for the design of experiments at the cellular and biochemical level that might aid in the elucidation of the mechanism responsible for the increased susceptibility to infections generally experienced by patients with neoplastic disorders (Viola, 1967; Armstrong et al., 1971).

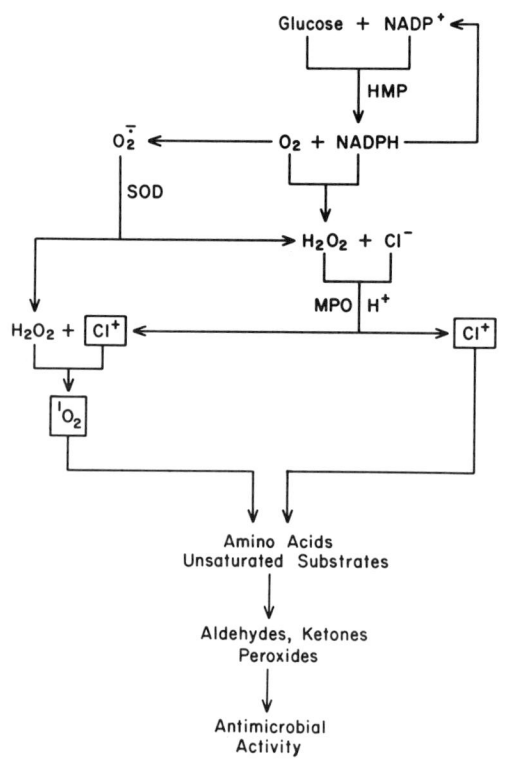

FIG. 2. Brief resume of the biochemical events that are activated when particulate materials are incubated with polymorphonuclear leukocytes. The possible relationship of these stimulated activities with antimicrobial activity is indicated. Abbreviations: O_2^-, superoxide; $^1O_2$, singlet oxygen; SOD, superoxide dismutase; MPO, myeloperoxidase; HMP, hexose monophosphate shunt.

See text for additional details.

D. Relationships between Metabolic and Bactericidal Activities

A brief resume of the biochemical events that appear related to the antimicrobial activities of the cell is diagrammed in Fig. 2. Briefly, incubation of PMN with particulate material results in a number of different metabolic stimulations. These enhanced metabolic events function to activate a potent antimicrobial system in the cell. The generation of MPO–H_2O_2–Cl^- has at least two major consequences: decarboxylation and deamination of free amino acids, resulting in microbicidal aldehyde formation; and equally important, chlorination of peptide bonds in the protein structure of the microbial cell, leading to unstable chloramines and effective disintegration of protein. Chlorination of the bacterial surface may be the first step in the eventual destruction of the microorganisms. A postulated by-product of the MPO–H_2O_2–Cl^- system, singlet oxygen, may also participate in additional peptide cleavage through oxidation. Finally, the superoxide anion, resulting from the oxidation of NADPH, may also be involved with microbicidal activity through its effect on H_2O_2 production.

The microbicidal activity of macrophages and lymphocytes also involves a peroxidase–H_2O_2–halide system. In the lymphocyte, actual engulfment is not evident, and bacterial killing probably occurs on or near the cell surface. The peroxidative activity of the alveolar macrophage is different from that noted in the lymphocyte and PMN, particularly in its halide requirement in that iodide appears to be the functional halide.

The evidence presented suggests that a peroxidase–H_2O_2–halide antimicrobial system is present in different cell types. The system is latent, and particle contact and/or entry activates it. In PMN and lymphocytes, chlorination of bacteria resulting in peptide cleavage, and/or aldehyde formation appears to be a plausible mechanism of action. In alveolar macrophages, production of "active" iodine appears to be involved.

VII. Alterations and Decreased Resistance to Infections

It has been pointed out in the Introduction that many different factors can be involved in protecting a host against infections. For example, production of cells in bone marrow, storage of phagocytes, delivery to the blood, margination, and actual microbial contact are all of obvious importance in the host–parasite interactions. A failure of any one parameter can favor the parasite and decrease host resistance. Owing to the complexity of host–defense relationships, the precise pinpointing of a specific failure in a particular facet of the total phagocytic process *in vivo* is difficult. With this in mind, we will, nevertheless, attempt to describe some disorders in chemotaxis, recognition, biochemical and microbicidal activities of phagocytes that appear to be related to increased susceptibility to infections.

A. Altered Chemotaxis

Defective chemotaxis has been found to be associated with absence, dysfunction, or inhibition of complement factors. Altered chemotactic activity has been noted in neonatal serum. This serum has often been found to be deficient in components of the classic or alternative complement pathways. Such deficiency would result in a failure to produce the chemotactic agents C3a and C5a. Individuals deficient in C3 or C5 show increased susceptibility to infection and their serums exhibit decreased chemotactic activity (Alper et al., 1970; Miller and Nilsson, 1970).

Although altered chemotactic responses have been described for PMN in a variety of disorders, the exact basis of the cellular abnormality remains unclear. For example, in patients with rheumatoid arthritis, immune complexes inhibit PMN movement. In other disease states, similar complexes may be responsible for decreased PMN motility. In these conditions, the immunoglobulin levels are high and the patients experience recurrent infections (Hill and Quie, 1974).

Many reports have appeared describing defective leukocyte movement in patients with recurrent infections. However, to date, any therapeutic manipulation of the chemotactic process must await the discovery of the biochemical and biophysical events that are associated with leukocyte locomotion. Therapeutic intervention will certainly be a realistic goal once this information becomes available.

B. Altered Recognition Activity

Generally, PMN and mononuclear cells ingest opsonized bacteria more efficiently than nonopsonized ones. Activation of C3 is essential for optimal serum opsonization. Failure of C3 activation in different disease states has been associated with recurrent pyogenic infections. These states include low-birth-weight infants, systemic lupus erythematosus, hepatic cirrhosis, acute glomerulonephritis, and genetic absence of C3.

Many patients with sickle-cell anemia have been reported to have diminished amounts of heat-labile opsonins for pneumococci type 25. The possibility that this deficiency coupled with the functional asplenia of the patient may be responsible for susceptibility of these patients to pneumococeal sepsis and meningitis has been suggested (Winkelstein and Drachman, 1968; Pearson et al., 1969).

Defective opsonization generally results in defective ingestion. However, other factors may similarly account for poor ingestion. Thus, serum with high opsonic activity may not support efficient ingestion. This may be due to hyperosmolar conditions, as in the case of the serum of patients with diabetes mellitus. The increased glucose levels actually inhibit phagocytosis.

C. Altered Biochemical and Microbicidal Activity

1. *Chronic Granulomatous Disease and Hereditary MPO Deficiency*

Recently different disease states have been instrumental in providing significant information relative to the relationship between the biochemical and antimicrobial activities of phagocytes. Patients with chronic granulomatous disease suffer from severe and recurrent infections. Both, the PMN and the monocytes from these patients fail to develop the burst of oxidative metabolic activity generally associated with phagocytosis. They are unable to oxidize glucose through the HMS and unable to produce hydrogen peroxide. Recently it has been shown (Hohn and Lehrer, 1974) that the specific defect in these leukocytes is a deficiency in NADPH oxidase. A deficiency in this enzyme would of course result in decreased HMS activity (due to a limiting of NADP) and decreased H_2O_2 production. Some support for the above is that the microbicidal defect of these leukocytes can be, at least partially, corrected by providing an exogenous source of hydrogen peroxide or by stimulating endogenous oxidative metabolism with redox dyes (Baehner, 1972). Also, these leukocytes will efficiently kill hydrogen peroxide-producing bacteria such as streptococci, lactobacilli, and pneumococci.

Another disorder, hereditary MPO deficiency, a syndrome characterized by the complete absence of peroxidase activity in PMN and monocytes, has contributed to our understanding of the role of peroxidase in the antimicrobial activity of the phagocyte (Lehrer and Cline, 1969). Peroxide-deficient neutrophils, a common finding in these patients, are unable to kill certain bacteria. Neutrophils from a patient with hereditary MPO activity required approximately 3 hours to kill a variety of *Staphylococcus* or *Serratia marcescens*. Normal neutrophils would have achieved the same killing efficiency in less than 1 hour.

Glucose-6-phosphate dehydrogenase deficiency of red cells is associated with decreased levels of the enzyme in PMN. The leukocytes from these patients, however, do not generally show a decreased bactericidal activity. However, if the level of enzyme is less than 1% of normal, hydrogen peroxide formation is interferred with, bactericidal activity is subsequently decreased, and persistant bacterial infections pervail (Cooper *et al.*, 1972).

Chediak–Higashi disease is another hereditary (autosomal recessive) entity, characterized by repeated infection, which has been related to altered phagocytes. Children with this disorder generally die within the first few years of life. At least four different abnormalities in Chediak–Higashi disease have been reported: (1) a defect in chemotaxis; (2) a delay in killing; (3) giant abnormal lysosomes; and (4) a decrease in circulatory granulocytes. Recently it has been suggested that a delay in the rate of degranulation, coupled with a total decrease in the overall deposition of granule contents into the phagocytic vacuole, are major defects in this disorder leading to decreased resistance to infections (Stossel et al., 1972).

2. Leukemic Disorders

a. Chronic. The biochemical activities of leukemic cells have been extensively studied and excellent reviews adequately cover the field. The review of Seitz (1965) is particularly important as a serious attempt was made to review the literature on a worldwide basis. Relatively few studies have been published that were designed to investigate the metabolic activities of leukemic cells while these cells were performing a physiological function, i.e., phagocytosis. However, a considerable number of published studies have been directed toward establishing the effect of the leukemic state on particle entry from a morphological viewpoint.

We have investigated the phagocytic and bactericidal activities of leukocytes isolated from patients with a variety of lymphoproliferative disorders (Sbarra et al., 1964b). Results indicated that the phagocytic and bactericidal rates in these patients were decreased. In many of the cases studied, the substitution of homologous serum for autologous serum reversed the effect and suggested that humoral factors may be involved in controlling the extent of phagocytosis at least in some cases. It is interesting to note that most patients who showed abnormal phagocytic and bactericidal patterns also had some clinical complication. The converse, however, was not true; i.e., patients with complications did not always show an abnormal phagocytic pattern. At least two explanations may be presented that would account for this finding. First, the phagocytic defense mechanism per se may not have an important role in these disorders; second, the phagocytic system of the host will eventually become involved and result in decreased activity and consequently in an increased susceptibility to repeated infections. Finally, this work suggests that the phagocytes from patients on steroid therapy, specifically prednisone therapy, have a decreased bactericidal activity. This finding is in agreement with the work of Shaw et al. (1961), which showed that the administration of prednisone to patients with chronic lymphocytic leukemia (CLL) increased the severity of bacterial infections. It is also in agreement with our work in which we demonstrated that the inhibitory nature of sera from patients with CLL is no longer evident if the patients are undergoing prednisone therapy (Sbarra et al., 1964a).

In leukocytes isolated mainly from patients with myeloproliferative disorders, we have noted a generally normal phagocytic and bactericidal pattern (Sbarra et al., 1965). When an abnormality was noted, it was experienced mostly with the test organism *Pseudomonas aeruginosa*. This was not an unexpected finding as, when these patients come down with infections, *P. aeruginosa* is often the organism responsible. In a further study (McRipley and Sbarra, 1967a), we extended previous investigations to include a group of patients with a wider range of neoplastic disorders and have assessed the bactericidal activities of selected patients over a period of time. In general, this study revealed that patients with CLL, lymphoma, and various carcinomas have abnormal leukocytic activities. No correlation between γ-globulin levels, hemagglutinin titers, and leukocytic activities, however, could be made. Selvaraj *et al.* (1967) went on to study the metabolic activities of leukocytes from patients with lympho- and myeloproliferative disorders at rest and during phagocytosis. These activities studied included oxygen uptake, glucose-1-^{14}C and glucose-6-^{14}C oxidations, and lactate production, all of which had previously been shown to be affected by phagocytosis. In this relation, we shall use the term leukocyte to refer to the total white cell population of peripheral blood. This represents varying populations of granulocytes and mononuclear cells. The overall metabolism of leukocytes from patients with lymphoproliferative disorders was lower than normal on a per cell basis. However, some correlation was found to exist between peripheral blood leukocyte counts and metabolic activity. The higher the peripheral count, the more marked was the decrease in metabolic activity. Lymphocytes isolated from patients with lymphoproliferative disorders showed a metabolic stimulation that is consistent with phagocytizing cells. Bacteria were not detected in these cells; however, the presence of bacteria around these cells was striking. This phenomenon was not observed with lymphocytes isolated from normal people. Leukocytes isolated from myeloproliferative disorders generally showed somewhat reduced oxidative metabolic activity. Possibly these decreased activities were caused by the presence of high percentages of young and immature cells that do not contribute significantly to the total leukocyte metabolism. Leukocytes from multiple myeloma patients showed significantly elevated resting metabolic activities and decreased response to phagocytic stimulation. These patients are known to possess a number of abnormal proteins in their serum that could conceivably contribute to the stimulated metabolic state of the leukocyte. Finally, leukocytes isolated from some of the miscellaneous carcinoma patients studied showed decreased metabolic activity during phagocytosis. As a result, some of the leukocytes also showed decreased bactericidal activities. Hence, it is concluded that the cancerous growths in these patients somehow interfered with the phagocytic metabolism of the cells. The mechanism responsible for this interesting observation is still unknown.

Ohta (1965) has examined the matabolic phagocytic stimulation of leukocytes isolated from patients with chronic myelocytic, monocytic, chronic lymphatic, and acute myelocytic leukemias. Increased oxygen uptaken and HMS activity were noted in these cells upon the addition of bacteria. Ohta concluded from his study that these leukocytes were able to respond to the metabolic phagocytic stimulations that accompany phagocytosis, and that the magnitude of their response is determined by the maturity of the cell under study.

b. Acute. The phagocytic, bactericidal, and associated metabolic activities of peripheral blood leukocytes from children with acute lymphocytic leukemia in relapse and remission have been compared with similar parameters of leukocytes from nonleukemic control children. Leukocytes from children with acute lymphocytic leukemia in relapse had significantly less phagocytic activity than those from children in remission or nonleukemic controls. The bactericidal activity of leukocytes from the three groups indicates that samples from patients in remission had less activity than controls but more than those in relapse. The G6PDH, 6PGDH, and NADPH oxidase activities of circulating leukocytes from patients in relapse were less than those in remission or controls. The activities of these enzymes in leukocytes from patients in remission and controls are similar (Strauss et al., 1970b). Additional studies are necessary before one can fully understand the nature of the differences in the bactericidal activities of leukocytes between the latter two groups. Whether the decreased bactericidal activity of leukocytes from patients in relapse is related only to the decreased activity of the enzymes studied or to another enzyme, possibly MPO, remains to be established.

Obviously some significant differences in metabolic activities between phagocytizing cells in the different disorders exist. Future investigations directed along lines similar to those alluded to above should prove fruitful.

3. Kwashiorkor

Recently one of us (RJS) studied the phagocytic, metabolic, and bactericidal activities of peripheral blood leukocytes from children with protein-calorie malnutrition (PCM) (Selvaraj and Bhat, 1972a,b). These studies were conducted at the National Institute of Nutrition, Hyderabad, India. The HMS stimulation was significantly less in phagocytizing leukocytes isolated from PCM children compared with those from normal children. Bactericidal activity of leukocytes isolated from these children was also considerably decreased. These alterations were found to be due to changes within the leukocytes rather than to altered serum factors. Our studies have revealed that one biochemical lesion in these leukocytes is decreased NADPH oxidase activity. Also, the phagocytic stimulation of this critical enzyme noted in leukocytes isolated from well nourished children does not occur in the leukocytes from children with PCM (Table I). With treatment, which consisted of feeding a high-calorie, high-protein diet with multivitamin and iron supplements, the above parameters reverted toward a normal pattern. The children, who were severely malnourished, were deficient not only in calories and protein, but also in essential nutrients, especially vitamin A, vitamin B-complex and iron (Selvaraj and Bhat, 1972a). The altered phagocytic and bactericidal activities observed in these patients could be due to one or a combination of these deficiencies.

It is evident from the above that increased susceptibility to infections in certain disease states can be attributed to altered phagocytic activity of leukocytes. Further, it is suggested that in some cases this altered activity results from an intrinsic metabolic disturbance in the phagocyte. Obviously progress has been made in elucidating the mechanism of antimicrobial activity in the cell. There is

TABLE I
NADPH OXIDASE ACTIVITY IN LEUKOCYTE GRANDULES[a]

	Resting	During phagocytosis	P value for phagocytic effect
Control (9)	0.15 ± 0.03	0.25 ± 0.05	<0.05
Malnourished, before treatment (12)	0.07 ± 0.01	0.07 ± 0.01	NS
P, for control vs malnourished	<0.02	<0.001	–
Malnourished, after treatment (7)	0.09 ± 0.02	0.15 ± 0.04	<0.01
P, for effect of treatment	<0.07	<0.001	–

[a] Data taken from Selvaraj and Bhat (1972).
[b] Enzyme activities are expressed as nanomoles of NADPH oxidized per minute per 10^5 leukocytes (means ±SEM of the number of observations in parentheses). P values were determined by one-tailed pair test. NS: not significant.

every reason to believe that greater advances will be forthcoming in the near future.

REFERENCES

Allen, R.C., Stjernholm, R.L., and Steele, R.H. (1972). *Biochem. Biophys. Res. Commun.* **47**, 679.
Alper, C.A., Abramson, N., Johnson, R.B., Jr., Jandl, J.H., and Rosen, F.S. (1970). *New Engl. J. Med.* **282**, 349.
Armstrong, D., Young, L., Meyer, R.D., and Blevis, A.H. (1971). *Med. Clin. No. Amer.* **55**, 729.
Baehner, R.L. (1972). *Pediat. Clin. No. Amer.* **19**, 935.
Bainton, D.F., and Farquhar, M.D. (1966). *J. Cell Biol.* **28**, 277.
Bainton, D.F., and Farquhar, M.D. (1968). *J. Cell Biol.* **39**, 286.
Belding, M.E., Klebanoff, S.J., and Ray, C.G. (1970). *Science* **167**, 1951.
Boyden, S. (1962). *J. Exp. Med.* **115**, 453.
Cagan, R.H., and Karnovsky, M.L. (1964). *Nature (London)* **204**, 255.
Cline, M.J., and Lehrer, R.I. (1969). *Proc. Nat. Acad. Sci. U.S.* **62**, 756.
Cooper, M.R., DeChatelet, L.R., Lavia, M.R., McCall, C.E., Spurr, C.L., and Baehner, R. (1972). *J. Clin. Invest.* **51**, 769.
Daems, W.T., Poelmann, R.E., and Brederoo, P.J. (1973). *J. Histochem. Cytochem.* **21**, 93.
David, J.R. (1966). *Proc. Nat. Acad. Sci. U.S.* **56**, 72.
Gee, J.B.L. (1970). *Amer. J. Med. Sci.* **260**, 195.
Henson, P.M. (1971). *J. Immunol.* **107**, 1535.
Hill, H.R., and Quie, P.G. (1974). *Lancet* **1**, 183.
Hohn, D.C., and Lehrer, R.I. (1974). *Clin. Res.* **22**, 394A.
Jacobs, A.A., Paul, B.B., Strauss, R.R., and Sbarra, A.A. (1970). *Biochem. Biophys. Res. Commun.* **39**, 384.
Jacobs, A.A., Low, I., Paul, B.B., Strauss, R.R., and Sbarra, A.J. (1972). *Infect. Immun.* **5**, 127.
Kaplan, A.P., Kay, A.B., and Austen, K.F. (1972). *J. Exp. Med.* **135**, 81.

Kaplan, A.P., Goetzl, E.J. and Austen, K.F. (1973). *J. Clin. Invest.* **52**, 2591.
Klebanoff, S.J. (1967). *J. Exp. Med.* **126**, 1063.
Klebanoff, S.J. (1968). *J. Bacteriol.* **95**, 2131.
Klebanoff, S.J. (1970). In "Biochemistry of the Phagocytic Process" (J. Schultz, ed.), pp. 89–110. Wiley (Interscience), New York.
Kelbanoff, S.J. (1974). *J. Biol. Chem.* **249**, 3724.
Krinsky, N.I. (1974). *Science* **186**, 363.
Kvarstein, B., and Stormoken, H. (1971). *Biochem. Pharmacol.* **20**, 119.
Lehrer, R.I. (1969). *J. Bacteriol.* **95**, 1425.
Lahrer, R.I., and Cline, M.J. (1969). *J. Clin. Invest.* **48**, 1478.
McRipley, R.J., and Sbarra, A.J. (1967a). *Radiation Res.* **31**, 706.
McRipley, R.J., and Sbarra, A.J. (1967b). *J. Bacteriol.* **94**, 1425.
Mandell, G.L. (1970). *Proc. Soc. Exp. Biol. Med.* **134**, 447.
Miller, M.E., and Nilsson, V.R. (1970). *New Engl. J. Med.* **282**, 354.
Nichols, B.A., Bainton, D.F., and Farquhar, M.G. (1971). *J. Cell Biol.* **50**, 498.
Ohta, H. (1965). *Acta Haematol.* **33**, 28.
Ouchi, E., Selvaraj, R.J., and Sbarra, A.J. (1965). *Exp. Cell Res.* **40**, 456.
Paul, B.B., and Sbarra, A.J. (1968). *Biochim. Biophys. Acta* **156**, 168.
Paul, B.B., Strauss, R.R., Jacobs, A.A., and Sbarra, A.J. (1970a). *Infect. Immun.* **1**, 338.
Paul, B.B., Jacobs, A.A., Strauss, R.R., and Sbarra, A.J. (1970b). *Infect. Immun.* **2**, 414.
Paul, B.B., Strauss, R.R., Jacobs, A.A., and Sbarra, A.J. (1970c). *Bacteriol Proc.* p. 91.
Paul, B.B., Strauss, R.R., Jacobs, A.A., and Sbarra, A.J. (1972), *Exp. Cell Res.* **73**, 456.
Paul, B.B., Jacobs, A.A., Strauss, R.R., and Sbarra, A.J. (1973a). *J. Reticuloendothel. Soc.* **13**, 478.
Paul, B.B., Strauss, R.R., Selvaraj, R.J., and Sbarra, A.J. (1973b). *Science* **181**, 849.
Pearson, H.A., Spencer, R.P., and Cornelius, E.A. (1969). *New Engl. J. Med.* **281**, 923.
Rebuck, J.W., and Crowley, J.H. (1955). *Ann. N.Y. Acad. Sci.* **59**, 757.
Reed, P.W. (1969). *J. Biol. Chem.* **244**, 2459.
Roberts, J., and Quastel, J.H. (1964). *Nature (London)* **202**, 85.
Romeo, D., Cramer, R., Marzi, T., Soranzo, M.R., Zabucchi, G., and Rossi, F. (1973). *J. Reticuloendothel. Soc.* **13**, 399.
Rossi, F., and Zatti M. (1964). *Brit. J. Exp. Pathol.* **45**, 548.
Rossi, F., Romeo, D., and Patriarca, F. (1972). *J. Reticuloendothel. Soc.* **12**, 127.
Sandberg, A.L., Synderman, R., and Frank, M.M. (1972). *J. Immunol.* **108**, 1227.
Sbarra, A.J., and Karnovsky, M.L. (1959). *J. Biol. Chem.* **234**, 1355.
Sbarra, A.J., Ouchi, E., and Rosenbaum, E. (1964a). *Cancer Res.* **24**, 498.
Sbarra, A.J., Shirley, W., Ouchi, E., and Rosenbaum, E. (1964b). *Cancer Res.* **24**, 1958.
Sbarra, A.J., Shirley, W., Selvaraj, R.J., McRipley, R.J., and Rosenbaum, E. (1965). *Cancer Res.* **25**, 1199.
Seitz, I.F. (1965). *Advan. Cancer Res.* **9**, 303.
Selvaraj, R.J., and Bhat, K.S. (1972a). *Amer. J. Clin. Nutr.* **25**, 166.
Selvaraj, R.J., and Bhat, K.S. (1972b). *Biochem. J.* **127**, 255.
Selvaraj, R.J., and Sbarra, A.J. (1966). *Nature (London)* **211**, 1271.
Selvaraj, R.J., McRipley, R.J., and Sbarra, A.J. (1967). *Cancer Res.* **27**, 2287.
Selvaraj, R.J., Paul, B.B., Strauss, R.R., Jacobs, A.A., and Sbarra, A.J. (1974). *Infect. Immunol.* **9**, 255.
Shaw, R., Boggs, D.R., Silberman, H.R., and Frei, E. (1961). *Blood* **17**, 182.
Simon, H.B., and Sheagren, J.N. (1972). *Cell. Immunol.* **4**, 163.
Skarnes, R.C. (1970). *Nature (London)* **225**, 1072.
Sorkin, E., Stecher, V.J., and Borel, J.F. (1970). *Ser. Haematol.* **3**, 131.
Spitznagel, J.K., Dalldorf, F.G., Leffell, M.S., Folds, J.D., Welsh, I.R.H., Cooney, M.H., and Martin, L.E. (1974). *Lab. Invest.* **30**, 774.

Stelmaszynska, T., and Zgliczynski, J.M. (1974). *Eur. J. Biochem.* **45**, 305–312.
Stossel, T.P. (1974). *New Engl. J. Med.* **290**, 774.
Stossel, T.P., Root, R.K., and Vaughan, M. (1972). *New Engl. J. Med.* **286**, 120.
Strauss, R.R., Paul, B.B., and Sbarra, A.J. (1968). *J. Bacteriol.* **96**, 1982.
Strauss, R.R., Paul, B.B., Jacobs, A.A., and Sbarra, A.J. (1969). *Arch. Biochem. Biophys.* **135**, 265.
Strauss, R.R., Paul, B.B., Jacobs, A.A., and Sbarra, A.J. (1970a). *J. Reticuloendothel. Soc.* **7**, 754.
Strauss, R.R., Paul, B.B., Selvaraj, R.J., and Sbarra, A.J. (1974). *Cancer Res.* **34**, 3220. **30**, 480.
Strauss, R.R., Paul, B.B., Jacobs, A.A., and Sbarra, A.J. (1971). *Infect. Immun.* **3**, 595.
Strauss, R.R., Paul, B.B., Jacobs, A.A., and Sbarra, A.J. (1972a). *Infect. Immun.* **5**, 120.
Strauss, R.R., Paul, B.B., Jacobs, A.A., and Sbarra, A.J. (1972b). *Infect. Immun.* **5**, 114.
Strauss, R.R., Paul, B.B., Selvaraj, R.J., and Sbarra, A.J. (1974). *Cancer Res.* (in press).
van Furth, R., and Thompson, J. (1971). *Ann. Inst. Pasteur* **120**, 337.
Viola, M.V. (1967). *Amer. Med. Ass.* **201**, 923.
Winkelstein, J.A., and Drachman, R.H. (1968). *New Engl. J. Med.* **279**, 459.
Zatti, M., and Rossi, F. (1966). *Experientia* **22**, 758.
Zigmond, S.H., and Hirsch, J.G. (1973). *J. Exp. Med.* **137**, 387.
Zgliczynski, J.M., Stelmaszynska, T., Ostrowski, W., Naskelski, J., and Szneja, J. (1968). *Eur. J. Biochem.* **4**, 540–547.
Zgliczynski, J.M., Stelmaszynska, T., Domanski, J., and Ostrowski, W. (1971). *Biochim. Biophys. Acta* **235**, 419.
Zgliczynski, J.M., and Stelmaszynska, T. (1975). *Eur. J. Biochem.* **56**, 157–162.
Zgliczynski, J.M., Selvaraj, R.J., Paul, B.B., Stelmaszynska, T., Poskitt, P.K.F., and Sbarra, A.J. (1976). Submitted for publication.

Transfer Amyloidosis

FINN HARDT[1] and POUL RANLØV[2]

University Institute of Pathological Anatomy, Copenhagen, Denmark

I. Introduction	273
II. Experimental Amyloidosis	274
A. The Biphasic Development	274
B. Morphological Characteristics	275
C. Immune Functional Characteristics	281
III. Transfer of Experimental Amyloidosis	289
A. Introduction	289
B. Amyloidosis as a Transferable Disease	289
C. Transfer with Cells	292
D. Source of Cells	302
E. Transfer with Subcellular Fractions	304
F. Donor–Recipient Combinations	311
G. Role of Specific Antigen	311
H. Nature of Amyloid-Inducing Factor (AIF)	312
I. Precursors of Amyloid in Serum	314
IV. Transfer of Amyloid-Enhancing Factor (AEF)	315
A. Transfer with Cells	315
B. Source of Cells	322
C. Transfer with Subcellular Material	323
D. Donor–Recipient Combinations	326
E. Role of the Antigen	327
F. Nature of the Amyloid-Enhancing Factor	328
V. Conclusions and Summary	329
References	330

I. Introduction

For writers of medical intelligence such as "Case Records of X-ville General Hospital" and suspense-loaded Clinicopathological Conferences, syndromes in-

[1] Present address: Department of Medicine II, Kommunehospitalet, 1399 Copenhagen K, Denmark.
[2] Present address: Department of Medicine B, Frederiksborg Amts Centralsygehus, 3400 Hillerød, Denmark.

volving amyloid degeneration have always carried a strange attraction. After having been dragged through a jungle of misleading clinical symptoms and contradictory laboratory findings, a confused Dr. Watson will ultimately be confronted with the not-so-obvious solution by the triumphant pathologist. In these everyday situations all members of the cast will usually find themselves equally unrewarded: The clinician will most probably miss the diagnosis next time again and—having no proper therapy to offer—insult will be added to injury; the nonreflective type of pathologist will find the whole thing very elementary and a bit boring—after all, the amyloid deposit is easily recognized and could be mistaken for nothing else; the third party—the patient—is usually dead. Invariably, the spectator (the unwary reader) is left frustrated.

To maintain this rather defeatist attitude toward amyloid disease seems hardly justified in light of the considerable amount of experimental work on amyloidosis accumulated during the last decade. A few facts should be emphasized: amyloidosis is one of very few (if any) mesenchymal diseases of man which—for all we know—can be reproduced to identity in animal models; accordingly, the amyloidosis problem has been subject to investigations from many different angles, of which the immunological one has proved particularly profitable. Amyloidosis has been produced in many different animal species without much variation in the responses to modifying procedures, in patterns of tissue distribution, ultrastructural characteristics, etc., which suggests that results obtained in experimental animals may safely be projected to the human situation. We shall first review several features of experimental amyloidosis and then the present state of knowledge about transfer amyloidosis.

II. Experimental Amyloidosis

A. THE BIPHASIC DEVELOPMENT

As all known types of experimentally induced amyloidosis involve a certain period of treatment with the amyloidogenic agent (usually a substance with antigenic properties) before tissue amyloid can be detected, it is natural to distinguish between a period of latency—a primary phase—and the period during which amyloid is being laid down in the tissues—a secondary phase. A considerable number of functional and morphological features separate these two phases qualitatively and quantitatively. Maintaining this distinction has proved fruitful. The histologic characteristics of the biphasic development have been described by Teilum (1954, 1956, 1964a), and his observations have spearheaded a major part of subsequent research.

1. *The Primary Phase*

Depending on the species, the primary, preamyloid phase of experimentally induced amyloidosis will last from a few weeks to several months. In regional lymph nodes and later in the spleen, the liver, and the kidneys (not the thymus) vast numbers of cells will gradually appear, cells with large pale nuclei containing one or two nucleoli and with abundant pyroninophilic cytoplasm. These pyroninophilic cells are perifollicularly arranged in the splenic red pulp and line sinusoids or endothelium of small vessels within other organs. In the kidneys they are found in proximity to the mesangial cells of the glomerulus (Shimamura and Sorenson, 1965). Simultaneously, a gradual decrease in the number of small lymphocytes is noted.

2. *The Secondary (Amyloid) Phase (Figs. 1–6)*

The beginning of the second, or amyloid, phase is characterized by the appearance of increasing numbers of reticuloendothelial cells containing a finely granular periodic acid-Schiff (PAS)-positive cytoplasm. These cells are primarily found in the perifollicular zone of the spleen. Their appearance is preceded by, and runs parallel with, a rapid decrease in the number of infiltrating pyroninophilic cells in various tissues. Adjacent to the PAS-positive reticuloendothelial cells small amyloid deposits will appear, often coalescing with their cytoplasm (Teilum, 1956). The small amyloid deposits will become heaped up and will grow with the formation of new PAS-positive cells provided a continuous challenge of the organism with the amyloidogenic (= antigenic?) material takes place. It is noteworthy that one never finds amyloid deposits in the thymus or in the lymph nodes regional to the site(s) of injection.

B. Morphological Characteristics

1. *The Lymphoid Tissue*

A conspicuous feature of the preamyloid, pyroninophilic phase in the spleen is the increasing involution of the splenic white pulp. This lymphoid depletion is reflected by lymphopenia in the blood during the antigenic challenge leading to amyloidosis (Jaffe, 1926). This central lymphoid depletion is always present (Perasalo et al., 1950; Latvalahti, 1953; Christensen and Rask-Nielsen, 1962; Bradbury and Micklem, 1965) and chronologically and topographically it is invariably found to coincide with the increase in cells with pronounced pyroninophilia in the same tissue. Moreover, an inverse relationship between the time needed for induction of amyloidosis and the degree of lymphoid depletion and pyroninophilia in spleen and lymph nodes has been shown to exist (Druet and Janigan, 1966): The shorter the induction period, the heavier the pyroninophilia. However, none of these features are disclosed by the thymus which remains morphologically (though not functionally) unaffected all through the amyloid-inducing regimen (Claesson et al., 1974).

However, in electron micrographs of spleens from casein-treated mice in the preamyloid phase the pyroninophilic cells containing exclusively "free" ribosomes or polyribosomes far outnumbered those also containing ergastoplasmic

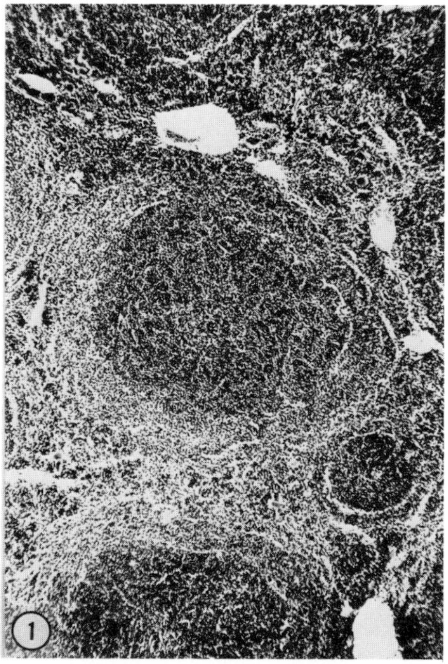
1

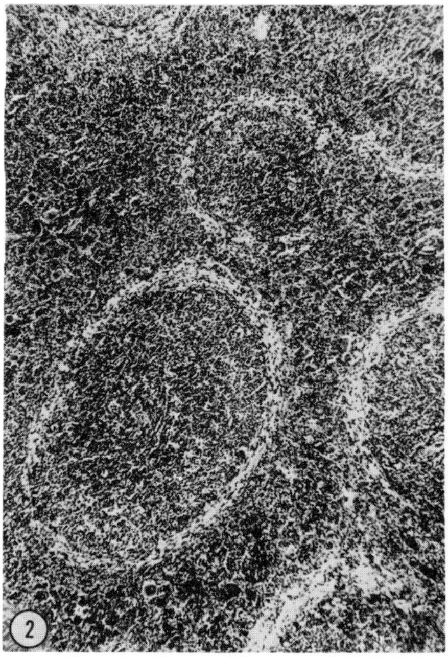
2

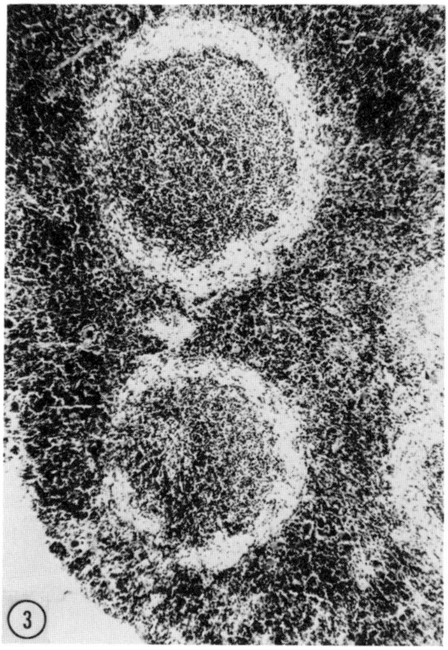
3

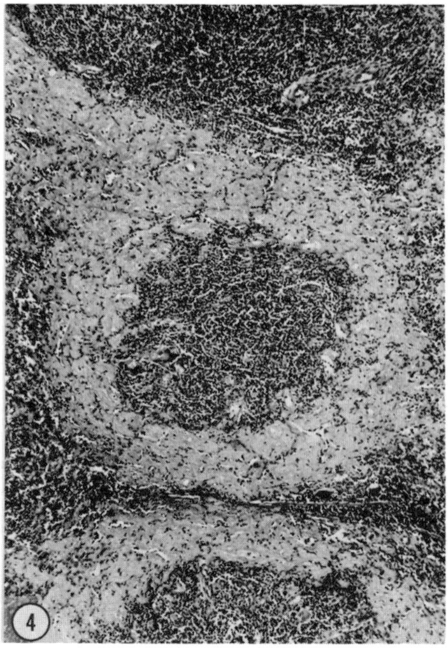
4

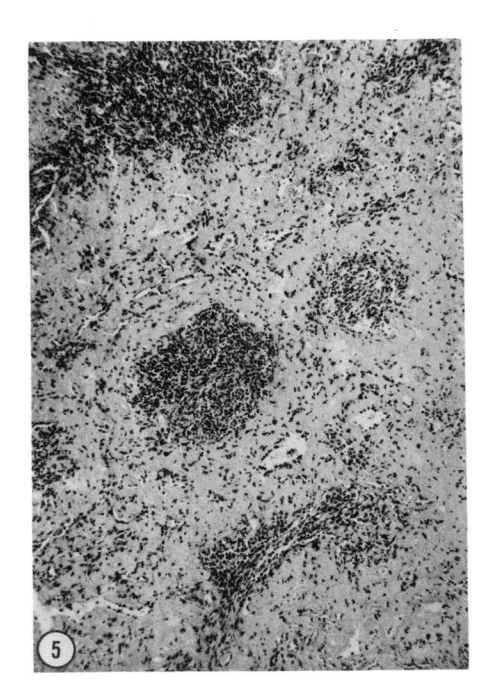

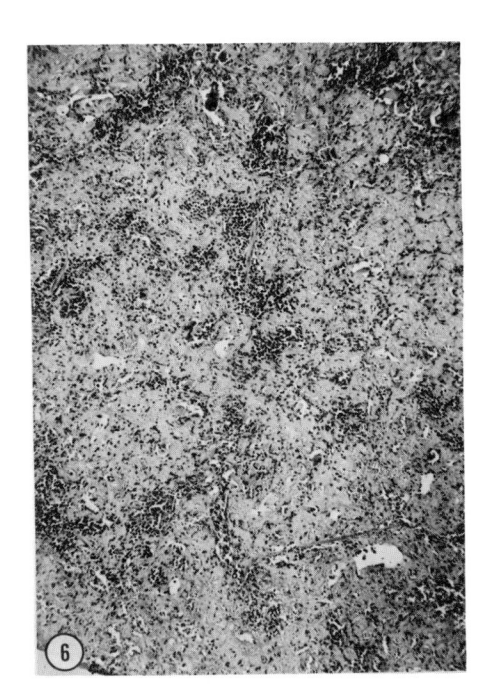

FIGS. 1–6. An illustration of the grading of experimental amyloidosis in the mouse from sections of spleen. Grade 1 (Fig. 1) is characterized by the appearance of periodic acid-Schiff positive cells perifollicularly and only occasional small amyloid deposits. In grade 2 (Fig. 2) a thin, though continuous, ring of amyloid has formed perifollicularly. Grades 3 and 4 (Figs. 3 and 4) exhibit increasing thickness of these rings—in grade 4 several rings show partial fusion. In grade 5 (Fig. 5) amyloid deposits appear to be widespread in the red pulp, and in grade 6 (Fig. 6) a total loss of splenic structure is evident, more than 90% of the tissues being replaced by amyloid. From Christensen and Hjort (1959).

channels, i.e., plasma cells (B lymphocytes). By comparison, θ-positive cells (T lymphocytes) comprise approximately 40% of the lymphoid cell population of the normal mouse spleen (Raff, 1971). The relative numbers of plasma cells are reduced in casein-treated preamyloid mice. The functional implications of this will be dealt with later in relation to the role of immunity in the pathogenesis of amyloidosis.

When the pyroninophilic tissue phase is at its maximum and until its cessation, an increasing number of pyknoses and accumulation of cellular debris are regularly noted within the splenic red pulp. That a considerable cell destruction is one of the characteristics of the pyroninophilic phase is supported by the demonstration of a doubling of the normal lymphoid cell decay in spleens and thymi from mice undergoing amyloidogenic treatment (Claesson and Hardt,

1972a); it is noteworthy that no such increase occurred in other lymphoid organs.

In a cytokinetic study of the spleen cell populations during an amyloid-inducing regimen in mice, Hardt and Claesson (1972a)—using anti-θ serum and electronic cell-size determination—found a doubling of the number of θ-bearing cells (T lymphocytes) during the pyroninophilic phase, followed by a marked decrease with the onset of the second, amyloid phase. These observations strongly suggest that the increased decay of lymphoid cells that accompanies the onset of amyloidosis (Claesson and Hardt, 1972a) involves mainly T cells. After the decrease of θ-bearing cells, an increase of large cells (11–17 μm in diameter or larger) was recorded, reflecting an increase in reticuloendothelial cells.

2. *The Reticuloendothelial Tissue*

Owing in particular to the work of Teilum (1952, 1956, 1964a) the relation of amyloid deposits to PAS-positive reticuloendothelial (RE) cells is well established. Since then, further evidence for local production of amyloid has been accumulated in conventional histological studies (Christensen and Rask-Nielsen, 1962; Druet and Janigan, 1966; Werdelin and Ranløv, 1966), by *in vitro* experiments (Cohen *et al.*, 1965; Ben-Ishay and Zlotnick, 1968), and by electron microscopy (Gueft and Ghidoni, 1963; Sorenson *et al.*, 1964; Cohen, 1965). Strong evidence was obtained by the demonstration of intracytoplasmatically located amyloid fibrils (Ranløv and Wanstrup, 1967), later confirmed and extended by immunofluorescent methods (Ben-Ishay and Zlotnik, 1968; Zucker-Franklin and Franklin, 1970). From these ultrastructural studies it appeared that amyloid formation may occur either by excretion from the RE cell of a substance (preamyloid) which, in the extracellular environment, precipitates in the form of the characteristic amyloid microfibrils or by (premature) intracytoplasmatic formation. The evidence available at present suggests that the amyloid-producing RE cell runs through phases, from extra- to intracellular amyloid synthesis, followed by cell degeneration leading to ultimate destruction (Ranløv and Wanstrup, 1967) (Figs. 7 and 8)

The RE nature of the amyloid-forming cell is indicated by its metalophilia (Christensen, 1960) and its phagocytic properties (Smetana, 1927; Ranløv, 1966b). In several combined cytochemical and electron micrographic studies, Kazimierczak (1969, 1972) has been able to demonstrate a markedly increased lysosome content within macrophages concurrent with the appearance of amyloid fibrils within the same cells. Recently, Zucker-Franklin (1974) elegantly

FIG. 7. Reticuloendothelial cell in amyloidotic mouse spleen, closely related to surrounding amyloid substance (A). This substance appears clearly fibrillar and is characteristically arranged at right angles to the cell border, which appears to be intact. The nucleus (N) is large and has a moderate amount of chromatin. Apart from a prominent vesicular Golgi area (G) the cytoplasm seems to be poorly differentiated. From Ranløv and Wanstrup (1967).

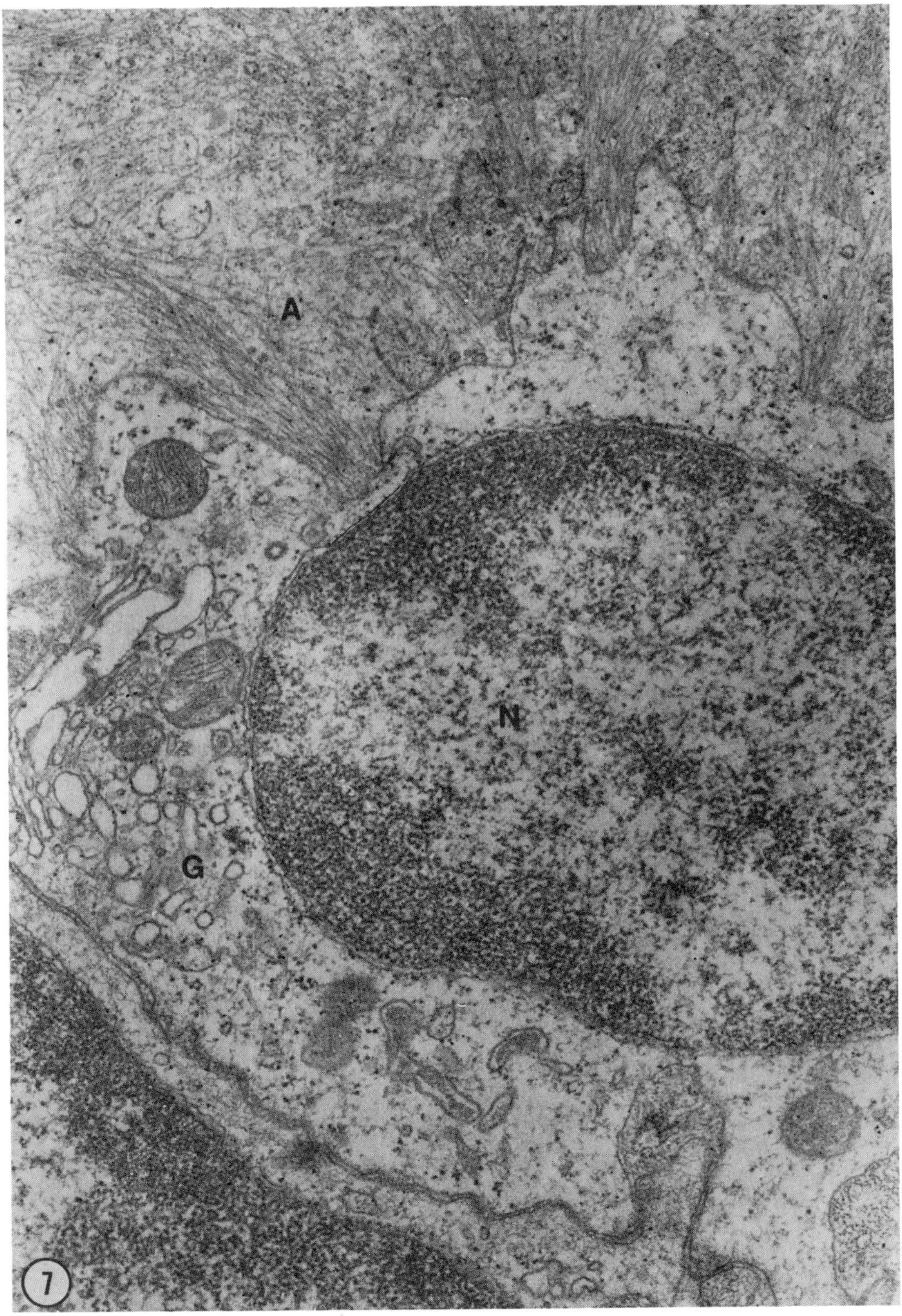
A
N
G
7

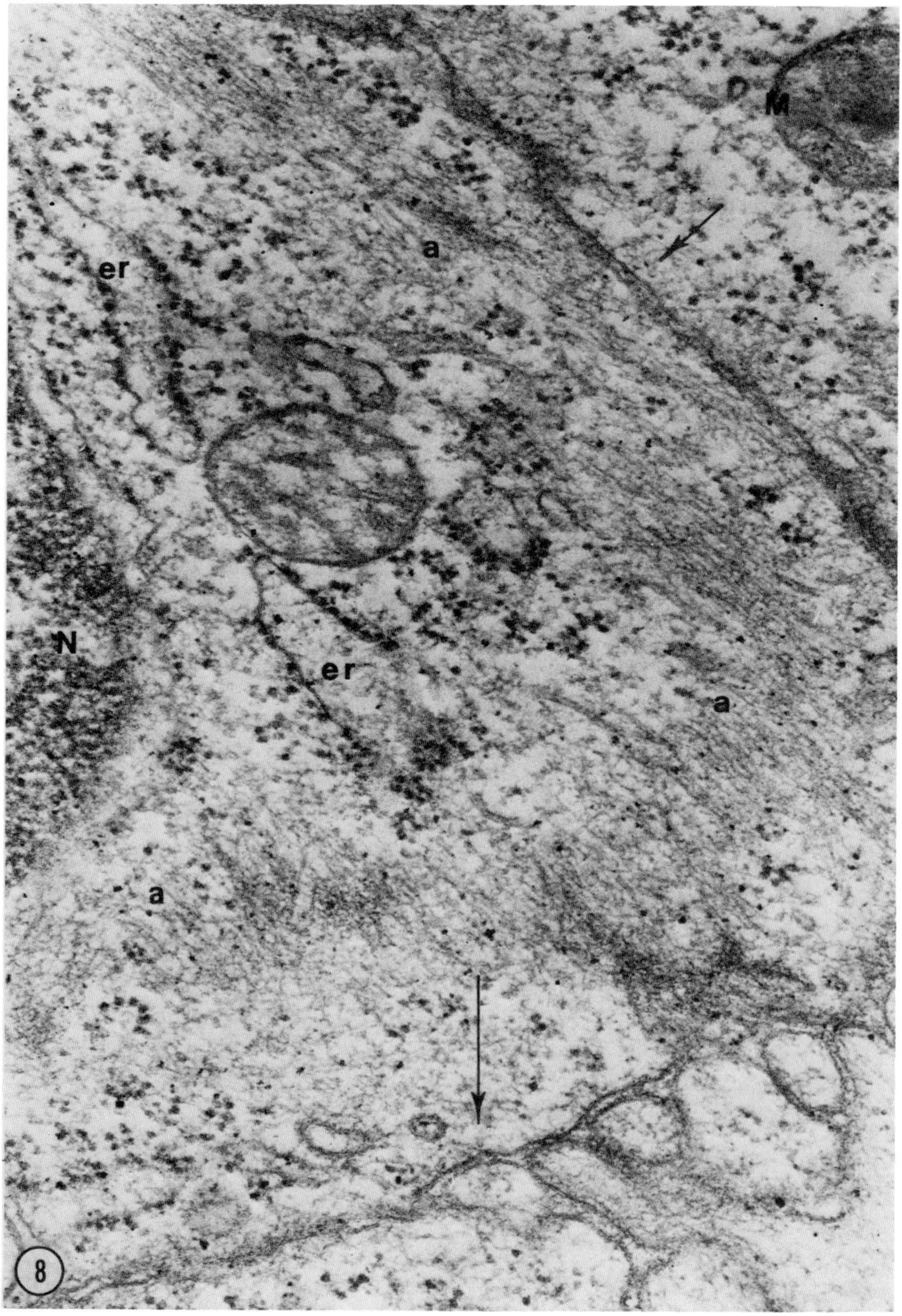
M
a
er
N
er
a
a
8

demonstrated the exclusive occurrence of immunologically characterized amyloid precursor substance within monocytes from peripheral blood obtained from patients with amyloidosis.

C. Immune Functional Characteristics

1. T Cells

The role of the T cell in the pathogenesis of amyloid has lately been the subject of investigation in several laboratories. In experimental models this role has been approached by means of three different procedures: (1) by examining the course of an experimentally induced amyloidosis in an animal after artificial modification of its immune apparatus, i.e., induced lymphopenia; (2) by examining, *in vivo* and *in vitro*, T cell function in the experimental animal during the development of amyloid disease; and (3) by means of amyloid transfer experiments with lymphoid tissues or tissue extracts in syn-, allo-, and xenogeneic combinations.

Induced lymphopenia has been brought about in a variety of ways. The graft-vs-host (GVH) reaction (Simonsen, 1957, 1962), induced by injection of parental strain lymphocytes into F_1 hybrid mice leads to the development of "runt disease," the severity of which is positively correlated with the degree of histoincompatibility between donor and recipient. A prominent feature of the GVH reaction is a severe lymphopenia, and this has been found in several instances to be combined with development of amyloidosis (Fiscus *et al.*, 1962). In a somewhat similar model, lethally irradiated mice, after being restored by injections of allogeneic bone marrow cells, will subsequently develop "secondary disease." This is also characterized by lymphopenia and, often, by amyloidosis (Bradbury and Micklem, 1965). "Wasting disease" is produced in neonatally thymectomized mice and is practically indistinguishable from the GVH reaction and from runt disease. In adult mice a pronounced lymphopenia may be produced by combining thymectomy with sublethal irradiation (400 rad). Such treated animals may sometimes develop spontaneous amyloidosis (Kellum *et al.*, 1965; Sutherland *et al.*, 1965), and casein-induced amyloidosis in mice has been markedly accelerated after adult thymectomy plus irradiation (Ranløv, 1966a), after neonatal thymectomy in mice (Ebbesen, 1971), and after combined thymectomy—bursectomy—irradiation in chickens (Druet and Janigan, 1966).

While lymphopenia is a common denominator of all the above-mentioned

---

FIG. 8. Section of reticuloendothelial (RE) cell from amyloidotic mouse spleen. This RE cell is adjacent to similar cells, and the plasmalemma (arrow) appears well demarcated. There is abundant ergastoplasm (er), and there are clusters of free ribosomes. Conspicuous is a large cytoplasmic area containing a fibrillar, nonmembrane-lined amyloidlike substance (a) which extends close to the nucleus (N). From Ranløv and Wanstrup (1967).

experimental designs, other experiments seem to indicate that lymphopenia in itself is not enough to bring about or to facilitate an experimentally induced amyloidosis. Treatment of mice with antilymphocyte antiscrum (ALS) simultaneous with daily injections of casein delays or even abolishes the development of amyloid disease in the majority of the animals (Ranløv, 1967b). Likewise, nitrogen mustard may inhibit amyloidosis (Ranløv, 1967c). However, it is of decisive importance that both ALS and cytostatics be given both before and during the amyloidogenic treatment; when given after the pyroninophilic phase has been fully developed, cytostatics and adrenocorticosteroids may, at least in experimental models, cause a rapid increase in the amount of amyloid substance being laid down in the tissues (Teilum, 1952, 1954; Ranløv and Christensen, 1968). All these observations illustrate the complexity of the problems related to the role of lymphopenia in amyloidogenesis, but they have also provided us with useful tools for the design of a number of experiments. Thus, experimental transfer of amyloidosis—which will be dealt with in detail below—owes part of its success to the fact that experimentally induced amyloidosis may be markedly accelerated by nitrogen mustard. Further, the observation that experimental amyloidosis may be abolished by immunosuppressives has already proved to have clinical relevance, leading to kidney transplantation in human amyloidotic patients (Cohen et al., 1971). A unique experiment of nature, the nude mouse mutant, is a feasible model for induction of amyloid. This animal, which is hairless, shows retardation of growth, reduced fertility, and a congenital thymic aplasia, is the end product of an autosomal, recessive mutation and is usually referred to as "nu/nu" (Flanagan, 1966; Pantelouris, 1968). The nu/nu mouse has a markedly reduced number of circulating lymphocytes (Pantelouris, 1968), a reduced level of serum immunoglobulins (Rygaard, 1969), which differ qualitatively from those in normal mice (Wortis, 1971). The peripheral lymphopenia has been shown to be due to a reduction in the number of T cells (Raff and Wortis, 1970) and, as anticipated, the nude mouse will readily accept xenogeneic skin transplants (Rygaard, 1969). Other T cell-mediated immune reactions are depressed or abolished: postpertussis lymphocytosis, phytohemagglutinin (PHA)-induced lymphocyte transformation, allograft rejection, and the appearance of plague-forming cells after stimulation with sheep red blood cells (Pantelouris, 1971; Wortis, 1971).

In experiments with mice of the nu/nu strain it has been possible to induce amyloidosis after prolonged treatment with casein (Hardt and Claesson, 1974). Controls were heterozygotes possessing an acceptable degree of histocompatibility with the experimental nu/nu mice (sharing more than 90% of the major tissue antigens). The main observation was a considerable increase in induction time in the nu/nu group; further, the nu/nu mice invariably failed to produce circulating antibodies to casein, while all controls did so in amounts proportionate to the number of casein injections administered. This latter observation led to the rather interesting conclusion that casein is one antigen that requires T cell cooperation in order to exert its immunogenicity in the humoral system. The immunologic capacities of T lymphocytes during the development of experimental amyloidosis have been looked into *in vivo* as well as *in vitro*. We have employed skin graft survival times in a murine allogeneic combination of St/a donors and casein-treated C3H recipients as parameter for the functional capacity of the cellular immune apparatus (Ranløv and Jensen, 1966). After 8 weeks of casein treatment, skin graft survival in severely amyloidotic mice was doubled compared to untreated controls, an observation that was interpreted as signifying a depression of the thymus-dependent immune system. Further substance was lent to this interpretation by observations in a similarly designed experiment using the local GVH reaction designed by Ford et al. (1970). Hardt and Claesson (1971) recorded the increase in the number of nucleated cells in the regional, popliteal lymph node of F_1 hybrid mice injected in the footpad with spleen cells of the parental strains taken from donors in various stages of the induction phase of amyloidosis. The number of cells in the lymph nodes showed a linear relationship to logarithmically spaced numbers of cells injected. A marked depression of this local GVH reaction was observed when the injected spleen cells were derived from donors pretreated with 10 or 20 daily injections of casein. On the assumption that this early depression of GVH reactivity might be due to antigenic competition (Liacopoulos et al., 1967) by nontransplantation antigens administered to the donors, control experiments were performed. In these the donor mice, prior to the casein treatment, were presensitized with two consecutive allogeneic skin grafts (from the other parental strain). The anticipated depression of the GVH reaction was now found only with spleen cells from amyloidotic donors, i.e., donors that had received 20 injections of casein. With the same experimental protocol, GVH reactivity of mixtures of thymus and bone marrow cells from casein-treated parental strain donor mice in the lymph nodes were investigated (Claesson et al., 1974). The combined thymus and bone marrow cells exhibited complete loss of GVH reactivity following 10 casein injections in the donors, and this reactivity could be completely restored by adding thymocytes from untreated donors while bone marrow cells from the same, normal, donors were ineffective in this respect. Quantitative comparison of GVH reactivity of normal thymocytes and thymocytes from casein/cortisol-treated donors gave evidence—in parallel line assays—that the reduced capability of thymocytes to induce the local GVH reaction was caused by a decrease in the number of cortisol-resistant T cells. These experiments have all indicated a markedly reduced cellular immune reactivity in amyloidotic animals, and this reduction is likely to be related to the induced formation of amyloid.

Based on *in vitro* experiments, a similar depression of cellular immune reactivity in the course of casein-induced amyloidosis has been reported by Rodey and Good (1969). Using mice, they found inhibition of blast transformation when spleen cells from amyloidotic animals were exposed to azocasein and PHA.

In human patients with amyloid disease the lymphocyte response to PHA was found to be normal, though the response to certain virus antigens was reduced (Lehner et al., 1970).

The leukocyte migration test (LMT), originally discovered by Rich and Lewis in 1932, has in recent years been given renewed interest. In current usage, the migration of white blood cells, spleen cells or peritoneal macrophages from the mouth of a capillary tube is assayed after placement in tissue culture medium, where it may be inhibited by the presence of specific antigen. A prerequisite is presensitization of the donor animal. The mechanism of the inhibition of migration is not entirely clear, but is believed to depend on the production, by sensitized T cells, of various substances termed "lymphokines." These are soluble proteins with molecular weights between 30,000 and 80,000, resistant to RNase and DNase, but easily destroyed by various proteolytic enzymes. They are generally classified according to their biological activity, mostly in vitro, i.e., as "migration inhibition factor" (MIF), mitogenic factor, cytotoxic factor, etc. (Dumonde et al., 1969). We have modified this assay for use with mouse spleen cells (Ranløv and Hardt, 1970). We found that after 7 days of casein treatment, mice showed a marked cellular immune response in vitro toward casein, judged by MIF production. In similar experiments with guinea pigs, Cathcart et al. (1970, 1971) likewise found cellular immune reactivity directed against casein after 2 weeks of stimulation by casein. However, during the following weeks—in face of prolonged administration of casein—this anti-casein immune response gradually disappeared. Thus, in amyloidotic guinea pigs, cellular immune reactivity toward the amyloid-inducing antigen was lost, while reactivity directed against a number of other antigens was intact. These findings were interpreted as a state of selective tolerance toward casein, and hence amyloid was regarded as one end result of antigen-mediated inactivation of a specific clone of lymphocytes. As a consequence, Cathcart et al. believed that the sustained presence of the amyloid-inducing antigen was a prerequisite for the continued laying-down of amyloid in the tissues.

As the question of the necessity of sustained antigenic presence during formation of amyloid has some bearing on the subject of transfer amyloidosis, the concept of a pathogenetic significance of specific tolerance in experimental amyloidosis deserves further consideration. Letterer and Kretschmer (1966) examined the degree of amyloidosis in mice previously made tolerant toward casein. Their in vivo studies showed a markedly decreased incidence of amyloidosis in mice rendered tolerant toward casein by administration of massive doses of this antigen during the neonatal period. However, they did not produce evidence that their experimental animals were actually still tolerant at the time of the amyloidogenic casein treatment. Although their results were highly significant, their interpretation must be looked upon with caution. Somewhat similar experiments by others included control of the state of tolerance: lack of circulating anti-casein antibodies and lack of immune elimination of ^{131}I-labeled casein from plasma (Clerici et al., 1965). Clerici et al. failed to detect any difference in the degree of amyloidosis between tolerant and nontolerant casein-treated mice. Furthermore, it is well known that the rate of production of anti-casein antibodies is independent of the length of treatment and of the degree of amyloidosis, observations that are not particularly favorable to the tolerance hypothesis (Ebbesen, 1971; Willerson et al., 1969a). A strong argument against the concept of a pathogenetic role of tolerance toward the amyloid-inducing antigen is presented in a report (Hardt et al., 1972) describing unhampered production of amyloid in C3H mice after multiple infusions of normal syngeneic lymphoid cells during the course of amyloidogenic injections of casein. If—as claimed by Cathcart and co-workers—specific tolerance toward casein were of major pathogenetic importance, the infusions of lymphocytes should have prevented or broken the tolerance, and thus have abolished formation of amyloid in the recipient. This did not happen.

Of considerable importance in the evaluation of the functions and kinetics of T and B lymphocytes are the findings of specific surface antigens on mouse T cells, the so-called θ-antigens (Reif and Allen, 1963; Raff, 1969). Allogeneic anti-θ antiserum can be produced by immunizing, for example AKR mice with thymocytes from C3H mice (Raff, 1971). Employing a rather simple cytotoxicity test, the T cells in a given cell suspension (from C3H mice) can thus be recognized. In experiments by Hardt and Claesson (1972a) this method has been used in order to follow the fluctuations of the T cell populations in lymphoid organs of C3H mice undergoing casein treatment. In the pyroninophilic tissue phase, after 5–10 injections of casein, the number of T cells in the spleen rose significantly, corresponding to the increased T cell-mediated immunity toward casein characteristic of this stage (Ranløv and Hardt, 1970). After 15–20 injections of casein (i.e., at the beginning of the amyloid phase proper), a marked reduction in the number of T cells set in. After 30 injections of casein, when amyloidosis was fully developed, T cells were absent from the spleen.

These findings offer a sufficient explanation of the systemically reduced cell-mediated immunity found in severely amyloidotic mice (Ranløv and Jensen, 1966; Hardt and Claesson, 1971). The fact, that RE cell production of amyloid is initiated concurrently with a massive decay of T cells is highly suggestive of a release of an amyloid-inducing factor (AIF) from disintegrating lymphoid cells. This AIF—in conjunction with specific macrophage-processed antigen—may have been responsible for the transfer of amyloid-producing potency to the RE cells.

2. B Cells

In the pyroninophilic phase of casein-induced amyloidosis, only a small increase in the number of plasma cells can be found (Teilum, 1964a; Scholten et al., 1968). Proliferation of plasma cells can thus be responsible for only part of the observed increase in lymphoid cells with markedly pyroninophilic cytoplasm, while the major part of this increase is probably due to proliferation of T lymphocytes and/or macrophages. Ranløv (1968) also noted that the mature plasma cells found during this phase bore no relation to the duration or the intensity of the treatment with antigen and had no topographic relation to the areas of the RE system in which pyroninophilia was or had been maximal, and where amyloid was eventually deposited.

Histological studies of casein-induced amyloidosis have not supported the concept of plasma cells playing any significant role in the formation of amyloid. This is in accord with the findings of Druet and Janigan (1966), who managed to induce amyloidosis with casein in bursectomized chickens "despite the total absence of mature plasma cells."

However, a relationship between plasma cell neoplasia and the occurrence of amyloidosis in man has been noted in many studies (Bayrd and Bennet, 1950; Osserman et al., 1964; Isobe and Osserman, 1974; review: Franklin and Zucker-Franklin, 1972). Likewise, similar relationships have been found in mice with transplanted plasma cell leukemia (Dunn, 1957; McIntire and Potter, 1964; Lehner et al., 1966; review: Ebbesen, 1968) as well as in mice with spontaneous plasma cell leukemia (Rask-Nielsen et al., 1961; Ebbesen and Rask-Nielsen, 1967). It may be added that Rask-Nielsen et al., (1960) showed that transplantation of reticulosarcomas that had arisen spontaneously in old (CBA × DBA/2)F_1 hybrid mice were followed by amyloidosis in the recipients. In this particular tumor some of the tumor cells exhibited differentiation into plasma cells.

In other experiments along these lines, Ebbesen and Rask-Nielsen (1967) found that 50% of mice that had received acellular extracts from mice with plasma cell leukemia remained aleukemic; and of these the males, and only the males, developed amyloidosis. This observation does not support the suggestions made by many authors (Glenner et al., 1971; Isobe and Osserman, 1974) that protein synthesis in plasma cells is directly and causally involved in amyloid fibril formation. Ebbesen and Rask-Nielsen proposed a mechanism by which a virus could directly induce production of amyloid fibrils in infected cells. Virus could also be acting either by prolonged antigen stimulation or by inducing defects in the immune system.

Ebbesen and co-workers found in 1969 that BALB/c mice inoculated with subcellular leukemic material from mice with plasma cell leukemia developed plasma cell neoplasia with and without paraproteinemia. In both these groups amyloidlike fibrils were found by electron microscopy, while light microscopy of alkaline Congo red-stained sections did not reveal the presence of amyloid. The fibrils were found in lymph nodes, both extracellularly and within cells that were described as "malignant plasma cells." Lehner and Rosenoer (1968) have described similar findings in BALB/c mice that had received plasma cell tumor transplants subcutaneously. In this experiment fibrillar material was found by both electron and light microscopy. However, the amyloid nature of the partly amorphous substance described by Lehner and Rosenoer has been questioned. Thus both reports suggest that formation of the fibrils is related to abnormal plasma cells, but the evidence for production of amyloid by plasma cells is not convincing.

Although the normal plasma cells do not seem to produce amyloid, there is a correlation of abnormal plasma cells and amyloidosis. The demonstration by Glenner et al. (1971) that some forms of human amyloid fibrils contain fragments of light chains supports the concept of Ebbesen et al. (1969) that abnormal plasma cells can produce amyloidlike fibrils from light chains.

Letterer (1926, 1934) postulated that an increase in the amount of circulating serum globulin was an important factor in the pathogenesis of amyloidosis and elaborated this theory by postulating that amyloid is a precipitate of antigen and normal γ-globulin (Letterer, 1934). Others later proposed that amyloid is altered nonspecific γ-globulin (Latvalahti, 1953) or is an altered abnormal specific protein (Bence–Jones) by itself (Osserman et al., 1964; Isobe and Osserman, 1974).

That experimentally induced amyloid should be a product of the injected antigen (casein) and circulating antibodies to casein is not likely, as amyloid can be formed without the presence of plasma cells (Druet and Janigan, 1966) and without concurrent formation of circulating casein-precipitating antibodies. The latter point has been demonstrated by Clerici et al. (1965) in mice tolerant toward casein and by Hardt and Claesson (1974) in "nude" mice. In experiments in which the injections of casein promote the formation of circulating antibodies, the antibody level could not be correlated with the incidence or the severity of the resulting amyloidosis (Giles and Calkins, 1958; Ebbesen, 1971). This point has been further looked into by Willerson and collaborators (1969a), who showed injections of casein into six different strains of mice to provoke amyloid formation in all but one strain, though in variable degrees and with different induction times. In this experiment no relationship was found between the serum level of immune globulins and the production of amyloid; also production of amyloid could proceed without simultaneous or prior occurrence of circulating antibodies to casein. It was further shown that infusion of immune globulin from ascites fluid obtained from other mice with a plasma cell tumour could not induce formation of amyloid, even though the amount of circulating immune globulin in the recipient became as great as the level found in mice of the same strain injected with casein in doses sufficient to induce amyloidosis.

More directly arguing against the theory of hypergammaglobulinemia in man being the sole causal factor is the well known report by Teilum (1964b, 1968) describing amyloidosis in patients with hypogammaglobulinemia.

In mice given various numbers of injections of casein, Ranløv (1967d) measured the humoral immune reactivity toward an unrelated antigen, ferritin. He found the capacity to produce circulating antibodies against ferritin markedly decreased in mice treated with casein for less than 4 weeks. The antibody response had become normal at the time the mice became amyloidotic, and it remained normal until the last observation, after 8 weeks of casein treatment, at which time the mice had severe amyloidosis. Ranløv interpreted the early depression of the antibody response as due to antigen competition, and the normalization as a result of a nonspecific proliferation of B lymphocytes during prolonged antigen stimulation. This experiment showed that the humoral part of the immune system remained intact, in contrast to the heavy depression of the cellular part, reported elsewhere (Ranløv and Jensen, 1966; Hardt and Claesson, 1971; Claesson et al., 1974).

3. *Macrophages*

The phagocytic capacity of murine macrophages during the induction of experimental amyloidosis has been investigated by Zschiesche and Ghatak (1965). Employing intravenously administered India ink, they found carbon clearance from the blood to vary between AB/Jena and C57BL mice. While the former showed a steady rate of carbon clearance, the latter exhibited an increased clearance rate through the preamyloid phase, followed by a decrease to normal values concurrent with the deposition of amyloid substance in the spleen and liver. The same year, Shearing and co-workers repeated these observations in rabbits made amyloidotic by continued injections of casein (Shearing et al., 1965). Similar experiments were carried out by us and reported the following year. We also found that phagocytosis of intravenously injected colloidal carbon varied with the stage of amyloidosis in St/a mice. Carbon clearance increased gradually during the pyroninophilic tissue phase and decreased toward normal levels after production of amyloid had begun (Ranløv, 1966b).

Hardt and Claesson (1972a) described the fluctuations in the number of lymphocytes and macrophages in spleens of mice subjected to increasing numbers of casein injections. It was found that both lymphocyte and macrophage total counts rose significantly during the pyroninophilic phase. These findings were all in line with those obtained by conventional histologic examinations of tissues from casein-treated mice (Teilum, 1954, 1956; Christensen, 1960; Druet and Janigan, 1966; Werdelin and Ranløv, 1966; Kazimierczak, 1969). Further, Hardt and Claesson (1972a) found the increase in the amount of tissue amyloid formed during prolonged casein stimulation to be accompanied by a simultaneous decrease in the total number of lymphocytes and macrophages. The decrease of lymphocytes was particularly conspicuous, but that of macrophages was also significant and explains the reduction in total phagocytic capacity during the formation of amyloid.

Another approach to the evaluation of the possible functional role of macrophages in amyloidogenesis is to employ either blockade or stimulation of macrophages during an amyloid-inducing regimen. Smetana (1927) made an attempt to block the RE system by injecting massive doses of India ink simultaneously with casein treatment. Even though he did not check the effectiveness of the blockade, he managed to demonstrate that mice so treated only reluctantly developed amyloid in comparison to controls treated with casein alone. The RE system may be stimulated with Bacillus Calmette-Guérin (BCG). This has been tried in experimental mouse amyloidosis by Zschiesche (1968; Zschiesche et al., 1967), who injected 0.5 mg of BCG intravenously prior to a series of injections of sodium caseinate. Pretreatment with BCG resulted in a considerable delay in the development of amyloid within the various organs examined. When multiple doses of BCG were injected later during the course of the casein treatment, delay in formation of amyloid was usually more pronounced, and in some instances amyloidosis was even prevented. In these experiments the stimulating effect of BCG on the mouse RE system was reflected in a 3- to 5-fold increase in carbon clearance expressed as phagocytic indices.

III. Transfer of Experimental Amyloidosis

A. INTRODUCTION

In 1965 evidence accumulated from several years of work on experimental amyloidosis in our laboratory indicated unequivocally a cellular morphogenesis of the amyloid substance and strongly suggested a participation of immune reactions in the events leading to its formation. These combined observations led us to the working hypothesis that amyloid disease might be transferable with cells from one experimental animal to another. In the following year we found that the transfer of spleen cells from casein-treated C3H mice into syngeneic normal mice induced significant amyloidosis in the recipients within 3–5 days (Werdelin and Ranløv, 1966). These observations have later been consistently reproduced and extended in our laboratory and in those of others.

On the following pages we shall discuss two methods, differing in principle, by which amyloidosis has been transferred from one animal to another. We shall describe and evaluate a number of reported experiments that all have in common the feature that amyloidogenic treatment had been restricted to the donor animal. This model we term "transfer of amyloidosis." In Section IV yet another type of experimental amyloidosis will be dealt with. Although this type also involves transplantation of cells or tissues in experimental animals, it depends, in addition, upon continued antigenic challenge of the recipients of the transplants. For this and other reasons we do regard it not as amyloid transfer in the strict sense, but as a transfer of immunity to the amyloidogenic agent.

B. AMYLOIDOSIS AS A TRANSFERABLE DISEASE

When one is confronted with a disease that can be transferred from one animal to another, its etiology or pathogenesis should be searched for among the following: (a) infection, (b) neoplasm, (c) disorder of the immune system.

1. *The Role of Infection*

Virchow (1854) considered infection to be a direct causal factor in amyloidogenesis. Later experiments showed that killed bacteria or parasites had identical effects, suggesting that the role of infection in amyloidosis may be that of heavy antigenic stimulation. From time to time, however, the question has been raised whether the formation of amyloid was directly due to a generalized infection, facilitated by injections of antigen, GVH-reactions, wasting phenomena, or avitaminosis, all known to promote, under some circumstances, formation of amyloid. That an interaction between amyloid-producing cells, e.g., macrophages, and bacteria or parasites should be the common pathway of all amyloidogenesis is not likely since Dunn (1967) has pointed out that spontaneous amyloidosis appears in germfree mice and Claesson and Hardt (1972b) found that germfree mice develop amyloidosis to the same degree as controls after stimulation with sterilized casein.

In several electrophoretic and morphologic studies Rask-Nielsen and co-workers have analyzed many aspects of the coincidence of murine leukemia and amyloidosis (see below). In one of their experiments Ebbesen and Rask-Nielsen (1967) found an amyloidogenic effect of an acellular agent in tissue extracts causing plasma cell leukemia in mice, indicating the presence of a virus having both oncogenic and nononcogenic properties. That cells infected with a specific (?) virus should, as a result of the infection, produce amyloid fibrils is a very attractive hypothesis. However, in electron microscopic studies so far no evidence has been produced for the presence of virus particles in cells producing amyloid fibrils.

2. *Neoplasia*

The connection between malignant diseases and amyloidosis is well recognized in clinical medicine. In particular, amyloid appears in such systemic malignancies of the lymphoreticular tissues as Hodgkin's disease, multiple myeloma, and Waldenstrøm's disease (Ranløv and Elling Nielsen, 1966). Certain solid tumors are also represented: the medullary thyroid carcinoma, the calcifying epithelial odontogenic tumor (Ranløv and Pindborg, 1967) and hypernephroma (Teilum, 1964a). In animal experiments a number of transferable tumors have been found to be associated with formation of amyloid, again mainly tumors of the lymphoreticular system (review: Ebbesen, 1968). In such experiments the tumor-bearing animals develop considerable amounts of amyloid diffusely throughout spleen, liver, and kidney. Although amyloidlike fibrils have been found in neoplastic plasma cells (Ebbesen *et al.*, 1969; Lehner and Rosenoer, 1968), conclusive evidence for tumor cells as a source of amyloid fibrils is still lacking. The coincidence of tumors and amyloidosis has therefore been explained as a result of sustained challenge with tumor antigens.

Transfer amyloidosis experiments with subcellular fractions do not support the concept that amyloidosis is a neoplastic disorder unless one accepts the hypothesis that oncogenic viruses can be amyloidogenic.

3. *Immune Disorders*

Another group of diseases that may be transferred in experimental animals are the immune disorders.

Analysis of the immunologic injuries found in immune disorders indicates two principal mechanisms: (1) a direct form resulting from the action of the specific antibody or sensitized cell directed against target cells or tissue constituents; (2) an indirect form in which cells or tissues are injured because, by chance, antigen—antibody or antigen—cell reactions happen in their environment.

The antibody-elicited injuries are again divided into (1) precipitinogenic, (2) cytotropic, and (3) cytolytic types.

The antibody-elicited injury of the precipitinogenic type is the one demonstrated by Arthus in 1903, in which the antigen—antibody complex triggers a multitude of mechanisms that all tend to disturb the function and integrity of surrounding cells and structures.

The cytotropic type of immune injury depends on the presence of homocytotropic antibodies, which in man probably belong to the immunoglobulin class IgE. Their presence in man was first demonstrated by Prausnitz and Küstner in 1921 in their passive transfer experiments. In such experiments the "recipient" is injured by a reaction between IgE and antigen. The lesion in the "recipient" is transitory and does not alter the reactivity of the "recipient."

The third form of damage elicited by antibodies is the cytolytic type, where circulating antibody reacts with cell surface components, and via the serum complement system severely damages the cell membrane.

The idea that cells could be directly responsible for an immune injury has its roots in Robert Koch's classic description (1890) of the tuberculin-type skin reaction in guinea pigs. Zinsser (1925) later demonstrated this reaction to be a hypersensitive reaction taking place without demonstrable circulating antibodies.

Further support for a cell-mediated immune reaction was given by Landsteiner and Chase (1942) and later more definitely by Chase (1945), who succeeded in transferring a delayed hypersensitive skin reaction in guinea pigs with leukocytes from the peritoneal exudate of sensitized animals. It was later found that not only the leukocytes from the peritoneal exudate, but also leukocytes from the peripheral blood and from the lymph nodes were effective in transferring delayed-type hypersensitivity. It has been difficult, if not impossible, to rule out that transfer of delayed hypersensitivity is due to a simultaneous transfer of cell-bound antibody. However, the demonstration of a thymus-dependent population of lymphocytes (Miller, 1961, 1962) led to experiments that showed that delayed skin reactions are solely elicited via sensitization of thymus-dependent lymphocytes (T lymphocytes) (Arnason *et al.*, 1964); and in mice anti-θ-serum can inhibit this transfer of hypersensitivity by selective killing of T lymphocytes in mice (Raff and Wortis, 1971).

Experiments with passive transfer of cellular hypersensitivity by means of subcellular components have convincingly confirmed that the cell-derived principle, which determines the specific alteration of cellular behavior, can be adopted by noncommitted lymphocytes of a nonreactive organism.

This passive transfer of cellular hypersensitivity by means of subcellular fractions was shown by Lawrence in humans to be due to a protein with a molecular weight of possibly less than 10,000 (Lawrence et al., 1963). Many different experiments have given evidence that the transfer of specific reactivity from one cell to another may be due not to one single factor, but rather to a system of interacting macromolecules possibly representing alternative pathways (review: Bloom and Chase, 1967). These mechanisms seem to differ from species to species as Lawrence's "transfer factor" has been shown only in humans. It has been claimed, however, that RNA is able to confer on syngeneic nonsensitive guinea pig lymphoid cells the ability to activate delayed hypersensitivity to various antigens (Jureziz et al., 1970).

One of the main questions about transfer amyloidosis has been to what extent amyloidosis can be considered an autoimmune disease, as amyloidosis has many features in common with this type of immune disorder. The autoimmune diseases may, in principle, be elicited by any one of the above-mentioned types of immune injuries. But it is generally agreed that a disease should be called autoimmune only if it fulfills Witebsky's four criteria (Witebsky, 1959; Milgrom and Witebsky, 1962): (1) circulating or cell-bound antibodies reactive with the autoantigen must be detectable; (2) the autoantigen must be identified; (3) mononuclear inflammation must be present in the target tissue; (4) passive transfer of the disease must be possible either with lymphoid cells or with serum.

From what has been said amyloidosis certainly does not qualify as an autoimmune disease. Neither criterion 1 or 2 is met. Perhaps criterion 3 is fulfilled. On the following pages we shall endeavor to clarify the applicability of criterion 4 to experimental amyloidosis.

C. Transfer with Cells (Table I)

1. *The Hypothesis*

The preconception that experimental mouse amyloidosis might be transferable between syngeneic animals by means of injections of lymphoid cells had three bases: (1) studies pointing to RE cells, especially those in the spleen, as being directly engaged in the synthesis of amyloid or amyloid microfibrils *in loco* (Teilum, 1956, 1964a; Christensen, 1963; Cohen et al., 1965); (2) the reports discussed in the preceding section, which indicate that immune mechanisms of the cellular type play an important role in the commencement and maintenance of the initial, pyroninophilic tissue phase; and (3) the fact that lymphoid cells—

TABLE I
AMYLOID TRANSFER EXPERIMENTS WITH WHOLE CELLS

Authors	Donors				Transfer material			Recipients			
	Mouse strain	Treatment	Amyloidotic	Source	No. of cells	Route of administration	Mouse strain	Treatment prior to transfer	Treatment post transfer	Incidence of amyloidosis	Interval transfer to sacrifice (days)
Werdelin and Ranløv (1966)	C3H	17 Casein injections	30%	Spleen	100×10^6	i.v.	C3H	None	Nitrogen mustard, 0.05 mg × 3	68/74	2–6
Ranløv (1967a)	C3H	17 Casein injections	34%	Spleen	100×10^6	i.v.	C3H	None	Nitrogen mustard, 0.05 mg × 2	19/19	4
Ranløv and Werdelin (1967)	C3H	17 Casein injections + tritiated thymidine	50%	Spleen	100×10^6	i.v.	C3H	None	Nitrogen mustard, 0.05 mg × 2	10/15	2–4
Hardt (1968)	C3H	21 Casein injections	100%	Whole spleen graft	ca. 25 mg	Tissue graft to kidney	C3H	None	Nitrogen mustard, 0.05 mg × 2	20/20	14
Clerici et al. (1969)	C57BL	30 Casein injections	100%	Thoracic duct lymphocytes	$5–30 \times 10^6$	i.v. or i.p.	C57BL	Irradiation (500 rad)	None	2/42[a]	5–20
Willerson et al. (1969b)	White Swiss	6–20 Casein injections	75%	Spleen	300×10^6	i.v.	White Swiss	None	None	50/55	4–12
	White Swiss	14–20 Casein injections	?	Liver	?	i.v.	White Swiss	None	None	6/16	5
	White Swiss	14–20 Casein injections	?	Liver	?	i.v.	White Swiss	None	Nitrogen mustard, 0.05 mg × 2	10/12	5

Continued

TABLE 1—*Continued*

Authors	Donors				Transfer material			Recipients			
	Mouse strain	Treatment	Amyloidotic	Source	No. of cells	Route of administration	Mouse strain	Treatment prior to transfer	Treatment post transfer	Incidence of amyloidosis	Interval from transfer to sacrifice (days)
	White Swiss	14–20 Casein injections	?	Lung	?	i.v.	White Swiss	None	None	3/17[a]	5
	White Swiss	14–20 Casein injections	?	Lung	?	i.v.	White Swiss	None	Nitrogen mustard, 0.05 mg × 2	5/13	5
	C3H	32 Casein injections	?	Spleen	300 × 10⁶	i.v.	C3H	None	None	1/9[a]	5
	C3H	32 Casein injections	?	Spleen	300 × 10⁶	i.v.	C3H	None	Nitrogen mustard, 0.05 mg × 2	6/8	5
	C57BL	19 Casein injections	?	Spleen	300 × 10⁶	i.v.	C57BL	None	None	3/11	4
	C57BL	19 Casein injections	?	Spleen	300 × 10⁶	i.v.	C57BL	None	Nitrogen mustard, 0.05 mg × 2	12/12	4
Dreher and Letterer (1970)	White Swiss	*Escherichia coli* endotoxin 0.5 mg × 21	100%	Spleen	300 × 10⁶	i.v.	White Swiss	None	None	8/10	5
	NMRI, C3H, C57BL	7 Casein injections	32%	Spleen	300 × 10⁶	i.p.	NMRI, C3H, C57BL	None	None	23/75[a]	5
Hardt (1971)	C3H	17 Casein injections	100%	Spleen	100 × 10⁶	i.v.	C3H	None	Nitrogen mustard, 0.05 mg × 3	37/37	6
	C3H	17 Casein injections	100%	Thymus	100 × 10⁶	i.v.	C3H	None	Nitrogen mustard, 0.05 mg × 3	0/9	6

	C3H	17 Casein injections	100%	Bone marrow	50×10^6	i.v.	C3H	None	Nitrogen mustard, 0.05 mg × 3	0/5	6
	C3H	17 Casein injections	100%	Bone marrow + thymus	$50 \times 10^6 + 50 \times 10^6$	i.v.	C3H	None	Nitrogen mustard, 0.05 mg × 3	0/9	6
	C3H	17 Casein injections	100%	Lymph node	100×10^6	i.v.	C3H	None	Nitrogen mustard, 0.05 mg × 3	0/10	6
	C3H	17 Casein injections	100%	Peritoneal macrophages	25×10^6	i.v.	C3H	None	Nitrogen mustard, 0.05 mg × 3	0/11	6
	C3H	17 Casein injections	100%	Blood lymphocytes	100×10^6	i.v.	C3H	None	Nitrogen mustard, 0.05 mg × 3	0/17	6
Hardt and Hellung-Larsen (1972)	C3H	21 Casein injections	?	Spleen	100×10^6	i.v.	C3H	None	Nitrogen mustard, 0.05 mg × 3	56/60	6
Hardt and Claesson (1974)	C3H	40 Casein injections	100%	Spleen	100×10^6	i.v.	C3H	None	Nitrogen mustard, 0.05 mg × 3	4/4	6
	C3H	40 Casein injections	100%	Spleen	100×10^6	i.v.	nu/nu-C3H	None	Nitrogen mustard, 0.05 mg × 3	0/8	6
	nu/nu-C3H	40 Casein injections	100%	Spleen	100×10^6	i.v.	nu/nu-C3H	None	Nitrogen mustard, 0.05 mg × 3	0/8	6
	nu/nu-C3H	40 Casein injections	100%	Spleen	100×10^6	i.v.	C3H	None	Nitrogen mustard, 0.05 m; × 3	3/3	6
Hardt et al. (1975)	C3H	21 Casein injections	75%	Splenic T cells, (B-cell deprived)	100×10^6	i.v.	C3H	None	Nitrogen mustard, 0.05 mg × 3	0/20	6

[a] Not significant.

including those in the spleen—can transfer several experimental diseases that are presumed to involve cellular immune mechanisms at one stage or another (Felix-Davies and Waksman, 1961; Åstrøm and Waksman, 1962; Hess et al., 1962).

Werdelin and Ranløv (1966) postulated that the primary pyroninophilic phase, having commenced and completely developed in an animal after several weeks of treatment with casein, must be transferable by means of spleen cells to another syngeneic animal. Thus the recipient animal is rapidly brought into the actual amyloid phase. Several reasons for choosing spleen cells as donor material are obvious. The spleen is the most frequent primary site of amyloid formation in experimental animals and in man. Spleen cells are known mediators of cellular immunity. Finally, there are sufficient spleen cells in one animal (mouse) for transfer into several recipients.

2. *Spleen Cells*

The hypothesis was confirmed by Werdelin and Ranløv (1966), who found regular development of amyloidosis in normal C3H mice 2–5 days after intravenous administration of 10^8 spleen cells from syngeneic donors that had previously been given a series of injections of casein. It was found necessary to subject the donor mice to at least 14, preferably 17, injections of casein, given as daily subcutaneous doses of 25 mg of bovine sodium caseinate. This treatment rendered approximately 20% of the donor animals slightly amyloidotic, with a thin perifollicular collar of amyloid in the spleen, graded as + or ++ according to Christensen and Hjort (1959). After the cell transfer, the recipient mice were treated with nitrogen mustard in order to accelerate formation of amyloid (Teilum, 1954); serial necropsies 1, 2, 3, 4, and 5 days after the spleen cell transfer showed amyloid in the spleens of recipients, beginning 48 hours after transfer, when some of the recipients developed thin, incomplete rings of amyloid in the perifollicular regions of the Malpighian corpuscles. During the following days the incidence and severity of the amyloid lesions increased. On the fifth day after cell transfer all spleens of recipients showed marked amyloidosis. Control experiments employing (1) the transfer of spleen cells from normal, nonimmunized donors followed by nitrogen mustard treatment of the recipients, (2) treatment of C3H mice with nitrogen mustard alone, and (3) transfer of spleen cells from donors given multiple injections of casein into mice that were not treated with nitrogen mustard, all failed to produce amyloid in the respective recipients.

In this experiment care was taken to ensure that the transferred cells were viable. The pooled donor spleens—usually derived from 15–20 casein-treated mice—were gently teased apart in a loose-fitting Potter-Elvehjem homogenizer while suspended in Ringer's solution, then filtered through a stainless steel sieve (1600 holes per cm^2), washed three times in Ringer's solution (sedimentation at approximately 800 g), and finally adjusted to a cell density of 200×10^6 nucleated cells per milliliter, the volume injected into the recipient then being

0.5 ml. In these and similar experiments done in our laboratory Trypan blue tests have consistently revealed cell viability in the transferred suspensions to exceed 80%, usually 90—95%. Cells were transferred into each recipient mouse through a tail vein. It is of paramount importance to use well-washed cell suspensions and to inject the desired volume (0.5 ml) at a slow rate (over approximately 15 seconds). In many instances heparin has caused agglutination of the cells and thus rendered the material uninjectable or caused rapid death of the recipients and should be avoided in this type of transfer experiments. Apart from that, some cell suspensions cause instant and dramatic exitus of all the recipients, for no obvious reasons. We have not been able to find explanations for this by autopsies.

3. Nitrogen Mustard

Though it is not invariably necessary (Ranløv, 1967a; Willerson et al., 1969b), we prefer to speed up formation of amyloid in our recipients by treating them after the cell transfer with a short course of nitrogen mustard. This accelerating procedure was described originally by Teilum in 1954. Teilum's protocol is still being used. Starting on the day of the transfer, a subcutaneous injection of 0.05 mg of nitrogen mustard (Erasol®), solubilized in distilled water, was given. This procedure was repeated on day 3 and, if the experiment extended beyond that day, on day 5. In most transfer experiments 2 injections were given. In the classic, casein-treated mouse the amyloid-enhancing effect of nitrogen mustard is indisputable (Ranløv and Christensen, 1968), but the mechanism is not understood. It is tempting to correlate the cytolytic action of nitrogen mustard and the consequent lymphopenia with the phenomenon of lymphoid depletion in experimental amyloidosis, as discussed in the previous section.

4. Preformed Amyloid

Werdelin and Ranløv (1966) have acknowledged that in their original experiment the inoculum may have contained, apart from spleen cells and Ringer's solution, small lumps of amyloid derived from the 20% of donors that usually are slightly amyloidotic at the time of sacrifice. Relatively larger lumps were found in the small vessels of the recipients' lungs (Fig. 9). However, it cannot be excluded that small particles of preformed amyloid may have passed the lungs and reached the spleen in the recipient. The fact that amyloid is never found in the recipient spleen until at least 48 hours after the cell transfer and that recipients not treated with nitrogen mustard only occasionally develop amyloidosis, offers conclusive evidence against any significant part of such a mechanism in the establishment of the amyloidotic lesions in the recipients. This has also been stated in the comprehensive report by Willerson and co-workers (1969b).

5. Number of Cells and Route of Transfer

Among the various factors critical for a successful outcome of an amyloid transfer experiment employing whole cells are the number of cells employed and

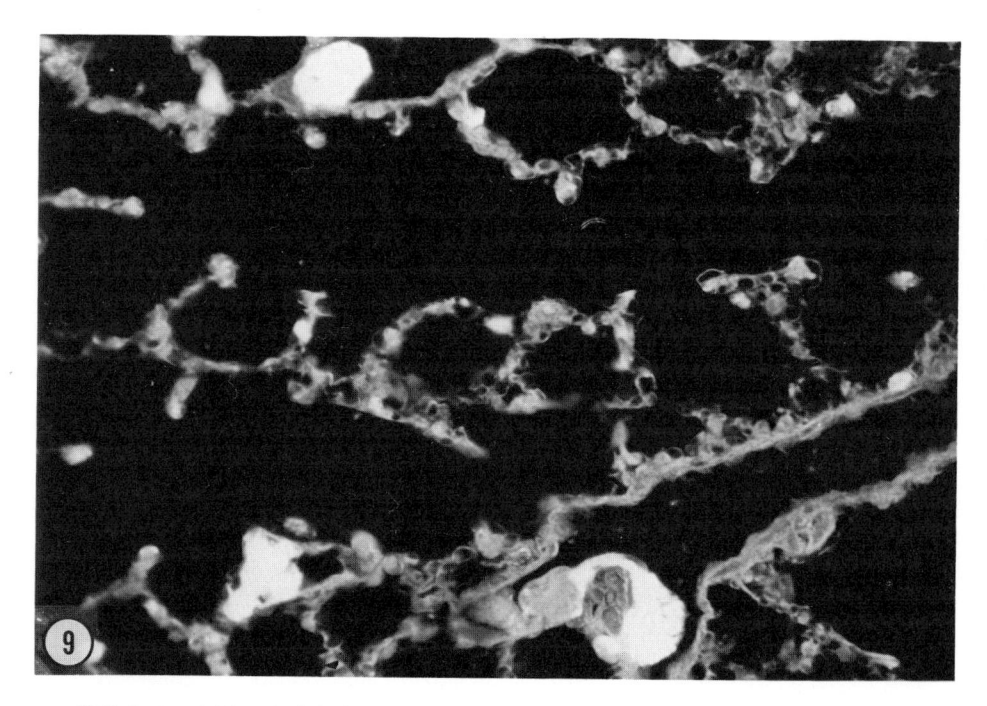

FIG. 9. Amyloid emboli in lung vessels of mouse treated with nitrogen mustard for 6 days after "cell" transfer. Some of the donor mice contributing to this cell suspension had developed amyloidosis. Thioflavine T-stain, fluorescence in ultraviolet light. × 350. From Werdelin and Ranløv (1966).

the route of injection into the recipient (Table I). Reliable guidelines do not exist, as systematic experiments on the methodology of transfer amyloidosis have not been published. It is our impression that 100×10^6 spleen cells are necessary in order to get consistent and reproducible "takes," e.g., at least an incidence of 90% amyloidosis in any group of recipients. Hardt (unpublished) injected, respectively, 25×10^6 and 50×10^6 spleen cells. Approximately 20% of recipient mice showed amyloid lesions and then only to a minor degree. It is also our impression that the intravenous route of administration is to be preferred, although Hardt and Hellung-Larsen (1972) obtained positive results after intraperitoneal administration of spleen cells. The apparent superiority of intravenous transfer is, however, to be weighed against the greater mortality linked to this procedure. Intravenous transfer was also preferred by Willerson et al. (1969b), who found the equivalent of one mouse spleen, approximately 10^8 cells, a suitable transfer dose. Using guinea pigs, Cathcart et al. (1972) gave 200×10^6 sensitized donor spleen cells by the intraperitoneal route. As already mentioned, intravenous transfer will cause donor amyloid emboli in the capillaries of the recipient lungs. The interpretation of such findings is facilitated by the fact that amyloidosis of the lungs is not a regular feature of ordinary experimentally induced mouse amyloidosis. By contrast, a potential source of confusion is the presence of amyloid deposits along the lymphatic drainage pathways of the peritoneal cavity after intraperitoneal transfer of cells, e.g., in lymph nodes of the omentum and mesentery (Hultgren et al., 1967). In transfer experiments in which only slight deposits of amyloid in the recipients are expected, such findings may cause difficulties.

6. Pathology

The pathological anatomy and the histological findings in recipients of cells from amyloidotic or preamyloidotic donors are not conspicuously different from those encountered in the classic type of experimental amyloidosis. This goes for the location in the tissues and the organ distribution and for the tinctorial properties of the amyloid substance. For ordinary light microscopy, hematoxylin-eosin (Fig. 10) or PAS-stained paraffin sections are suitable; more specific is the fluorescence of amyloid when stained by the thioflavine T-stain and excited by ultraviolet light (Vassar and Culling, 1959) or when stained by Congo red and viewed through polarizing optics (green birefringence of amyloid). These procedures allow the detection of minute amounts of amyloid. Morphologically the spleen amyloid is found in irregular rings with shaggy borders in the perifollicular zone round the splenic follicles. The amyloid is somewhat vacuolated and a netlike pattern is visible, which appears to be comprised of remnants of the splenic reticulum. The red and white pulp may be shrunken and depleted of cells, usually after nitrogen mustard has been given. Great numbers of PAS-positive reticuloendothelial cells with vacuolated and granular cytoplasm are found in the red pulp close to the borders of the amyloid rings, and sometimes there is direct transition from PAS-positive cells to amyloid (Figs. 11 and 12). In such areas the amyloid is heavily PAS-positive. In those (few) mice of our transfer experiments which failed to develop amyloid, abundant PAS-positive RE cells were found in the same locations. The amount of amyloid found in the mice 3–4 days after cell transfer averaged grade 3, according to the semiquantitative method of Christensen and Hjort (1959). Liver and kidney amyloid was usually scarce though significant (Werdelin and Ranløv, 1966; Willerson et al., 1969b, Cathcart et al., 1972). In autoradiographic investigations (thymidine-^{3}H label) of the casein-sensitized donor mice (Ranløv and Werdelin, 1967), most labeled cells in the donor spleens were found in the perifollicular regions of the spleens. A large proportion of these cells showed cytoplasmic pyroninophilia. In the recipients, immediately after transfer, all labeled cells were confined to the lungs. One day after the cell transfer practically all the injected, labeled cells had disappeared from the lungs and reappeared within the Malpighian corpuscles of the recipients' spleens, with a tendency to accumulate near and around the central vessel. At this stage only an occasional labeled cell could be found in the perifollicular zone, but never in the

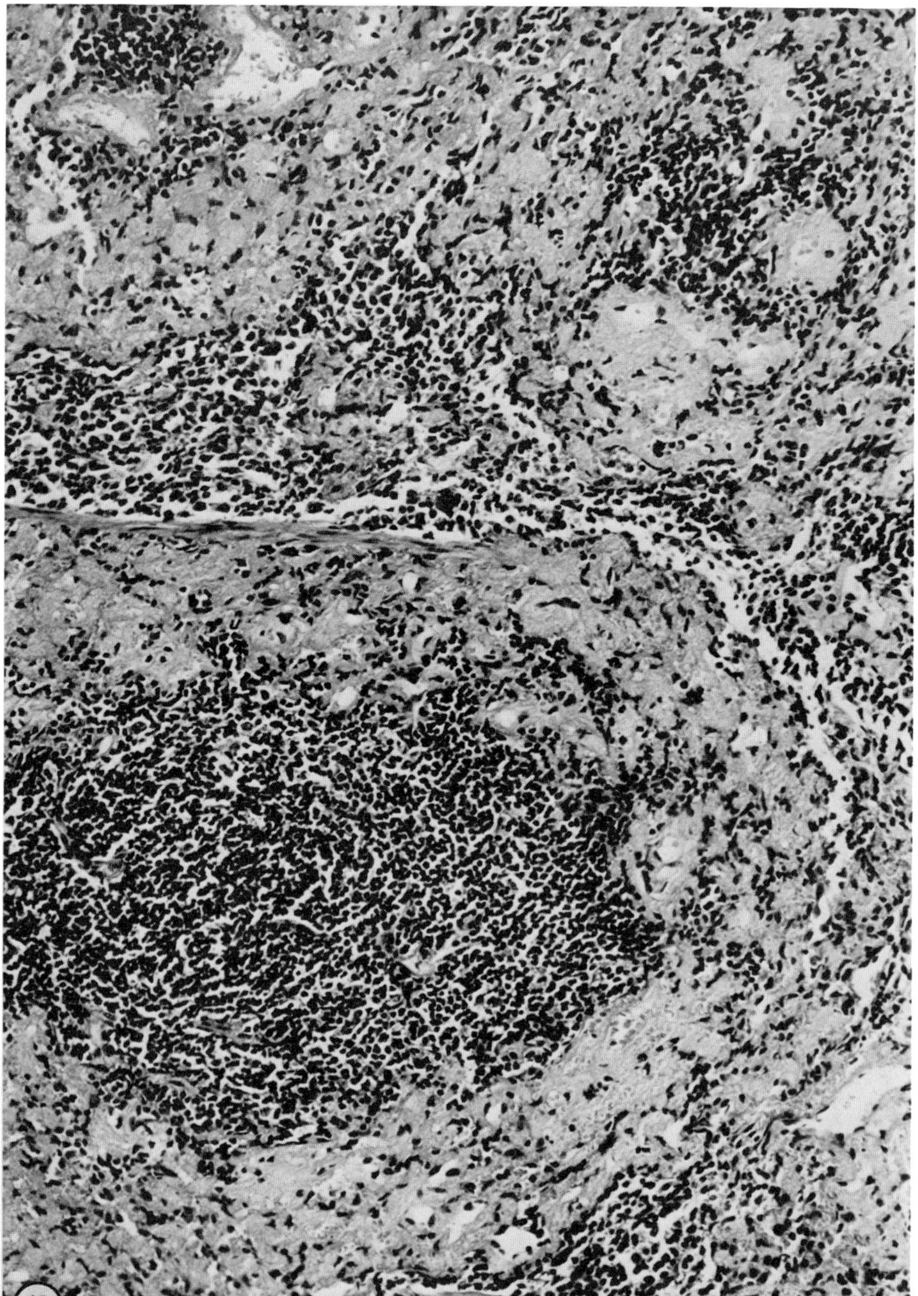
10

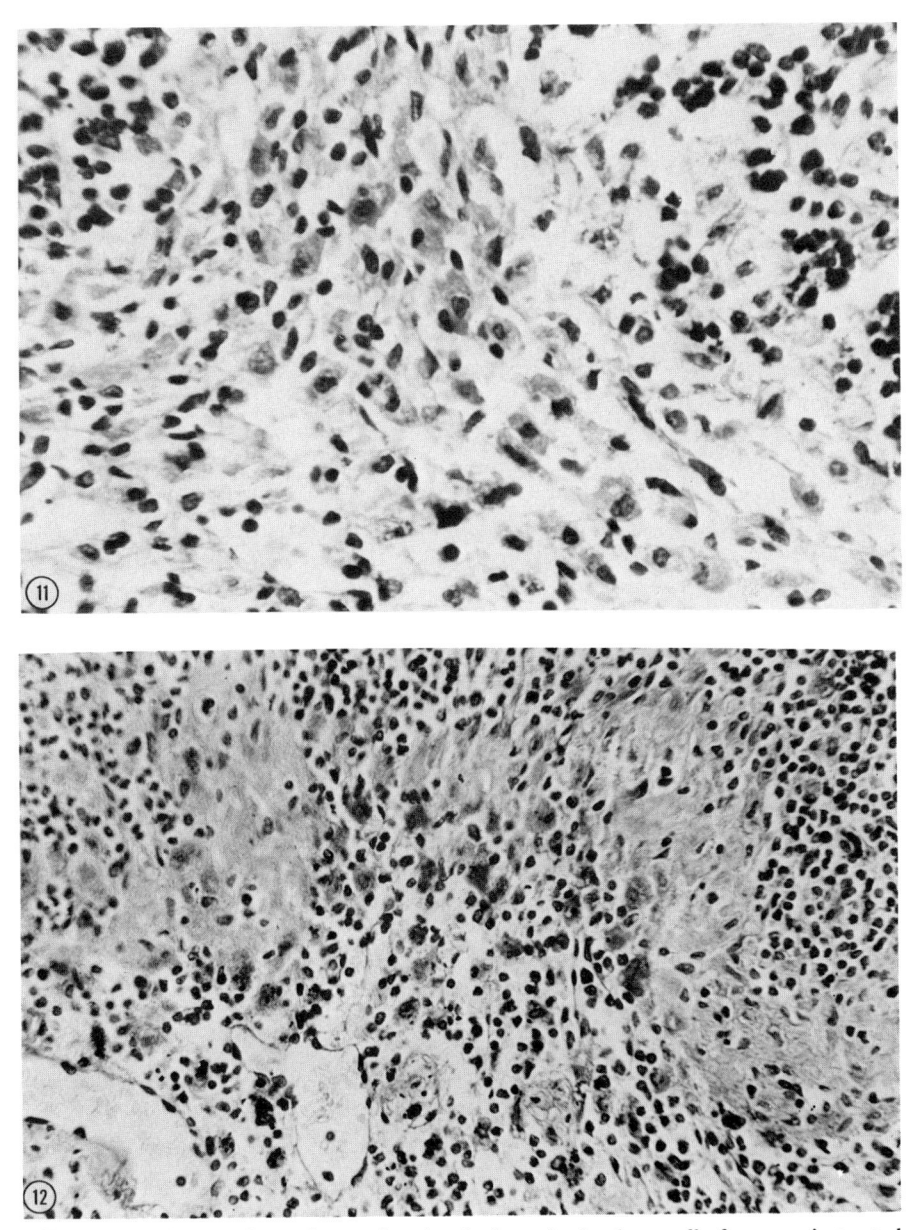

FIGS. 11 and 12. Spleens from mice that had received spleen cells from casein-treated donors and then had been treated with nitrogen mustard. Fig. 11 shows perifollicular periodic acid-Schiff (PAS)-positive cells in a recipient, which has not yet developed amyloidosis. PAS stain × 238. Fig. 12 shows PAS-positive cells on the border of the amyloid deposits. PAS stain × 238.

FIG. 10. Amyloidosis of spleen, degree 4. Mouse treated with nitrogen mustard for 6 days after transfer of sensitized cells. Note the well-defined amyloid rings. Hematoxylin-eosin. × 100. From Werdelin and Ranløv (1966).

red pulp. At 2 and 3 days after transfer the labeled cells had migrated farther out into the splenic red pulp and were now found in the same sites as the newly formed amyloid.

7. *Whole Spleen Grafts*

Hardt (1968) reported a modification of the cell transfer system which gave a better picture of the histological changes in the recipient mouse. After having been subjected to the usual course of 17–20 daily injections of casein, the donor spleens were isolated and cut into small slices. Each slice was immediately grafted onto the decapsulated surface of a recipient kidney. The syngeneic recipient mice were allowed 10 days to recover following the operation. Then the usual course of two injections of nitrogen mustard was given and later the recipients were sacrificed. As before, none of the recipients was treated with casein. Examination of the recipients showed amyloidosis, grade 3–4, in the spleens of all of 20 recipients and to a lesser extent in the grafted spleen slice. A noteworthy finding was extensive deposition of amyloid in the graft-bearing kidney in contrast to an almost normal contralateral host kidney. Another pertinent observation, made in the controls of this experiment, was that resorption of the amyloid from amyloidotic grafts did not take place in normal syngeneic recipients.

The type of experimental transfer amyloidosis just described is sometimes referred to as "the Copenhagen model," which is characterized by the use of spleen cells. Next we shall consider a number of basically similar transfer experiments with other kinds of cells and also experiments with isolated subtypes of spleen cells.

D. SOURCE OF CELLS

1. *Lymphoid and Reticular Tissues*

There have been but few reports of experiments on transfer amyloidosis in which cells from sources other than the spleen were used. In one of a series of papers on negative experiments, Clerici *et al.* (1969) reported failure to transfer casein-induced amyloidosis with thoracic duct cells in syngeneic mice. The numbers of cells transferred were rather modest, ranging between 5 and 30 × 10^6, and the cells were given either intravenously or intraperitoneally. No further treatment was given to the recipient mice, which were subsequently sacrificed on days 5, 10, and 20. Although most of the donor mice were amyloidotic after 30 casein injections, only 2 out of 42 recipients of thoracic duct cells from donors became amyloidotic, an incidence not different from that in the control group. Clerici did not investigate the amyloid transfer capacity of the spleens from the same donors. Willerson *et al.* (1969b), however, seem to have met this objection. In a carefully planned study they reproduced earlier work on amyloid transfer with spleen cells from casein-treated and from endotoxin-treated donor mice. In addition, suspensions of liver and lung cells from the same donors were found amyloidogenic when likewise transferred, though to a somewhat less extent; lung cells were least effective. A number of interesting observations were made: (1) not all donor mice had microscopically detectable amyloid in the tissues from which transfer cells were derived, but a sufficiently prolonged antigenic treatment of the donor was essential; (2) the recipient mice did not require cytostatic agents or further injections of casein; and (3) there were strain differences in the ease with which the transfer was accomplished, C3H mice being less susceptible in this respect than C57BL and White-Swiss mice.

Hardt (1971) has published a detailed study on the transfer of various lymphoid cells from amyloidotic mice to syngeneic nonamyloidotic recipients. He compared—in the usual mouse amyloid transfer system—cells from spleen, thymus, lymph node, bone marrow, peritoneal cavity, and peripheral blood. The donors were pretreated with a total of 17 injections of casein, and the recipients were subjected to the usual course of nitrogen mustard (over two injections) followed by sacrifice on day 5. All of 37 mice given spleen cells developed amyloid, but no recipient out of a total of 61 mice receiving lymphoid cells from other sources in equivalent doses (50 or 100×10^6) did so. Of particular interest—in light of the discussion in the previous section—was the failure to induce transfer amyloidosis with 25×10^6 peritoneal macrophages or with 50×10^6 bone marrow cells mixed with an equal number of thymus cells: a mixture mimicking the B cell and T cell composition of the spleen. Hardt interpreted these negative effects as evidence against autoimmune mechanisms in amyloidogenesis, since lymphoid cells are essential to the development of autoimmunity (Claman et al., 1966). Hardt suggested that the findings pointed toward macrophages in the spleen, and indicated a specific role of this organ in amyloidosis in general, and in transfer amyloidosis in particular.

2. The Mouse Mutant "Nude"

Recently, it has been demonstrated that the development of amyloidosis may be induced with suspensions of spleen cells presumably devoid of T lymphocytes, an observation of particular interest in the light of the immunological considerations discussed in Section I of this review. The thymus-deprived, T cell-deficient nude strain of mice (nu/nu-C3H) may be rendered amyloidotic by means of prolonged casein treatment (Hardt and Claesson, 1974). When spleen cells from nude, amyloidotic donors are transferred to related C3H recipients, amyloidosis is induced, while transfer of such spleen cells to nudes is ineffective. We have not yet been able to give an adequate explanation for this rather puzzling feature.

3. Cell Fractionation with Columns

We have explored the possibility of reducing or abolishing the transfer capacity of spleen cells by selectively removing from the suspension one or more of the functionally different cell classes that make up the spleen cell population. It is possible to remove quantitatively (lymphoid) cells carrying surface receptors of immunoglobulin type, believed to be the so-called B cells, by adherence to specific anti-immunoglobulin bound to particles. Hardt et al. (1975) have used activated Sephadex columns coated covalently with purified highly specific rabbit anti-C3H anti-IgG. In the cold, spleen cell suspensions from C3H mice pretreated with 20 injections of casein were passed through these columns. Recovery averaged 50%. The resulting cell suspension was examined by fluorescence microscopy after incubation with fluorescein-conjugated antimurine anti-light chain antisera. No immunoglobulin-bearing cells were found. Moreover, treatment of the cell suspension with anti-C3H-θ-serum from AKR mice followed by the nigrosin dye exclusion test revealed more than 98% of the cells to be T cells (e.g., carrying the θ antigen). The resulting cell suspension was injected intravenously into 20 syngeneic recipients, 100 × 10^6 cells each. The usual course of nitrogen mustard was given, and the recipients were sacrificed 6 days after transfer. None of the recipients developed amyloid, and the tentative conclusion was that splenic T cells alone—like peripheral lymphocytes, lymph node cells, thymus cells, and thoracic duct lymphocytes—cannot transfer experimental amyloidosis in the mouse.

4. *Parabiosis*

Somewhat in line with the transfer experiments described above was the attempt made by Hardt and Claesson (1973) to explore the suitability of a syngeneic mouse parabiosis system. They joined together, in lateral parabiosis, pairs of C3H mice of which only one parabiont was amyloidotic (after 30 injections of casein) while the other was normal. The mice were killed after 15 or 30 days in parabiosis without further treatment apart from a short course of nitrogen mustard to half the number of pairs. Unexpectedly, none of 8 "recipients" became amyloidotic. That this was not due to lack of vascular continuity between the two parabionts had been ascertained at the beginning of the experiments by injecting one of the partners intravenously with 0.2 ml of a 0.1% nigrosin solution. If systemic coloring of the uninjected partner failed to occur within a minute, the parabiosis was considered not established and the pair was excluded from the experiment. Thus, the parabionts must have had a common circulation including the blood cells. One interpretation was therefore that the transferring agent in amyloidosis was restricted to noncirculating cells in the amyloidotic spleen, the most likely cell being the RE cell.

E. TRANSFER WITH SUBCELLULAR FRACTIONS (Table II)

1. *Introduction*

After the cellular morphogenesis of both clinical and experimental amyloidosis had been well established, the transition of a pyroninophilic cell into an amyloid-producing, PAS-positive RE cell (Teilum, 1956, 1964a) was accepted by us. The original transfer experiment (Werdelin and Ranløv, 1966) did nothing to change that opinion; moreover, the huge numbers of PAS cells appearing in the recipient spleens as early as 2 days after the cell transfer were believed to be derived directly from the injected, predominantly pyroninophilic, donor spleen cells and were believed to be producing amyloid. In an additional transfer experiment in which nuclear labeling of the donor cells with thymidine-^{3}H was done, it was noted, 4 days after the transfer, that silver grains appeared over the perifollicular regions in the recipients' spleens and that there was well-defined nuclear labeling in the same areas (Ranløv and Werdelin, 1967). Most of the grains were apparently related to the cytoplasm of reticuloendothelial cells, "probably representing phagocytized nuclear material derived from the labelled donor cells" (Ranløv and Werdelin, 1967). The same year, Ranløv (1967a,e) found that experimental amyloidosis could also be induced by transfer of subcellular fractions of spleen cells or of X-irradiated cells.

For convenience, we shall consider transfer experiments with cells damaged by various physical means together with transfer by means of subcellular fractions. In doing so, we are well aware of the inherent difficulties in interpreting such terms as "dead" and "damaged" cells. It remains an open question to what extent the loss of vital cellular functions such as the ability to divide and proliferate, to synthesize protein, and to undergo transition into "blast" or "activated" forms should be considered synonymous with cell death. This is pertinent to evaluating reports on amyloid transfer with "dead" cells. Such claims should be dealt with skeptically, in particular if the alleged cell death has been brought about by irradiation *in vitro*. Several observations indicate sustained synthesis of RNA and protein in lymphoid cells in spite of irradiation doses averaging several thousand rad (Kaplan, 1966; Fliedner, 1967).

2. *Various Subcellular Fractions*

Having found that cells are mediators of transfer amyloidosis, it became necessary to determine whether the amyloid-inducing potency was dependent upon intact spleen cells of the donors. The experimental design (Ranløv, 1967a) was basically similar to that of Werdelin and Ranløv (1966), care being taken that every experimental run with subcellular material was accompanied by a parallel control run with intact donor cells from the pool which supplied the donor cell fractions. As a further control, mice were picked from the randomized recipient population and injected with either viable cells or cell fractions derived from normal, nonsensitized donors. In the controls, marked deposits of amyloid were found in the spleens of 12 out of 12 animals that had received sensitized, intact spleen cells and in 0 out of 29 animals that had received spleen cells or cell fractions from normal donors. The donor mice of the inbred C3H strain had been pretreated with 17 daily injections of casein. The spleen cell suspension had been prepared as usual, though entirely at 4°C. The donor spleen cells were fractionated largely according to the method for preparing

TABLE II
AMYLOID TRANSFER EXPERIMENTS WITH SUBCELLULAR FRACTIONS

Authors	Donors			Transfer material				Recipients				Interval from transfer to sacrifice (days)
	Species, strain	Treatment	Amyloidotic	Source	Fraction	Amount	Route of administration	Mouse strain	Treatment prior to transfer	Treatment post transfer	Incidence of amyloidosis	
Ranløv (1967a)	C3H mice	17 Casein injections	34%	Spleen	Whole homogenate	Eq.[a] 100×10^6 cells	i.v.	C3H	None	Nitrogen mustard, 0.05 mg × 2	15/15	4
	C3H mice	17 Casein injections	34%	Spleen	DNA-protein	Eq. 100×10^6 cells	i.v.	C3H	None	Nitrogen mustard, 0.05 mg × 2	18/18	4
	C3H mice	17 Casein injections	34%	Spleen	DNA-protein	Eq. 100×10^6 cells	i.v.	C3H	None	None	3/9	2–4
	C3H mice	17 Casein injections	34%	Spleen	DNA-protein	Eq. 100×10^6 cells	s.c.	C3H	None	Nitrogen mustard, 0.05 mg × 2	1/8	4
	C3H mice	17 Casein injections	34%	Spleen	DNase-treated DNA-protein	Eq. 100×10^6 cells	i.v.	C3H	None	Nitrogen mustard, 0.05 mg × 2	5/6	4
Willerson et al. (1969b)	White Swiss mice, C57BL mice	19 Casein injections	?	Spleen	Nuclear	0.3–0.5 mg	i.v.	White Swiss, C57BL (syngeneic transfer)	None	Nitrogen mustard, 0.05 mg × 2	11/53	4–5
	White Swiss mice, C57BL mice	19 Casein injections	?	Spleen	Mitochondrial	0.5–1.4 mg	i.v.	White Swiss, C57BL (syngeneic transfer)	None	Nitrogen mustard, 0.05 mg × 2	28/42	4–5
	White Swiss mice, C57BL mice	19 Casein injections	?	Spleen	Microsomal	0.2–1.3 mg	i.v.	White Swiss, C57BL mice (syngeneic transfer)	None	Nitrogen mustard, 0.05 mg × 2	15/37	4–5
	White Swiss mice, C57BL mice	19 Casein injections	?	Spleen	Ribosomes	0.1 mg	i.v.	White Swiss, C57BL mice (syngeneic transfer)	None	Nitrogen mustard, 0.05 mg × 2	1/34[b]	5

Reference	Strain	Pretreatment	Tumor take	Organ	Material	Dose	Route	Recipient strain	Irradiation	Other treatment	Takes	Weeks
	White Swiss mice, C57BL mice	19 Casein injections	?	Spleen	Supernatant	0.4 mg	i.v.	White Swiss, C57BL (syngeneic transfer)	None	Nitrogen mustard, 0.05 mg × 2	0/22	4–5
Shirahama et al. (1969)	Humans	None	100%	Spleen	Whole homogenate	?	i.p.	C3H	None	None	0/27	(?)
Hardt and Hellung-Larsen (1972)	C3H mice	21 Casein injections	?	Spleen	Whole homogenate	Eq. 100 × 10⁶ cells	i.v.	C3H	None	Nitrogen mustard, 0.05 mg × 2	25/30	6
	C3H mice	21 Casein injections	?	Spleen	Crude nuclear	Eq. 100 × 10⁶ cells	i.v.	C3H	None	Nitrogen mustard 0.05 mg × 2	22/30	6
	C3H mice	21 Casein injections	?	Spleen	DNase-treated crude nuclear	Eq. 100 × 10⁶ cells	i.v.	C3H	None	Nitrogen mustard, 0.05 mg × 2	0/5	6
	C3H mice	21 Casein injections	?	Spleen	Crude cytoplasm	Eq. 100 × 10⁶ cells	i.v.	C3H	None	Nitrogen mustard, 0.05 mg × 2	2/15[b]	6
	C3H mice	21 Casein injections	?	Spleen	Various RNA fractions	Eq. 100 × 10⁶ cells	i.v.	C3H	None	Nitrogen mustard, 0.05 mg × 2	0/20	6
Jakob and Hilgenfeld (1972)	Decin mice	None	50% (spontaneous)	Spleen	Whole homogenate	Eq. 1 spleen	i.p.	Decin	None	None	0/30	(?)
Ranløv (1967e)	C3H mice	17 Casein injections	?	Spleen	Lethally in vitro irradiated (1000 rad)	100 × 10⁶ cells	i.v.	C3H	None	Nitrogen mustard, 0.05 mg × 2	0/8	5
	C3H mice	17 Casein injections	?	Spleen	Lethally in vitro irradiated (1000 rad)	100 × 10⁶ cells	i.v.	C3H	None	Nitrogen mustard, 0.05 mg × 2	8/8	5
Werdelin (1968)	C3H mice	14 Casein injections	37%	Spleen	Heat-damaged 56°C/ 30 min	100 × 10⁶ cells	i.v.	C3H	None	Nitrogen mustard, 0.05 mg × 3	9/14	5
Lüders (1969)	C3H mice	17 Casein injections	?	Spleen	Lethally irradiated (1000 rad)	100 × 10⁶ cells	i.v.	C3H	None	Nitrogen mustard, 0.05 mg × 3	11/15	5

[a]Eq. = equivalent of. [b]Not significant.

antigenic tissue extracts described by Medawar (1963). The cells were repeatedly subjected to hypotonic lysis with iced water, then disrupted for 7 minutes in a Waring Blendor at top speed and afterward exposed to ultrasonic irradiation. After isotonicity had been restored, we were left with a sediment and a supernatant. The sediment was termed "DNA-protein" and was thought to contain all cellular DNA, DNA-linked enzymes, and histones. The supernatant, called "crude semisoluble extract" (or sometimes "cytoplasmic fraction") was thought to contain almost all cellular RNA, mitochondria, and microsomes. These fractions were injected intravenously into mice in doses approximating the equivalents of 100×10^6 spleen cells or 100 mg wet weight of donor spleen. Each dose was given in 0.5 ml and represented 2.0–2.5 mg of dry material. After transfer, the usual course of nitrogen mustard was given, and the recipient mice were sacrificed 2–4 days after transfer.

The results were highly significant and left no doubt: whole homogenate and DNA-protein from spleens of amyloidotic donors caused amyloidosis within 2–4 days in 33 out of 33 recipients if given intravenously. The cytoplasmic fraction was totally ineffective in all 14 recipients. When nitrogen mustard was not added, only 3 out of 9 recipients of DNA-protein became amyloidotic. Further, subcutaneous administration did not work, and, finally, treatment of the otherwise potent DNA-protein inoculum with beef pancreas DNase did not abolish the amyloid transfer activity. Morphologically, the amyloid deposits were similar to those usually seen in transfer amyloidosis and not much different from classical experimental amyloid, although the deposits in liver and kidney were somewhat more sparse.

The initial interpretation of the results was that the particulate DNA-protein suspension injected intravenously was phagocytized by RE cells in spleen and liver, i.e., the principle sites of amyloid. This would explain the ineffectiveness of subcutaneously administered material, and would fit the results of the previous autoradiographic study (Ranløv and Werdelin, 1967). It was tentatively concluded, that the results of the subcellular transfer experiment indicated that two different cell types operate specifically in the different phases of experimental amyloidosis in general. During the prolonged stimulation by casein "the increasing cell death or cell fragmentation results in the release of various nuclear and cytoplasmic fragments, some of them self-replicable nucleic acids or nucleotides carrying some kind of information from their metabolically highly active parental cells. These fragments of nuclear material are locally phagocytized in RE cells. Under the specific conditions of overloading, the ingested (self-replicable) material will impose protein-synthesizing information on the RE cell, thus causing a profound disturbance of its function. The visible results will be a cytoplasmic PAS positivity of "reticular" cells, indicating intracellular synthesis of glycoproteins and extracellular deposition of amyloid (Ranløv, 1967a).

Successful amyloid transfer with subcellular material was subsequently reported by Willerson and co-workers (1969b). Their results were largely the same as ours. They demonstrated differences in the ease with which transfer could be accomplished in various strains of mice, but their experimental mice were also syngeneic. They too used casein-sensitized donor mice and prepared cell fractions from spleens, but their fractionation procedure differed from ours. They used the method of Dounce et al. (1955), utilizing the technique of equilibrium fractionation (DeVenuto et al., 1962). The various fractions were injected intravenously; by dry weight the single doses were close to ours, in the range of 0.3–1.5 mg. They found the mitochondrial and microsomal fractions to be most effective, although nuclear fractions also had some activity. Their finding that several subcellular fractions were able to transfer the amyloid-accelerating substance led them to suggest that an inducer of amyloid or soluble amyloid rather than a specific functioning subcellular organelle was responsible for successful transfer. Like us, they further concluded that transfer of particulate amyloid could be ruled out as a significant contributing factor, mainly because of the lack of detectable deposits of amyloid in the majority of their donor groups. Their proposition that soluble amyloid might be the cause of the very early deposits of amyloid (within 4 days) is hardly warranted, mainly for quantitative reasons: in the majority of published reports on subcellular transfer the amount of material injected seldom exceeded 1 or 2 mg. In the spleens of our recipient mice, deposits of amyloid were estimated at 20 mg or more. Willerson et al. (1969b) suggested, further, that an inducer of amyloid may be operative at a later stage, when the soluble amyloid has been used up. This postulate is still not substantiated.

Shirahama et al. (1969) failed to induce amyloidosis by transfer in a xenogeneic system. They injected homogenates of human amyloidotic spleens intraperitoneally into untreated C3H mice, which were subsequently killed after 3–7 days without having received further treatment. In the same experiments they noted transfer of an amyloid-enhancing factor which—being a quite different phenomenon—will be dealt with later.

In an attempt to define the principle responsible for the amyloid transfer, Hardt and Hellung-Larsen (1972) reproduced the findings of Ranløv (1967a) and of Willerson et al. (1969b) in detail. This study yielded much information on the role of the methods and the importance of proper control of the various procedures involved in handling the cell suspensions. They separated the spleen cell suspensions into "crude nuclei" and cytoplasm by three different methods. The nuclear fractions were checked by electron and light microscopy. Crude cytoplasmic fractions were used, as well as cytoplasmic fractions extracted with hot or cold phenol. The extraction efficiency of the different procedures with respect to RNA varied from 70% to 90%, and none of the cold extracts showed any degradation of the RNA on polyacrylamide gel electrophoresis, while the RNA extracted with hot phenol showed slight degradation of the ribosomal component. Some preparations of DNA were treated with diethylpyrocarbonate, a very potent RNase-inhibitor. The various fractions were injected intravenously into syngeneic C3H mice which subsequently were given the standard course of nitrogen mustard. Hardt and Hellung-Larsen (1972) found that their spleen cell homogenates consistently transferred amyloidosis provided the donors had been treated with casein. Furthermore, positive transfer results were obtained after injections of crude nuclei. Treatment of the crude nuclei with DNase for a very short period led to complete loss of the transfer capacity, as did other types of treatment, such as incubation at 37°C for 2 hours or storage at 0 or 20°C for 3 days. This was in contrast to the result obtained by Ranløv (1967a) with DNase-treated "nuclear fraction." The discrepancy is explained by the more careful procedural controls of Hardt and Hellung-Larsen (1972). As was the case in Ranløv's experiment, crude cytoplasm was ineffective, a finding that argues against the findings of Willerson *et al.* (1969b) of an amyloid-transferring potency of a mitochondrial fraction. As might be expected, none of the various RNA preparations of Hardt and Hellung-Larsen were effective.

A potentially very interesting transfer model was explored by Jakob and Hilgenfeld (1972). They used mice of the strain Decin as donors. These mice have a high incidence of spontaneous amyloidosis. The donor group was selected so that approximately 50% of the mice were amyloidotic, thus not requiring pretreatment with casein. The transfer was syngeneic, and each recipient Decin mouse got an intraperitoneal injection of whole spleen homogenate, representing the equivalent of one donor spleen. No further treatment was given, and none of 30 recipients developed amyloid. Jakob and Hilgenfeld did not extend their studies by giving nitrogen mustard to recipient mice after transfer of spleen homogenate. It would also be of considerable interest to know the results of transfer of whole, viable spleen cells in Decin mice. From a clinical point of view, experiments exploiting spontaneously occurring amyloidosis are always of particular interest.

3. *Damaged Cells*

As indicated before, we shall briefly discuss some experiments with transfer of spleen cells damaged by various physical means. The first experiment of this sort was designed on the assumption that "lethal" X-irradiation would abolish the amyloid-transferring capacity of spleen cells from preamyloidotic donors. Using the "Copenhagen transfer model," Ranløv (1967e) found that this was not so. Spleen cell suspensions from C3H donor mice that had been pretreated by 17 daily injections of casein were subjected to X-irradiation *in vitro* (42.3 rad per minute to a total dose of 1000 rad). They were injected into syngeneic mice, and, as a control, untreated spleen cells from the same pool were injected into other syngeneic recipients. All recipients were subsequently treated with nitrogen mustard. The resulting amyloidosis in recipients that had received irradiated cells was comparable to that in controls which had received untreated cells from the same pool. Thus, irradiation did not influence the ability of cells to transfer amyloidosis. The experiment indicated that, within the host, proliferation of the transferred cells was not a prerequisite of amyloid-inducing potency. The results were also thought to indicate an interaction of a messenger function of material derived from the donor cells with reticular cells in the recipients, and thus to supplement the results obtained by means of subcellular fractions (Ranløv, 1967a). Simultaneously, Werdelin (1968) reached the same results. From donors pretreated with 14 injections of casein, he took spleen cells and irradiated them *in vitro*. With these cells he was able to produce amyloidosis in 11 of 15 syngeneic mouse recipients, while heat-damaged (56°C for 30 minutes) cells, obtained from comparable donors, induced amyloid in 9 out of 14 recipient mice.

F. Donor–Recipient Combinations

Apart from the unsuccessful attempts by Shirahama and co-workers (1969), all published experiments relating to transfer of amyloidosis have been conducted with inbred animals or at least animals of the same strain. One would, however, anticipate some positive results of transfer in most allogeneic animals for a number of reasons: first, the rapid onset of production of amyloid in the recipient would most probably precede the mounting of any significant degree of the recipient's immune reactivity against the injected allogeneic material; next, the presumed nucleic acid nature of the amyloidosis-conveying agent implies that the inoculum would have little if any antigenicity in the allogeneic host; finally, any hypothetical immune reaction of the recipient's lymphoid cells against the inoculum should be effectively abolished by the treatment with alkylating agents (nitrogen mustard). Indeed, in unpublished experiments we have transferred amyloidosis from C3H to St/a mice and *vice versa*, thus crossing the histocompatibility barrier.

In a later section the possible—but different—mechanisms involved in transfer of *amyloid-enhancing* factors that are operative in allogeneic combinations will be discussed.

G. Role of Specific Antigen

Little is known about the relation of the nature or specificity of the amyloidogenic agent (antigen) employed in the development of transfer amyloidosis. It seems that bovine casein has been used in the majority of published experiments, but Willerson *et al*. (1969b) have also tried *Escherichia coli* endotoxin, with sufficient results. In the experiments reported by Jakob and Hilgenfeld (1972) the development of amyloid in the donor mice was spontaneous and the antigen thus unknown. As a rule, one substance has been used throughout the period of induction of amyloid in the donor, and little is known about the role of antigenic specificity. In C3H mice, Hardt (unpublished) has investigated the amyloid-inducing potency of a series of different substances, given as alternating single courses of a few days' duration each (casein–albumin–tetanus toxoid–brucella antigen). These mice never developed amyloid, a finding that indicates a certain degree of specificity of the inducing agent (antigen?) in experimental amyloidosis.

In view of the existence of theories which postulate that formation of amyloid is a positive expression of tolerance toward the amyloidogenic agent (antigen) (Cathcart et al., 1970), it is important to deal with the question whether sustained presence of casein in the transferred material is necessary for the development of transfer amyloidosis. If the tolerance theory is true, then continued formation of amyloid in the transfer recipient should depend on the continued presence of antigen in the recipient's tissues. Since in the transfer model under consideration casein is never administered to the recipient mice, the only possible way in which the postulated need for casein could be met is if the inoculum were to contain sufficient amounts of casein to maintain the tolerant state. Otherwise, production of amyloid should cease (or never start). In order to clarify this issue, Hardt and Claesson (1974) injected two groups of mice, amyloidotic and normal C3H, with ^{3}H-labeled casein. After the usual three washings, 10^8 spleen cells were dissolved and counted in Dioxan scintillation fluid and gave 450 ± 68 cpm and 410 ± 37 cpm, respectively, as compared to a background (spleen cells from uninjected mice) of 212 ± 32 cpm. This experiment indicated that casein was present in the transferred material but gave no evidence regarding its role. Up to now, induction of transfer amyloidosis has not yet been tried in serial passages, in which—after several transfers—the casein would probably be diluted logarithmically so as to approach total removal. Apart from providing other valuable information, such experiments would probably shed some light on the unsolved question of antigenic specificity in amyloid transfer and, consequently, on amyloidosis in a broader sense.

H. Nature of the Amyloid-Inducing Factor (AIF)

The available data allow very few conclusions regarding the nature of AIF. Nor do they give any suggestions to what extent one may consider AIF to be a well defined chemical entity. Sporadic attempts have been made to clarify these issues. The morphological characteristics of the transferred subcellular material have been examined in the electron microscope by Wanstrup and Ranløv (1968). This "DNA-protein" appeared as a heterogeneous substance made up of more or less recognizable nuclear and cytoplasmic components. The dominating structures were highly osmiophilic, non-membrane-lined aggregations of a granular material—apparently nuclear chromatin, strongly Feulgen positive. In between, lamellar and vesicular bodies were found, some of which were coated with ribosomes. Only occasionally were mitochondria seen. Small bundles of amyloid microfibrils could now and then be seen dispersed in this material (Fig. 13).

Among other known characteristics of the AIF is its resistance to ultrasonic

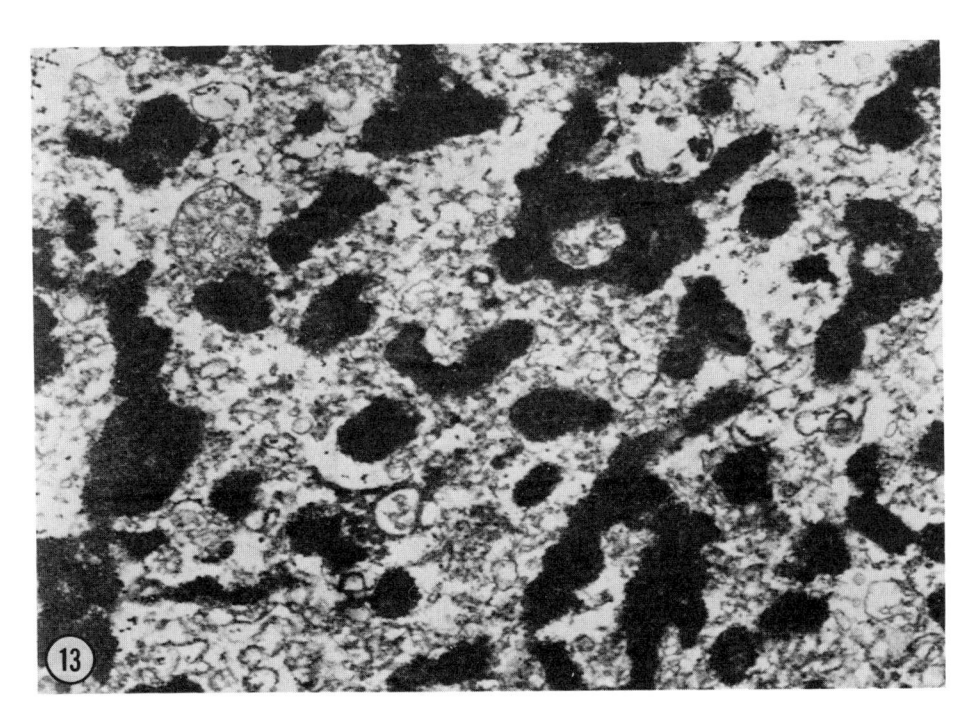

FIG. 13. The "DNA-protein" fraction of spleen cells from mice after 20 injections of casein. Ultrastructurally, this sediment is a heterogeneous substance, made up of more or less recognizable nuclear and cytoplasmic components. The dominating structure is strongly osmiophilic, non-membrane-lined aggregations of a granular material. From its morphology and the fact that this fraction is strongly Feulgen positive, it seems justified to interpret it as aggregates of nuclear chromatin. These conspicuous structures are dispersed in a mainly granular "matrix" containing a number of lamellar and vesicular bodies, some of which are coated with ribosomes. Occasionally a single mitochondrion has survived the experimental procedures. Sometimes small bundles of amyloid are seen "interstitially." No intact cells or larger cell fractions appeared in this sediment. From Wanstrup and Ranløv (1968).

(Ranløv, 1967a) and ionizing irradiation (Ranløv, 1967e) and to heating at $56°C$ for 30 minutes (Werdelin, 1968). AIF loses its activity completely after storage for 3 days at either $0°$ or $20°C$ (Hardt and Hellung-Larsen, 1972). AIF is apparently not circulating in the peripheral blood in any significant amounts, as evident from the negative attempts to transmit amyloidosis in a syngeneic parabiosis system (Hardt and Claesson, 1973); various attempts to establish transfer amyloidosis with a few bolus injections of donor serum have been negative, as might be expected.

Regarding the origin of AIF, all available data point toward tissues rich in RE cells, probably of the nonrecirculating type: first and foremost the spleen, but also—to a less extent—liver and lung (Willerson et al., 1969b).

Crude nuclei and various "nuclear fractions" readily transmit amyloidosis and, even though AIF activity is completely abolished by DNase-treatment, all attempts to obtain transfer with purified extracts of DNA have failed, as have those with RNA. At present, however, we are inclined toward regarding AIF as a rather unstable nucleoprotein, possibly depending on the presence of specific antigen within the macrophages or—under subcellular experimental conditions—on macrophage-processed antigen. The accelerating effect of nitrogen mustard on amyloid transfer might depend on the ability of alkylating agents to release cell-bound macrophage-processed antigens.

AIF is unlikely to be an analog of Lawrence's transfer factor (Lawrence et al., 1963). Although Lawrence's transfer factor is believed to be a polynucleotide and to be antigen-specific (Neidhart et al., 1973), its resistance to DNase treatment clearly indicates that it differs from AIF.

I. Precursors of Amyloid in Serum

The observations of Pras et al. (1968, 1969) that amyloid fibrils could be isolated from tissues by means of extraction with distilled water has led to a more direct approach to immunological and biochemical studies of purified amyloid fibrils.

Many results have been reported concerning the biochemical analysis of amyloid fibrils obtained from patients with amyloidosis. This subject is dealt with by Glenner and Page (1975) in detail.

Some groups of investigators have reported that the amino acid sequence of the proteins isolated from purified amyloid fibrils in cases associated with myeloma or other plasma cell disorders demonstrates the presence of fragments of immunoglobulin light chains (Glenner et al., 1971; Terry et al., 1973). Other groups have reported that a nonimmunoglobulin protein is the major component of amyloid fibrils (Benditt et al., 1971; Ein et al., 1972; Franklin et al., 1972; Husby et al., 1972). The latter groups obtained their amyloid fibrils from patients with amyloidosis associated with myeloma, macroglobulinemia, Hodgkin's disease, familial Mediterranean fever, and rheumatoid arthritis. It is not clear to what extent the nonimmunoglobulin protein is also present in those amyloid fibrils in which parts of light chains are believed to be the principal components, or whether immunoglobulins and their fragments might be present in amyloid fibrils having the nonimmunoglobulin protein as major constituent.

Independently, it has been reported by Levin et al. (1973) and by Husby et al. (1973) that a serum component with a molecular weight of about 100,000 and antigenically related to the nonimmunoglobulin protein in amyloid fibrils, was present in sera from patients with amyloidosis and also in sera from patients with other diseases known to be associated with amyloidosis. Husby and Natvig (1974) have studied this serum component (called ASC—amyloid-substance related component) further and found no structural relationship of the ASC to the plasma component of amyloid described by Cathcart et al. (1967). In some patients the protein ASC was found in the serum 2—3 years before the diagnosis of amyloidosis was established. Protein ASC was also frequently found in hypogammaglobulinemia. With immunoelectroosmophoresis ASC was found also in minor amounts in normal controls, with a noticeable increase with age and during pregnancy. Husby and Natvig suggested that ASC is a normal serum constituent, usually present only in minor quantities. Under certain conditions, ASC increases considerably in serum, and it may in such instances act as a precursor for the deposition of amyloid fibrils in tissues. This is, however, purely speculative. In none of the investigations hitherto published on serum components and amyloid has evidence for any cause—effect relation to amyloid disease been produced; for all we know, the simultaneous appearance of various "serum components" and amyloid deposits may be parallel or coincidental events lacking pathogenic significance.

In relation to experimental amyloidosis, it might be expected that the amyloid-inducing effect of an antigen challenge runs parallel with an increase in the amount of ASC in serum during antigenic stimulation. The ASC should thus in some unknown way be related to the immune system, being released from stimulated lymphocytes or macrophages, as AIF. If this is so, the amount of ASC should increase in the serum of recipients receiving AIF. Experiments based on this theory are under evaluation in our laboratory, in collaboration with Husby and Natvig (Oslo). Nevertheless, our parabiosis experiment (Hardt and Claesson, 1973) has failed to lend support to this theory, as parabiosis for 15 days of a heavily amyloidotic mouse and a normal mouse did not cause formation of amyloid in the latter.

Lately, yet another serum factor, the P component, has been isolated from sera of human patients with amyloidosis in amounts sufficient to allow further characterization (Skinner et al., 1974). The P-component has an MW of 180,000 and it is not known whether it is related to any known serum protein. It is quite distinct from the components described by Glenner et al. (1971) and by Husby et al. (1972) and from the "A-protein" of Benditt and co-workers (1971). Its amino acid sequence bears no likeness to those of immunoglobulin light chains. Skinner and co-workers have reserved judgment on the place of the P component in the pathogenesis of amyloidosis.

IV. Transfer of Amyloid-Enhancing Factor (AEF)

A. Transfer with Cells (Table III)

1. Introduction

In an elegant series of experiments on casein-induced amyloidosis, Janigan's group (Janigan, 1965; Janigan and Druet, 1968; Druet and Janigan, 1966)

TABLE III
TRANSFER OF AMYLOID ENHANCING FACTOR

Authors	Donors Species, strain	Donors Treatment	Transfer material Source	Transfer material No. of cells	Transfer material Route of administration	Recipients Species, strain	Recipients Treatment prior to transfer	Recipients Treatment post transfer	Incidence of amyloidosis	Interval from transfer to sacrifice
Hultgren et al. (1967)	C57BL/10J mice	12–14 Azocasein injections	Spleen	100 × 10⁶	i.p.	C57BL/10J mice	Irradiation 750 rad	2–7 Azocasein injections	30/50	3–8 Days
	C57BL/10J mice	12–14 Azocasein injections	Spleen fragments	?	i.p.	C57BL/10J mice	Irradiation 750 rad	2–7 Azocasein injections	13/20	3–8 Days
Hardt and Ranløv (1968)	C3H mice	10 Casein injections	Whole spleen grafts	ca. 25 mg	Tissue graft to kidney	C3H mice	None	10 Casein injections + nitrogen mustard	10/10	13 Days
Hardt (1971)	C3H mice	10 Casein injections	Whole spleen grafts	ca. 25 mg	Tissue graft to kidney	C3H mice	None	8–10 Casein injections	6/6	9–11 Days
	C3H mice	10 Casein injections	Whole thymus grafts	ca. 10 mg	Tissue graft to kidney	C3H mice	None	8–10 Casein injections	6/6	9–11 Days
	C3H mice	10 Casein injections	Whole lymph node grafts	ca. 10 mg	Tissue graft to kidney	C3H mice	None	10 Casein injections	8/8	11 Days
Cathcart et al. (1972)	Guinea pigs	15 Casein injections	Spleen	200 × 10⁶	i.p.	Guinea pigs	None	6–12 Casein injections	6/6	5 Weeks
	Guinea pigs	15 Casein injections	Peritoneal cells	200 × 10⁶	i.p.	Guinea pigs	None	12 Casein injections	2/2	5 Weeks
Hardt et al. (1975)	C3H mice	10 Casein injections	Splenic T cells (B-cell deprived)	50 × 10⁶	i.v.	C3H mice	None	10 Casein injections	10/10	2 Weeks

showed several significant relationships between antigenic challenge and amyloidosis: rapid induction of amyloidosis with higher doses of azocasein; a direct correlation between rate of induction of amyloid and depletion of small lymphocytes; a similarity of the lymphoid tissue changes occurring during rapid induction of amyloid to those found in states of immunological tolerance; and possible casein induction of amyloidosis in B lymphocyte-deficient chickens. These observations were interpreted as signifying a relationship between antigenic challenge and development of amyloidosis that may involve an immune mechanism other than increased production of specific immunoglobulins.

2. *Spleen Cells*

In order to explore this relationship further, experiments were carried out in which spleen cells or fragments from normal donor mice or from donors previously sensitized by multiple injections of azocasein were injected intraperitoneally into sublethally irradiated, isogeneic recipients (Hultgren et al., 1967). At the time of transfer the donor mice had received from 6 to 14 injections of azocasein, a dose insufficient to induce amyloidosis, as no amyloidosis was found in any of the donors used in this particular transfer system. The recipient mice were irradiated prior to the transfers and then treated with daily injections of azocasein for various lengths of time. Amyloidosis then developed in the recipients after far fewer injections of azocasein than were required for induction of amyloid in normal, intact mice.

The results of this experiment underlined the concept that sensitized lymphocytes played an indispensable and limiting role in the induction of amyloid.

It is important to stress that the experiment of Hultgren and co-workers involved transfer of tissue from casein-sensitized, preamyloidotic animals to irradiated recipients which subsequently received treatment with casein in order to provoke formation of amyloid. Some published experiments in which the same principles were applied have been discussed as though the transfer had been a direct transfer of the disease amyloidosis, and not, as was the case, a transfer of immunity toward a defined antigen, namely casein.

3. *Whole-Spleen Grafts*

While the experiments of Janigan's group mentioned above, in which spleen cells or small spleen fragments were administered intraperitoneally, left few opportunities to study the morphological relationships between amyloid in the recipients and tissues (cells) of donor origin, an experiment of Hardt and Ranløv (1968) was designed to keep the donor cells as a morphological entity within the host. The donor mice were given 10 daily injections of 0.5 ml of a 5% solution of sodium caseinate, and afterward two small slices (2×3×2 mm) of spleen tissue were removed from each donor under anesthesia and immediately transferred to the lateral margins of the right kidneys of two anesthetized syngeneic recipient mice, according to the method described by Wheeler et al. (1966). The remaining parts of the donor spleens were used for histological evaluation, the predominant picture being that of a marked pyroninophilia. Only in a small number of spleens were minor deposits of amyloid material detected.

The day after the transplantation, the first of a series of 10 daily injections of casein was given, and on the day of the last injection of casein the first of two injections of 0.05 mg of nitrogen mustard was given. All the recipients developed a severe and widespread amyloidosis, especially pronounced in the graft and in the spleen, in the latter often to the maximum degree according to the semiquantitative method described by Christensen and Hjort (1959). Not only did the graft show a severe degree of amyloidosis, but heavy amyloid infiltration was evident in the kidney tissue immediately adjacent to the graft, in contrast to the minor involvement of the rest of the recipient kidney and the contralateral kidney of the same animal. This local amyloid infiltration involved the tubular interstitial tissues as well as the glomeruli (Figs. 14 and 15).

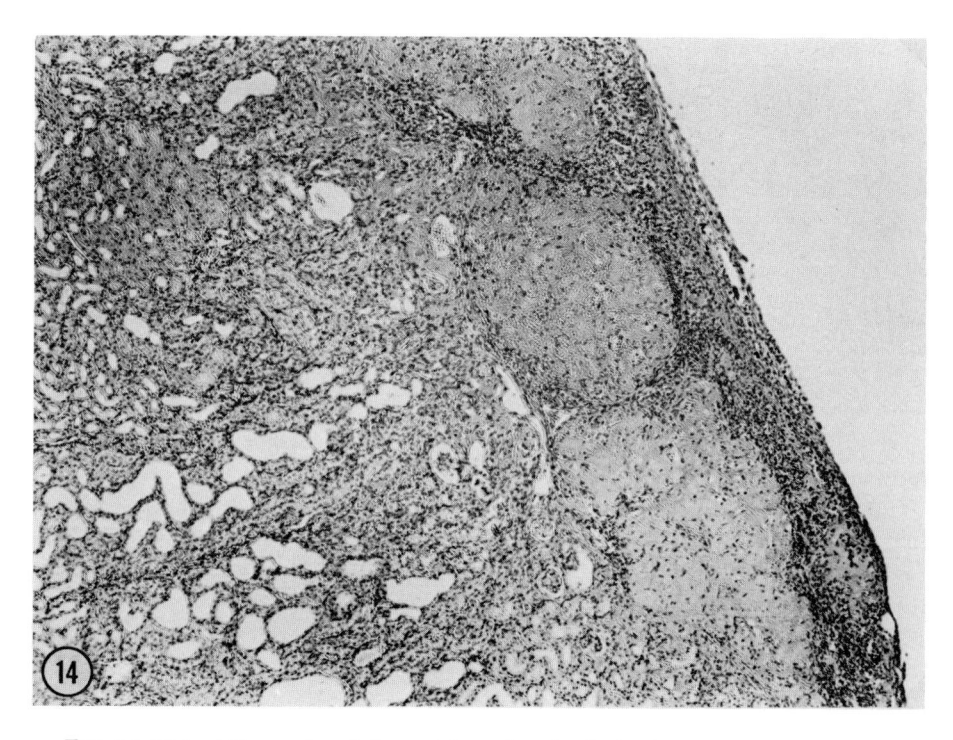

FIG. 14. Right kidney of recipient with graft of splenic tissue from donor that had received 10 injections of casein. The recipient had been treated for 10 days with casein, and had been given a short course of HN_2, the graft, as seen here, shows massive deposition of amyloid in contrast to the apparently amyloid-free adjacent host tissues. Alkaline Congo red . × 56. From Hardt and Ranløv (1968).

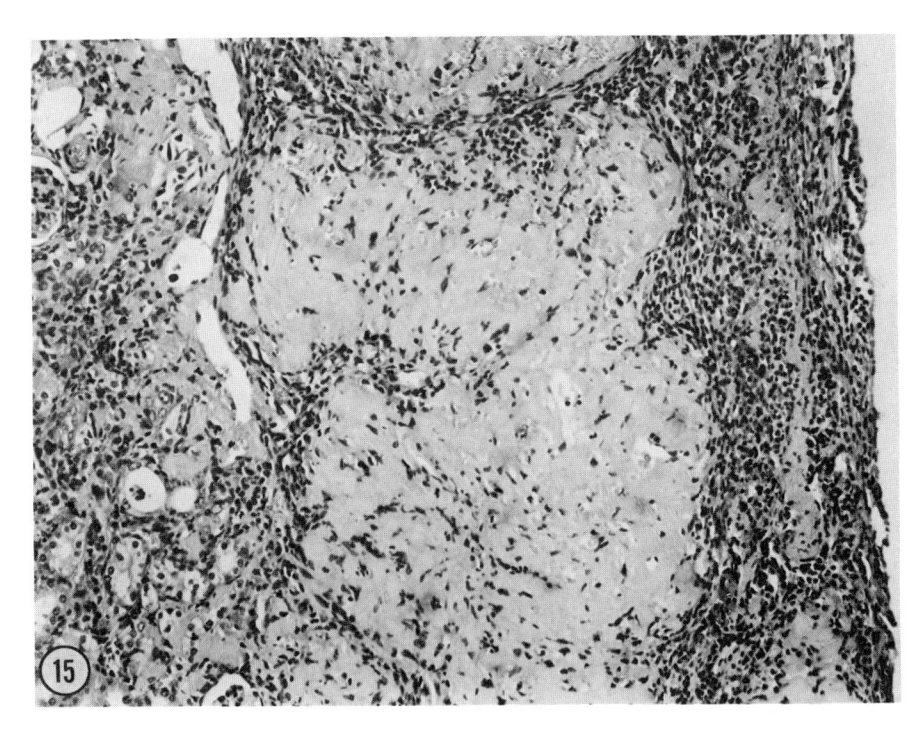

FIG. 15. Higher magnification of spleen graft shown in Fig. 14. The amyloid substance of the spleen graft extends into the adjacent host kidney, involving the tubular interstitial tissues and a few glomeruli. In contrast, no significant amyloid could be demonstrated in the remaining parts of this or the contralateral kidney. Hematoxylin-eosin. × 140. From Hardt and Ranløv (1968).

The degree of amyloidosis both in spleens and in grafts was significantly greater than that found in transfer experiments described earlier (Werdelin and Ranløv, 1966; Ranløv, 1967a), which is in accordance with the findings of Hultgren et al. (1967). The transfer of casein-sensitized spleen tissues or cells into a syngeneic organism thus enhanced the immune reaction, which is believed to play an essential role in the pathogenesis of amyloidosis.

This enhancement of the immune response has been described in an experiment under somewhat similar conditions by Moller and Moller (1966). They showed that the antibody titers rose to significantly higher levels in animals that had received sensitized lymphocytes prior to challenge with antigen than were obtained in animals challenged with antigen only. Moller and Moller believed that an antibody-induced inhibition of the immune response exists, and they proposed that such inhibition serves as a feedback control aimed at the maintenance of a stable level of immune reactivity in order to protect against excessive cellular multiplication in response to a single antigen. According to this theory, antigenic stimulation gives rise to production of antigen-sensitive cells, which in some unknown way give rise to the formation of antibody-producing cells. When the titers of antibodies rise to a certain level, they inhibit the division of antigen-sensitive cells, thereby reducing antibody production, until the antibody titer is decreased to such a degree that the inhibition of antigen-sensitive cells is broken. In this way a cyclic immune response is produced.

Hardt (1971) later showed that recipients of spleen tissue from donors treated with 10 injections of casein developed amyloidosis after only 8 injections of casein, without additional treatment with nitrogen mustard. This finding is additional evidence for the theory of a relationship between the intensity of the immune reaction and the time required for induction of experimental amyloidosis.

4. *The Mouse Mutant "Nude"*

Hardt and Claesson (1972a) suggested that stimulation of T lymphocytes might be the first step in the cellular events leading to the formation of amyloid fibrils. This hypothesis, however, has been questioned because Hardt and Claesson (1974) were able to induce amyloidosis in nude mice. To what extent the amyloid-enhancing effect of sensitized lymphoid tissue is or is not dependent on the presence of sensitized T lymphocytes has been studied by Hardt and Claesson (1974). In this experiment the two stocks of mice described in Section III, D, 2 were used: the nu/nu-C3H strains. Donors were nu/nu-C3H mice that had received 10 injections of casein. The recipients were C3H or nu/nu-C3H mice that had received either a nu/nu-C3H or a C3H spleen graft. All recipients were given 10 injections of casein after transplantation. The transfer of spleen grafts from C3H donors treated with casein for 10 days to either normal or nude recipients resulted in the development of amyloidosis, both in the spleens and in spleen grafts of the majority of the recipient mice. In contrast, only one nude and one normal C3H recipient which had received spleen grafts from casein-treated nude donors developed amyloidosis in their spleens, and no amyloid was found in any of the spleen grafts from these groups. These results open up the possibility that the acceleration is due to transfer of cell-mediated immunity to casein, since transfer of spleen grafts from nu/nu-C3H mice, which lack T lymphocytes, did not lead to acceleration of amyloid formation.

5. *Column Cell Fractionations*

In our laboratory (Hardt *et al.*, 1975) spleen cell suspensions have been depleted of B lymphocytes and macrophages by the method of immunoadsorbent columns described earlier. Spleen cell suspensions from donor mice treated with 10 injections of casein, were, after depletion of either B lymphocytes or macrophages, injected intravenously into syngeneic recipients. The recipients were, after the transfer, treated with 10 daily injections of casein, and it appeared that the same degree of amyloidosis developed in the recipients whether these had received an "untreated" cell suspension, a B lymphocyte- or a macrophage-depleted cell suspension from a casein-sensitized donor. This observation seems to provide additional evidence that T lymphocytes could play a significant role in the acceleration of amyloid formation.

Hardt and Claesson (1972b) found casein to be an antigen that needs cooperation between T and B lymphocytes in order to elicit an antibody response. The observed enhancing effect of T lymphocytes in the above-mentioned experiments is in line with suggestions made by Miller and Mitchell (1969) that the antibody-forming B cells alone can respond to a T-dependent antigen with a very weak response. Enhancement of the antibody production can be achieved only by the addition of T lymphocytes, not by increasing the dose of antigen. Hardt and Claesson (unpublished) found that the enhancing effect in transfer amyloidosis was dependent on the number of cells transferred: the transfer of 100×10^3 spleen cells from casein-treated donors enhanced the formation of amyloid to the same degree as did the transfer of 100×10^6 spleen cells, whereas a significantly lower degree of amyloidosis was found after 10×10^3 spleen cells were transferred.

6. *Guinea Pigs*

In outbred guinea pigs Cathcart *et al.* (1972) found that the induction time of casein-induced amyloidosis could be considerably reduced if spleen cells or peritoneal cells from casein-sensitized donors were transferred to a recipient subsequently subjected to casein treatment. White, outbred Hartley guinea pigs received 15 daily injections of casein. Spleen cells and peritoneal cells were harvested from these animals for subsequent transfer to non-casein-treated guinea pigs. When the recipients were afterward treated with casein, those which had received sensitized spleen cells needed only 6 injections of casein, and those which had received sensitized peritoneal cells only 12 injections of casein, in order to develop amyloidosis. In controls treated with casein only, about 30 injections of casein are usually needed to induce amyloidosis.

7. *Nonspecific Enhancement*

In all the experiments with transfer of sensitized spleen tissue or cells, performed by Janigan and co-workers, by the Boston (e.g., Cathcart *et al.*) and the Copenhagen groups, enhancing effect on antigen-induced amyloidosis was achieved only when sensitized donors were used whereas control experiments with transfer of material from normal donors were negative. However, Dreher and Letterer (1970) found 250 to 300×10^6 spleen cells from untreated normal donors nearly as effective in enhancing casein-induced murine amyloidosis as the same number of cells from casein-treated donors. Dreher and Letterer therefore claimed that formation of amyloid is due to an unspecific stimulation of the RE system, independent of an immune reaction.

This problem was further elucidated in an experiment set up by Hardt et al. (1972) in order to examine the influence of transfer of normal lymphoid cells to syngeneic mice undergoing casein-induced amyloidosis. The transfer of normal lymph node cells was supposed to inhibit formation of amyloid if the breakdown of the immune system was the major pathogenic mechanism in formation of amyloid (Teilum, 1964a). However, no such effect was found; to the contrary, transfer of normal lymph node cells caused a slight acceleration of the formation of amyloid, whereas no effect at all was obtained with other lymphoid cells. The enhancing effect of normal lymphoid cells in this experiment and in that of Dreher and Letterer (1970) could be due to a nonspecific immune stimulation by nucleoproteins released from the transferred cells. Such a phenomenon has been observed in several other transfer experiments (Johnson et al., 1968) and might, though in a circumstantial way, support the above-mentioned theory that a stronger immune response increases formation of amyloid.

B. Source of Cells

We have claimed that transfer of amyloidosis with material from amyloidotic animals without further treatment of the recipient with specific antigen is clearly distinguishable from the enhancing effect on amyloidosis obtained by transfer of tissue sensitized to an antigen followed by challenge of the recipients with the same antigen. This concept has been partly based on the results of Hardt (1971), who transferred slices from spleens, thymi, and axillary lymph nodes (regional to the casein injections) to the kidneys of syngeneic recipients. In donor mice treated with casein for 10 days, the spleens showed an increased cellularity, particularly perifollicularly, and many of these cells appeared to be of the pyroninophilic variety. In none of the donor spleens, however, could amyloid be detected. The axillary lymph nodes used as donor organs all showed hyperplasia with a marked pyroninophilia, and no amyloid was found. The transplanted thymi were histologically normal. After the transplantation the recipients received varying numbers of injections of casein, but in this experiment no nitrogen mustard was given.

All mice that had received a spleen graft from a casein-treated donor and then 8 or 10 injections of casein showed marked amyloidosis in their own spleen as well as in the spleen graft. The kidney bearing the spleen graft showed infiltration of amyloid in the area close to the graft bed.

Each mouse that had received a thymus graft from a casein-treated donor developed significant amyloid in the host spleen only if, after transfer, it was treated with 8 or 10 injections of casein. No local effect of the thymus graft on the kidney was observed. Also, transplantation of casein-stimulated lymph nodes led to formation of amyloid in the recipients' spleens when the recipients were treated with at least 10 injections of casein. No amyloid was found in the grafted lymph nodes, and no local reaction in the graft-bearing kidney was observed. No amyloid was found in transplant recipients that had been given either casein-sensitized lymphoid tissue and fewer than 8 injections of casein, or nonsensitized lymphoid tissue and casein treatment after the transfer, except for three mice (one from each group) in which an insignificant amount of amyloid was found in the spleens.

The finding that thymus grafts and lymph node grafts were as effective in enhancing formation of amyloid as spleen grafts, when all were derived from sensitized donors, supports our theory that the amyloid-enhancing effect observed in this model can be explained as a result of a transfer of immunity. However, in these experiments, also, the spleen seems to have had a unique role in amyloidogenesis, different from its role in immunity, since the spleen grafts were the only lymphoid tissues that showed formation of amyloid—sometimes to a high degree. Furthermore only the spleen grafts were able to induce formation of amyloid locally in the adjacent, graft-bearing kidneys. Cathcart *et al.* (1972) showed that peritoneal cells from casein-sensitized guinea pigs were likewise able to accelerate formation of amyloid in recipients treated with casein after having received the cells. The effect was weaker when peritoneal cells were transferred instead of spleen cells.

C. Transfer with Subcellular Material (Table IV)

Janigan and Druet (1968) believed that the transferred sensitized cells directly stimulated the RE cells in the recipients to form the amyloid fibrils. On the assumption that spleen homogenate preparations should be as effective as spleen cells, they prepared a spleen homogenate from casein-sensitized donor mice by extensively grinding the spleens. The homogenates were filtered through a 150 μm mesh wire screen, and then frozen and thawed. No intact nucleated cells were found in the homogenate. Donor mice were treated with seven injections of azocasein, and a dose of spleen homogenate equivalent to one spleen was transferred intraperitoneally into recipients which had been irradiated 2–4 hours previously. Nearly all mice treated with 4 injections of azocasein developed extensive amyloidosis, a result that paralleled the findings in recipients that had been given intact spleen cells instead of homogenate. In this experiment it was shown that in the strain used (C3H/Hej) 9 injections of azocasein was the minimum antigen challenge needed to induce amyloidosis. A significant reduction in the induction time was thus observed, both with transfer of spleen homogenates and with transfer of spleen cells.

Janigan (1968) extended the study on the enhancing phenomenon in experimental murine amyloidosis, using different fractions of spleen homogenates: (a) crude homogenate, (b) crude sediment, and (c) crude supernatant. The last two fractions were obtained by centrifugation of the crude homogenate. Furthermore, aliquots of the crude supernatant were subjected to ammonium sulfate precipitation. In the same study, nuclear fractions and cytoplasmic

TABLE IV
TRANSFER OF AMYLOID-ENHANCING FACTOR

Authors	Donors Species, strain	Treatment	Source	Transfer material Fraction	Amount	Route of administration	Recipients Species, strain	Treatment prior to transfer	Treatment post transfer	Incidence of amyloidosis transfer to	Interval from transfer to sacrifice (days)
Janigan and Druet (1968)	C3H/HeJ mice	7 Azocasein injections	Spleen	Whole spleen homogenate	Eq. 1 spleen	i.p.	C3H/HeJ mice	400–750 rad	4 Azocasein injections	72/79	5
	C3H/HeJ mice	7 Azocasein injections	Spleen	Whole spleen homogenate	Eq. 1 spleen	i.p.	C57BL/10J mice	750 rad	4 Azocasein injections	5/5	5
	C3H/HeJ mice	7 Azocasein injections	Serum		0.4 Ml	i.p.	C3H/HeJ mice	400–750 rad	4 Azocasein injections	6/9	5
Janigan (1968)	C3H/HeJ mice	7 Azocasein injections	Spleen	Crude homogenate	Eq. 1 spleen	i.p.	C3H/HeJ mice	Irradiation	4 Azocasein injections	?/10	5
	C3H/HeJ mice	7 Azocasein injections	Spleen	Crude sediment	Eq. 1 spleen	i.p.	C3H/HeJ mice	Irradiation	4 Azocasein injections	?/10	5
	C3H/HeJ mice	7 Azocasein injections	Spleen	Crude supernatant	Eq. 1 spleen	i.p.	C3H/HeJ mice	Irradiation	4 Azocasein injections	?/21	5
	C3H/HeJ mice	7 Azocasein injections	Spleen	Nuclear	Eq. 1 spleen	i.p.	C3H/HeJ mice	Irradiation	4 Azocasein injections	?/5	5
	C3H/HeJ mice	7 Azocasein injections	Spleen	Cytoplasmic	Eq. 1 spleen	i.p.	C3H/HeJ mice	Irradiation	4 Azocasein injections	?/5	5
	C3H/HeJ mice	7 Azocasein injections	Spleen	Whole spleen homogenate	Eq. 1 spleen	i.p.	C3H/HeJ mice	Irradiation	4 Albumin (32 mg) injections	10/10	5

Jakob and Hilgenfeld (1972)	Decin mice	Spontaneous amyloidosis	Spleen "Raw" homogenate	Eq. 1 spleen	i.p.	Decin mice (old)	None	5 Casein injections	19/19	7
	Decin mice	Spontaneous amyloidosis	Spleen "Raw" homogenate	Eq. 1 spleen	i.p.	A-B mice	None	5 Casein injections	10/15	7
	Decin mice	Spontaneous amyloidosis	Spleen "Raw" homogenate	Eq. 1 spleen	i.p.	Strong-A mice	None	5 Casein injections	14/15	7
	Decin mice	Spontaneous amyloidosis	Spleen Precipitate	Eq. 1 spleen	i.p.	Decin mice (old)	None	5 Casein injections	20/20	7
	Decin mice	Spontaneous amyloidosis	Spleen Supernatant	Eq. 1 spleen	i.p.	Decin mice (old)	None	5 Casein injections	20/20	7
	Decin mice	Spontaneous amyloidosis	Spleen Filtered supernatant	Eq. 1 spleen	i.p.	Decin mice (old)	None	5 Casein injections	19/19	7
Shirahama et al. (1969)	Human	Patients with amyloidosis	Spleen Whole spleen homogenate	300 Mg	i.p.	C3H mice	None	3–7 Casein injections	25/30	4–8
Keizman et al. (1972)	Human	Patients with amyloidosis	Spleen Glycoprotein MW 10,000	≥1 Mg	i.p.	White Swiss mice	None	4 Casein injections	28/30	5

[a] Eq. = equivalent of.

extracts from spleen cells were separated and used for transfer. All donors were C3H/Hej mice that had been treated with 7 daily injections of azocasein. Recipient mice of the same strain were injected, intraperitoneally (1) with spleen homogenates or (2) with spleen homogenate fractions, or (3) with lymph node homogenates, or (4) with the nuclear fraction, or (5) with the cytoplasmic fraction of spleen cells. Before the transfer, the recipients had been irradiated and afterward were all given 4 injections of azocasein. In all recipients—independent of the nature of inoculum received—amyloidosis was present.

Jakob and Hilgenfeld used a strain of mice (Decin) with a high incidence of spontaneous amyloidosis as donor mice to investigate whether spleens from these mice were able to enhance casein-induced formation of amyloid. They used 4 different fractions of spleen homogenates: (1) "raw" homogenate, (2) the precipitate after centrifugation of the "raw" homogenate (10 minutes at 5000–6000 rpm), (3) the supernatant, and (4) supernatant after filtration through a filter (pore <1.3 μm).

Donor mice were old Decin mice of whom about 50% had amyloidosis of the spleen; 1 ml of the different fractions of homogenates, equivalent to one and a half spleens, was injected intraperitoneally into each recipient, which then was given 5 injections of casein. It appeared that all spleen fractions obtained from the old amyloidotic Decin mice were effective in enhancing the formation of amyloid in young Decin mice, as 15 casein injections normally are needed to induce formation of amyloid in young mice of this strain. No amyloid was found in recipient mice when young Decin mice—without amyloidosis—were used as donors. These results indicate that the amyloid-enhancing factor should be related in time to the appearance of the amyloid fibrils, not to the preceding immune reactions.

D. Donor–Recipient Combinations

1. *Allogeneic*

The factor(s) responsible for amyloid enhancement seem to be active across allogeneic and xenogeneic barriers. Janigan and Druet showed that the same accelerating effect was obtained in C3H/Hej and in C57/10J mice when sensitized C3H/Hej mice were used as donors. With a similar allogeneic system, Cathcart *et al.* (1972) found that the accelerated induction of amyloid in guinea pigs was dependent on a factor that was capable of crossing histocompatibility barriers.

Jakob and Hilgenfeld (1972), in their experiment with spontaneous amyloidosis in Decin mice, showed that amyloid enhancement could be achieved in allogeneic combinations using old Decin mice as donors and AB mice or Strong A mice as recipients. Apparently, they did find a xenogeneic barrier, as no amyloid enhancement was observed in rats, hamsters, and guinea pigs when the old Decin mice served as donors.

2. *Xenogeneic*

A peculiar finding is that of Shirahama et al. (1969) who reported successful transfer—human to mouse—of amyloidosis. Three human spleens from patients with primary, secondary and myeloma-associated amyloidosis together with a normal human spleen as control were used as donor material. Aliquots of spleen homogenate were administered intraperitoneally in single doses to inbred C3H mice. The recipient mice were then treated with casein, and it was found that 5 injections of casein were sufficient to induce amyloidosis in the recipients of amyloidotic spleen homogenate, which is about one-third of the dose normally necessary for induction of amyloid in this strain of mice. Keizman et al. (1972) later confirmed that a factor from human amyloidotic spleens can enhance casein-induced amyloidosis in mice (see below).

E. Role of the Antigen

The amyloid-enhancing effect of a donor tissue can be estimated by its capacity to reduce the amount of casein necessary for induction of amyloid in normal animals. With the exception of Dreher and Letterer (1972), all authors of the above-mentioned papers seemingly agree that normal tissue has no inherent amyloid-enhancing potency. In these experiments the donors usually were sensitized with the same material that was later injected into the recipients. Hardt (unpublished) has noted that if recipients of casein-sensitized lymphoid tissue are treated with *Brucella* antigen instead of casein, no enhancement of *Brucella*-induced amyloidosis is observed. This observation may well indicate that the desired enhancement after this particular type of transfer depends on a transfer of specific immunity toward casein, consistent with the findings of Cathcart et al. (1972), who noted a specifically altered immune response to casein in guinea pigs that had received casein-sensitized lymphoid cells. This alteration of the immune response appeared prior to the amyloid formation in these animals.

Janigan (1968) postulated that it is not necessary that recipients be treated with the (same) antigen that was used to sensitize the donor. He based this conclusion on the finding that recipients of spleen homogenates from azocasein-treated mice exhibited amyloidosis of the same degree, whether treated with azocasein or with albumin after the transfer.

The mechanisms involved when amyloidotic tissue is used as donor material are more obscure. The amyloidotic tissue is derived either from mice with spontaneous amyloidosis (Jakob and Hilgenfeld, 1972) or from human amyloidotic spleens of patients with various diseases (primary amyloidosis, secondary amyloidosis, myeloma, familial Mediterranean fever) (Shirahama et al.,

1969; Keizman et al., 1972). Independent of origin, the spleen homogenates all enhanced the casein-induced amyloidosis in mice. It is rather difficult to fit these results into any other available data on transfer of immunity.

F. Nature of the Amyloid-Enhancing Factor

In principle, the enhancing effect of various lymphoid tissues and fractions thereof could be due to enhancement of the immune reactions believed to be the first step in the development of experimental amyloidosis. Also, the enhancing effect could be imagined mediated through a direct effect on the RE cells producing (actively or passively) the amyloid fibrils.

Druet and Janigan (1966) and Janigan (1968) reported an amyloid-enhancing factor (AEF) in viable spleen cells and in different fractions of spleen homogenate, as already described above. Of special interest is their finding that this factor was present in an ammonium sulfate-precipitated fraction of serum. The factor tolerated storage at $-20°C$ for 3 weeks and was effective across allogeneic histocompatibility barriers. Janigan (1968) pointed out that this factor differs from the factor involved in transfer of specific immunity by being present in the serum globulin fraction and by being effective in recipients later treated with antigens other than that used for sensitizing the donors. Janigan therefore suggested a direct "donor factor–recipient RE cell interplay."

We (Hardt and Ranløv, 1968; Hardt, 1971) have advanced the theory that the amyloid-enhancing factor (AEF) observed in our experiments most likely was a superantigen, namely, antigen (casein) in a highly immunogenic complex with RNA. Such superantigens have in many experiments (review: Bloom and Chase 1967) proved capable of transferring a high degree of immunity, both on the cellular and on the humoral level. In accordance with this concept we found, in contrast to Janigan, that the recipients had to be treated with the same antigen as the donors in order to provoke amyloidosis. The resulting reduction of the induction time should thus be due solely to a transferred acceleration of the immune reaction toward the specific antigen.

In their guinea pig transfer experiments, Cathcart et al. (1972) also obtained evidence that the AEF is related to immunity, but they believe that the factor enhances specific cellular immune tolerance toward casein, which they suggested to be the trigger mechanism in amyloidosis. However, they ventured no propositions about the nature of this factor.

As the results of Shirahama et al. (1969) and of Jakob and Hilgenfeld (1972) gave negative evidence for the antigen and species specificity of the AEF in amyloidotic spleens, these investigators proposed that the factor consisted either of amyloid fibrils or of their precursors.

Keizman et al. (1972) also used amyloidotic spleens (from humans) as their source of an AEF and showed in a careful analytical study (1) that amyloid fibrils, isolated by the method of Pras et al. (1968), did not contain AEF, and

(2) that an AEF could be isolated from the supernatant, obtained when crude spleen homogenate was centrifuged 20 minutes at 15,000 g. The AEF was extracted from the supernatant by a procedure based on differential solubility in acetone and passage through membranes of known porosity. In 50% acetone, AEF was extracted from the tissue, leaving behind amyloid filaments and other protein components; in 95% acetone, however, AEF was precipitated from solution. Its molecular size enabled it to pass through a regular dialysis membrane, but not through an Amicon UM-10 filter. It was also retained in a Sephadex G-25 column. These properties suggest a molecular weight of about 10,000, much less than that of the amyloid fibril. The amino acid and carbohydrate contents of this low-molecular-weight substance suggest that it is a glycopeptide. The factor did not show antigenic relation to any of the normal human serum components. The factor was not able in itself to induce formation of amyloid, that is, without concurrent antigenic challenge of the recipient.

V. Conclusions and Summary

In relation to experimental amyloidosis, two principally differing transfer systems have been developed during the last decade. The first model has enabled us to study the transfer of actual, fully developed amyloid disease (Werdelin and Ranløv, 1966; Ranløv, 1967a). Even though no definite conclusions regarding the nature of the transferable amyloid-inducing factor have as yet been reached, a considerable amount of evidence points toward a nucleoprotein, operating with, and depending on, the sustained presence of specific antigen. The amyloid-inducing factor has proved not to be strain specific, but is probably specific within species. A prominent feature is its close relation to the spleen, as successful transfer of amyloid in this model has been only achieved with cells or subcellular fractions derived from tissues rich in RE cells, first and foremost the spleen, but also liver and lung. This amyloid-inducing factor apparently does not circulate in the peripheral blood; many observations suggest that it exerts its effect at a rather restricted intercellular level, and very likely it is responsible for the transmission of information from hyperimmunized lymphoid cells to RE cells, forcing upon the latter a pattern of abnormal protein synthesis, among which is the production of amyloid.

In contrast, the second model of amyloid transfer (Hultgren et al., 1967), described in Section IV, presents a number of less specific characteristics, which are all suggestive of a transfer of immunity rather than of amyloidosis. First, the capacity to form amyloid may be transferred with all types of lymphoid cells, and even, it has been claimed, with serum. Second, an unavoidable prerequisite for success is continued treatment of the recipient animal with the amyloidogenic antigen that had been used in the donor from which the transferred material was prepared. Third, this alleged amyloid-enhancing factor has a number of physicochemical characteristics different from those of the amyloid-inducing factor described above. Thus, it seems to operate by enhancing the immune mechanisms necessary for the induction of amyloidosis under experimental conditions. Further, it provides us with additional evidence for the concept of immunity as a mandatory pathogenetic factor in amyloid disease.

During a century of research on amyloidosis, clinical observations alone have failed to produce material for a convincing theory of pathogenesis, and research on amyloidosis has from the very beginning benefited from results achieved in the field of experimental immunology.

The characteristic clinical and cellular reaction pattern of amyloidosis can be found in a variety of other diseases of the mesenchymal tissues, such as granulomatous diseases in animals and in humans, and in experimental autoimmune diseases, such as thyroiditis and nephritis. As amyloidosis is the only mesenchymal ("collagen") disease which, with any reasonable degree of certainty, can be reproduced in experimental animals, a more thorough understanding of the nature of this disease can be of importance for the understanding of the pathogenetic mechanisms of a larger group of mesenchymal diseases.

Transfer amyloidosis—as we see it—has made it possible to approach pathogenetic problems from a new angle. It has provided us with a new tool capable of "breaking up" the pathogenetic pathways into well defined stages differing from one another with regard to cell types involved and immune functional characteristics. Hence, the different stages of the disease may be induced in individual animals and thus analyzed separately. Further, mechanisms operating in the transition between stages may be defined more easily and, we hope, modified, and thus the road may be paved toward the ultimate goal: clinical treatment.

ACKNOWLEDGMENTS

Grants in support of the investigations reported from the authors' laboratory were received from The Danish League Against Rheumatism, Ingeniør af Frederikssund Søren Alfred Andersen's Legacy, Gårdejer af Stenløse Peder Laurits Pedersen's Legacy, The Daell Foundation, and King Christian X Foundation.

The authors further wish to acknowledge the participation of those colleagues who were involved in the experiments reported from this laboratory. These include: M. H. Claesson, P. Ebbesen, C. Koch, J. Wanstrup, and O. Werdelin. Indispensable technical assistance was provided by Mrs. Inge Nøhr Børgesen, Mrs. Lilly Rasmussen, and Miss Hanne Hansen. We are indebted to Mr. Bent Børgesen for the excellent photographic work.

REFERENCES

Arnason, B.G., DeVaux St.Cyr, C., and Shaffner, J.B. (1964). *J. Immunol.* 93, 915.
Åstrøm, K.E., and Waksman, B.H. (1962). *J. Pathol. Bacteriol.* 83, 89.
Bayrd, E.D., and Bennett, W.A. (1950). *Med. Clin. N. Amer.* 34, 1151.
Benditt, E.P., Eriksen, N., Hermodson, M.A., and Eriksson, L.H. (1971). *FEBS Lett.* 19, 169.

Ben-Ishay, Z., and Zlotnick, A. (1968). *Israel J. Med. Sci.* 4, 987.
Bloom, B.R., and Chase, M.W. (1967). *Progr. Allergy* 10, 151
Bradbury, S., and Micklem, H.S. (1965). *Amer. J. Pathol.* 46, 263.
Cathcart, E.S., Wolheim, F.A., and Cohen, A.S. (1967). *J. Immunol.* 99, 376.
Cathcart, E.S., Mullarkey, M., and Cohen, A.S. (1970). *Lancet* 2, 639.
Cathcart, E.S., Mullarkey, M., and Cohen, A.S. (1971). *Immunology* 20, 1001.
Cathcart, E.S., Rodgers, O.G., and Cohen, A.S. (1972). *Ann. Rheum. Dis.* 31, 303.
Chase, M.W. (1945). *Proc. Soc. Exp. Biol. Med.* 59, 134.
Christensen, H. E. (1960). *Acta Pathol. Microbiol. Scand.* 50, 29.
Christensen, H.E. (1963). Ph.D. Thesis, Copenhagen,
Christensen, H.E., and Hjort, G.H. (1959). *Acta Pathol. Microbiol. Scand.* 47, 140.
Christensen, H.E., and Rask-Nielsen, R. (1962). *J. Nat. Cancer Inst.* 28, 1.
Claesson, M.H., and Hardt, F. (1972a). *Acta Pathol. Microbiol. Scand., Sect. A* 80, 125.
Claesson, M.H., and Hardt, F. (1972b). *Clin. Exp. Immunol.* 11, 277.
Claesson, M.H., Hardt, F., and Røpke, C. (1974). *Acta Pathol. Microbiol. Scand., Sect. B* 82, 719.
Claman, H.N., Chaperon, E.A., and Triplett, R.F. (1966). *J. Immunol.* 97, 828.
Clerici, E., Pierpaoli, W., and Romussi, M. (1965). *Pathol. Microbiol.* 28, 806.
Clerici, E., Mocarelli, P., De Ferrari, F., and Villa, M.L. (1969). *J. Lab. Clin. Med.* 74, 145.
Cohen, A.S. (1965). *Int. Rev. Exp. Pathol.* 4, 159.
Cohen, A.S., Gross, E., and Shirahama, T. (1965). *Amer. J. Pathol.* 47, 1079.
Cohen, A.S., Bricetti, A.B., Harrington, J.T., and Mannick, J.A. (1971). *Lancet* 2, 513.
DeVenuto, F., Kelleher, P.C., and Westphal, U. (1962). *Biochim. Biophys. Acta* 63, 434.
Dounce, A.L., Witter, R.F., Monty, K.J., Pate, S., and Cottone, M.A. (1955). *J. Biophys. Biochem. Cytol.* 1, 139.
Dreher, R., and Letterer, E. (1970). *Virchows Arch. Abt. B. Zellpathol.* 5, 236.
Druet, R.L., and Janigan, D.T. (1966). *Amer. J. Pathol.* 49, 911.
Dumonde, D.C., Wolstencroft, R.A., Panayi, G.S., Matthew, M., Morley, J., and Howson, W.T. (1969). *Nature (London)* 224, 38.
Dunn, T.B. (1957). *J. Nat. Cancer Inst.* 19, 371.
Dunn, T.B. (1967). *In* "Pathology of Rats and Mice" (E. Cotchin and F.A.C. Roe, eds.), p. 181. Blackwell, Oxford and Edinburgh.
Ebbesen, P. (1968). Ph.D. Thesis, Copenhagen.
Ebbesen, P. (1971). *Virchows Arch. B* 7, 263.
Ebbesen, P., and Rask-Nielsen, R. (1967). *J. Nat. Cancer Inst.* 39, 917.
Ebbesen, P., Schiødt, T., and Christensen, H.E. (1969). *Cancer Res.* 29, 1851.
Ein, D., Kimura, S., and Glenner, G.G. (1972). *Biochem. Biophys. Res. Commun.* 46, 498.
Felix-Davies, D., and Waksman, B.H. (1961). *Arthritis Rheum.* 4, 416.
Fiscus, W.G., Morris, B.T., Session, J., and Trentin, J.J. (1962). *Ann. N.Y. Acad. Sci.* 99, 355.
Flanagan, S.P. (1966). *Genet. Res.* 8, 295.
Fliedner, T.M. (1967). *In* "The Lymphocyte in Immunology and Haemopoiesis" (J.M. Yoffey, ed.), p. 198. Arnold, London.
Ford, W.L., Burr, W., and Simonsen, M. (1970). *Transplantation* 3, 258.
Franklin, E.C., and Zucker-Franklin, D. (1972). *Advan. Immunol.* 15, 249.
Franklin, E.C., Pras, M., Levin, M. and Frangione, B. (1972). *FEBS Lett.* 22, 121.
Giles, R.B., and Calkins, E. (1958). *J. Clin. Invest.* 37, 846.
Glenner, G.G., and Page, D.L. (1975). *Int. Rev. Exp. Pathol.* 15 (in press).
Glenner, G.G., Terry, W., Harada, M., Isersky, C., and Page, D. (1971). *Science* 172, 1150.
Gueft, B., and Ghidoni, J.J. (1963). *Amer. J. Pathol.* 43, 837.
Hardt, F. (1968). *Acta Pathol. Microbiol. Scand.* 72, 446.

Hardt, F. (1971). *Amer. J. Pathol.* 65, 411.
Hardt, F., and Claesson, M.H. (1971). *Transplantation* 12, 36.
Hardt, F., and Claesson, M.H. (1972a). *Immunology* 22, 677.
Hardt, F., and Claesson, M.H. (1972b). *Acta Pathol. Microbiol. Scand.* 80, 471.
Hardt, F., and Claesson, M.H. (1973). *Acta Pathol. Microbiol. Scand.* 81, 770.
Hardt, F., and Claesson, M.H. (1974). *Acta Pathol. Microbiol. Scand.* (B) 82, 403.
Hardt, F., and Hellung-Larsen, P. (1972). *Clin. Exp. Immunol.* 10, 487.
Hardt, F., and Ranløv, P. (1968). *Acta Pathol. Microbiol. Scand.* 73, 549.
Hardt, F., Ebbesen, P., and Moesner, J. (1972). *Acta Pathol. Microbiol. Scand., Sect. A* 80, 468.
Hardt, F., Koch, C. Ranløv, P., and Claesson, M.H. (1975). In press.
Hess, E.W., Ashworth, C.T., and Ziff, M. (1962). *J. Exp. Med.* 115, 421.
Hultgren, M.K., Druet, R.L., and Janigan, D.T. (1967). *Amer. J. Pathol.* 50, 943.
Husby, G., and Natvig, J.B. (1974). *J. Clin. Invest.* 53, 1054.
Husby, G., Sletten, K., Michaelsen, T.E., and Natvig, J.B. (1972). *Nature (London)* 238, 187.
Husby, G., Michaelsen, T., Sletten, K., and Natvig, J.B. (1973). *Scand. J. Immunol.* 2, 319.
Isobe, T., and Osserman, E.F. (1974). *N. Engl. J. Med.* 290, 473.
Jaffe, R.H. (1926). *Arch. Pathol.* 2, 149.
Jakob, W., and Hilgenfeld, M. (1972). *Zentralbl. Allg. Pathol. Pathol. Anat.* 116, 94.
Janigan, D.T. (1965). *Amer. J. Pathol.* 47, 159.
Janigan, D.T. (1968). In "Amyloidosis" (E. Mandema, L. Ruinen, J.H. Scholten, and A.S. Cohen, eds.), p. 303. Excerpta Medica Found., Amsterdam.
Janigan, D.T., and Druet, R.L. (1968). *Amer. J. Pathol.* 52, 381.
Johnson, A.G., Schmidtke, J., Merritt, K., and Han, I. (1968). In "Nucleic Acids in Immunology" (O.J. Plescia and W. Braun, eds.). Springer-Verlag, Berlin and New York.
Jureziz, R.E., Thor, E.E., and Dray, S. (1970). *J. Immunol.* 105, 1313.
Kaplan, H.S. (1966). In "Thymus" (G.E.W. Wolstenholme and R. Porter, eds.), p. 176. Churchill, London.
Kazimierczak, J. (1969). *Acta Pathol. Microbiol. Scand.* 77, 201.
Kazimierczak, J. (1972). *Acta Pathol. Microbiol. Scand., Sect. A, Suppl.* 233, 141.
Keizman, I., Rimon, A., Sohar, E., and Gafni, J. (1972). *Acta Pathol. Microbiol. Scand., Sect. A, Suppl.* 233, 172.
Kellum, M.J., Sutherland, D.E.R., Eckert, E., Petersen, R.D.A., and Good, R.A. (1965). *Int. Arch. Allergy Appl. Immunol.* 27, 6.
Koch, R. (1890). *Deut. Med. Wochschr.* 16, 1029.
Landsteiner, K., and Chase, M.W. (1942). *Proc. Soc. Exp. Biol Med.* 49, 688.
Latvalahti, J. (1953). *Acta Endocrinol., Suppl.* 16.
Lawrence, H.S., Al-Askari, S., David, J., Franklin, E.C., and Zweiman, B. (1963). *Trans. Ass. Amer. Physicians* 81, 248.
Lehner, T., and Rosenoer, V.M. (1968). In "Amyloidosis" (E. Mandema, L. Ruinen, J.H. Scholten, and A.S. Cohen, eds.), p. 344. Excerpta Medica Found., Amsterdam.
Lehner, T., Rosenoer, V.M., and Topping, N.E. (1966). *Nature (London)* 209, 930.
Lehner, T., Cameron, J.S., and Ward, R.G. (1970). *Clin. Exp. Immunol.* 6, 439.
Letterer, E. (1926). *Zentralbl. Allg. Beitr. Pathol. Anat.* 75, 486.
Letterer, E. (1934). *Virchows Arch. Pathol. Anat.* 293, 34.
Letterer, E., and Kretschmer, R. (1966). *Nature (London)* 210, 290.
Levin, M., Pras, M., and Franklin, E.C. (1973). *J. Exp. Med.* 138, 373.
Liacopoulos, P., Merchant, B., and Harrell, B.E. (1967). *Transplantation* 5, 1423.
Lüders, K. (1969). *Z. Immunitaetsforsch., Allerg. Klin. Immunol.* 137, 474.
McIntire, K.R., and Potter, M. (1964). *J. Nat. Cancer Inst.* 33, 631.
Milgrom, F., and Witebsky, E. (1962). *J. Amer. Med. Ass.* 181, 706.

Miller, J.F.A.P. (1961). *Lancet* **2**, 748.
Miller, J.F.A.P. (1962). *Nature (London)* **195**, 1318.
Miller, J.F.A.P., and Mitchell, G.F. (1969). *Transplant. Rev.* **1**, 3.
Moller, G., and Moller, E. (1966). *In* "Antibodies to Biologically Active Molecules," p. 349. Pergamon, Oxford.
Neidhart, J.A., Schwartz, R.S., Hurtubise, P.E., Murphy, S.G., Metz, E.N., Balcerzak, S.P., and LoBuglio, A.F. (1973). *Cell Immunol.* **9**, 319.
Osserman, E.F., Takatsuki, K., and Talal, N. (1964). *Semin. Hematol.* **1**, 3.
Pantelouris, E.M. (1968). *Nature (London)* **217**, 370.
Pantelouris, E.M. (1971). *Clin. Exp. Immunol.* **20**, 247.
Perasalo, O., Kuusisto, A., and Halonen, P.L. (1950). *Ann. Med. Intern. Fenn.* **39**, 34.
Pras, M., Schubert, M., Zucker-Franklin, D., Rimon, A., and Franklin, E.C. (1968). *J. Clin. Invest.* **47**, 924.
Pras, M., Zucker-Franklin, D., Rimon, A., and Franklin, E.C. (1969). *J. Exp. Med.* **130**, 777.
Prausnitz, C., and Küstner, H. (1921). *Zentralbl. Bacteriol. (Orig.) Abt. 1* **86**, 160.
Raff, M.C. (1969). *Nature (London)* **224**, 378.
Raff, M.C. (1971). *Transplant. Rev.* **6**, 52.
Raff, M.C., and Wortis, H.H. (1970). *Immunology* **18**, 931.
Ranløv, P. (1966a). *Acta Pathol. Microbiol. Scand.* **67**, 42.
Ranløv, P. (1966b). *Acta Pathol. Microbiol. Scand.* **68**, 19.
Ranløv, P. (1967a). *Acta Pathol. Microbiol. Scand.* **70**, 321.
Ranløv, P. (1967b). *Acta Pathol. Microbiol. Scand.* **69**, 534.
Ranløv, P. (1967c). *Acta Pathol. Microbiol. Scand.* **70**, 19.
Ranløv, P. (1967d). *Acta Pathol. Microbiol. Scand.* **69**, 375.
Ranløv, P. (1967e). *Acta Pathol. Microbiol. Scand.* **71**, 316.
Ranløv, P. (1968). Ph.D. Thesis, Copenhagen.
Ranløv, P., and Christensen, H.E. (1968). *Acta Pathol. Microbiol. Scand.* **72**, 233.
Ranløv, P., and Elling Nielsen, P. (1966). *Acta Pathol. Microbiol. Scand.* **66**, 154.
Ranløv, P., and Hardt, F. (1970). *Clin. Exp. Immunol.* **8**, 163.
Ranløv, P., and Jensen, E. (1966). *Acta Pathol. Microbiol. Scand.* **67**, 161.
Ranløv, P., and Pindborg, J.J. (1966). *Acta Pathol. Microbiol. Scand.* **68**, 169.
Ranløv, P., and Wanstrup, J. (1967). *Acta Pathol. Microbiol. Scand.* **71**, 575.
Ranløv, P., and Werdelin, O. (1967). *Acta Pathol. Microbiol. Scand.* **70**, 249.
Rask-Nielsen, R., Christensen, H.E., and Clausen, J. (1960). *J. Nat. Cancer Inst.* **25**, 315.
Rask-Nielsen, R., Heremans, J.R., Christensen, H.E., and Djurtoft, R. (1961). *Proc. Soc. Exp. Biol. Med.* **107**, 632.
Reif, A.E., and Allen, J.M.V. (1963). *Nature (London)* **200**, 1332.
Rich, A.R., and Lewis, M.R. (1932). *Bull. Johns Hopkins Hosp.* **50**, 115.
Rodey, G.E., and Good, R.A. (1969). *Proc. Soc. Exp. Biol. Med.* **131**, 457.
Rygaard, J. (1969). *Acta Pathol. Microbiol. Scand.* **77**, 761.
Scholten, J.H., van den Broek, A.A., Ruinen, L., Mandema, E., and Keunig, F.J. (1968). *In* "Amyloidosis" (E. Mandema, L. Ruinen, J.H. Scholten, and A.S. Cohen, eds.), p. 52. Excerpta Medica Found., Amsterdam.
Shearing, S., Comerford, F.R., and Cohen, A.S. (1965). *Proc. Soc. Exp. Biol. Med.* **119**, 673.
Shimamura, T., and Sorenson, G.D. (1965). *Amer. J. Pathol.* **46**, 645.
Shirahama, T., Lawless, O.J., and Cohen, A.S. (1969) *Proc. Soc. Exp. Biol. Med.* **130**, 516.
Simonsen, M. (1957). *Acta Pathol. Microbiol. Scand.* **40**, 480.
Simonsen, M. (1962). *Progr. Allergy* **6**, 349.
Skinner, M., Cohen, A.S., Shirahama, T., and Cathcart, E.S. (1974). *J. Lab. Clin. Med.* **84**, 604.
Smetana, H. (1927). *J. Exp. Med.* **45**, 619.

Sorenson, G.D., Heefner, W.A., and Kirkpatrick, J.B. (1964). *Amer. J. Pathol.* **44**, 629.
Sutherland, D.E.R., Peterson, R.D.A., Archer, O.K., Eckert, E., and Good, R.A. (1965). *Lancet* **1**, 130.
Teilum, G. (1952). *Ann. Rheum. Dis.* **11**, 119.
Teilum, G. (1954). *J. Lab. Clin. Med.* **43**, 367.
Teilum, G. (1956). *Amer. J. Pathol.* **32**, 945.
Teilum, G. (1964a). *Acta Pathol. Microbiol. Scand.* **61**, 21.
Teilum, G. (1964b). *J. Pathol. Bacteriol.* **88**, 317.
Teilum, G. (1968). *In* "Amyloidosis" (E. Mandema, L. Ruinen, J.H. Scholten, and A.S. Cohen, eds.), p. 37. Excerpta Medica Found., Amsterdam.
Terry, W.D., Page, D.L., Kimura, S. Isobe, T., Osserman, E.F., and Glenner, G.G. (1973). *J. Clin. Invest.* **52**, 1276.
Vassar, P.S., and Culling, C.F.A. (1959). *Arch. Pathol.* **68**, 487.
Virchow, R. (1854). *Arch. Pathol. Anat. Phys.* **6**, 416.
Werdelin, O. (1968). *Acta Pathol. Microbiol. Scand.* **72**, 23.
Werdelin, O., and Ranløv, P. (1966). *Acta Pathol. Microbiol. Scand.* **68**, 1.
Wanstrup, J., and Ranløv, P. (1968). *Acta Pathol. Microbiol. Scand.* **74**, 303.
Wheeler, H.B., Gerson, J.M., and Gamin, G.J. (1966). *Ann. N.Y. Acad. Sci.* **129**, 118.
Willerson, J.T., Asofsky, R., and Barth, W.F. (1969a). *J. Immunol.* **103**, 741.
Willerson, J.T., Gordon, J.K., Talal, N., and Barth, W.F. (1969b). *Arthritis Rheum.* **12**, 232.
Witebsky, E. (1959). *In* "Immunopathology" (P. Grabar and P. Miescher, eds.), p. 1. Schwabe, Basel.
Wortis, H.H. (1971). *Clin. Exp. Immunol.* **8**, 305.
Zinsser, H. (1925). *Proc. Soc. Exp. Biol. Med.* **22**, 35.
Zschiesche, W. (1968). *In* "Amyloidosis" (E. Mandema, L. Ruinen, J.H. Scholten, and A.S. Cohen, eds.), p. 327. Excerpta Medica Found., Amsterdam.
Zschiesche, W., and Ghatak, S. (1965). *Verh. Deut. Ges. Pathol.* **49**, 284.
Zschiesche, W., Heinecke, H., and Klaus, S. (1967). *Beitr. Pathol. Anat.* **135**, 277.
Zucker-Franklin, D. (1974). In press.
Zucker-Franklin, D., and Franklin, E.C. (1970). *Amer. J. Pathol.* **59**, 23.

Subject Index

A

Acid phosphatase-positive cells, in Marek's disease, 80, 82
Actinomycin D, in detection of endogenous reverse transcriptase activity, 17
  in hybridization assay, 27
Aggregation, of viral reverse transcriptase, 23
AKR murine leukemia virus, 13
Allogeneic system, in transfer of amyloid-enhancing factor, 326
Alveolar macrophage, 252, 260
Amino acid chloramines, 257, 258
cAMP, in chalone activity, 168
Amyloid
  disease, transfer, 329
  enhancement, nonspecific, 321
  precursors, in serum, 314
  preformed, in amyloid transfer, 297
Amyloid-enhancing factor (AEF), "donor factor–recipient RE cell interplay," 328
  nature of, 328
  transfer, 315–329
    with cells, 315, 316
    donor–recipient combinations, 326
    source of cells, 322
    with subcellular material, 323–325
Amyloid-inducing factor (AIF), 285, 309
  nature of, 312
Amyloidogenic agent. See Antigen, specific, in transfer amyloidosis
Amyloidosis
  experimental, 274–289
    biphasic development
      primary phase, 274
      secondary (amyloid) phase, 275–277
    morphological characteristics, 275
    specific tolerance, pathogenetic significance, 284
  transfer, 273–334
    cells, 292, 293
      damaged, 310
      fractionation, column, 303
      number, 297
      route of transfer, 297
      source of, 302
      subcellular fractions, 304–307
      donor–recipient combinations, 311
      pathology, 299, 300–301
Amyloid-substance related component (ASC), 314
Angiogenesis, 208. See also Neovascularization
  biology, 214–227
  by control tissues and extracts, 233
  inhibition, 238
  tumor. See Tumor angiogenesis
Antibodies in Marek's disease
  complement-fixing, 131
  fluorescing, 130
  haemagglutinating, 131
  precipitating, 129
  protective effect, 127
  virus neutralizing, 130
θ-Antigens, 285
Antigens. See also Casein
Antigens, in feather follicle epithelium, 88
  immunofluorescent, in Marek's disease, 70, 130
  Marek's disease virus, in fluorescent antibody tests, 78
  specific, in transfer amyloidosis, 311
  surface, MD tumor-associated (MATSA), 125
  in transfer of amyloid-enhancing factor, 327
  tumor-specific, on HPRS cell lines, 123
  viral. See Viral antigen
Antimicrobial activities, in phagocytosis, 255–263
Aorta, endothelial turnover, 209
  injury to, endothelial regeneration following, 210, 211
  rat, endothelial cell turnover *in vitro*, 211, 212
ART. See RNA tumor, avian
Autoimmunity
  in amyloidosis, 292
  in Marek's disease, 109, 124
    mechanism, 303
Azurophilic granules, 251, 252, 254

335

B

Baboon endogenous virus, 10, 12
Bactericidal activity of leukocytes, in chronic leukemic states, 266
Bactericidal and metabolic cell activities, in phagocytosis: relationship, 263
B cells, in experimental amyloidosis, 285
BCG, in experimental mouse amyloidosis, 289
Blood leukocytes, crude extract, composition, 173, 174
Blood vessels, of tumors. See Angiogenesis
Bone marrow, chalone activity, 164, 182, 198
  infectivity, in Marek's disease, 85
Brain cells, human, finite life-span, 160
Breast tissue, RNA, 31
Burkitt lymphoma, cell lines, lymphoblastoid, 118
  cells, Epstein–Barr virus of, 3, 4–5
  extra virus-specific nucleotide sequences, 35
Bursa of Fabricius, in Marek's disease, 75, 78, 79, 83, 87, 131, 138
  origin of lymphoma cells, 116
Bursectomy, effect on Marek's disease, 131

C

Cancer, and chalones, 194–198
  definition, 194
  human, tumor viruses, molecular probes, 1–58
  of uterine cervix, *in situ,* avascular state, 232
Capillaries, proliferation, of chorioallantoic membrane, 222
  pathologic stimuli, 210
Capillary endothelium, tumor-stimulated migration, 244
Cartilage, diffusible factor, inhibition of tumor angiogenesis, 238, 239
Casein, cell-mediated immunity to, transfer of, 320
  induction of amyloidosis, 282
Cells
  B, in experimental amyloidosis, 285
  brain, human, finite life-span, 160
  classification, 158
  communication apparatus, in cancer, 195
  components, virus-related, intracellular localization, 13
  cycle, 165, 166
  growth, potential, 159
    strategy, 157–162
    three-dimensional, 243
  HeLa, 161
  invading, in demyelination of Marek's disease, 104
  leukemic. See Leukemic cells
  lines, indefinite growth potential, 161
    specificity of chalone action, 182
  lymphoid, in experimental amyloid transfer, 302
    in Marek's disease, 112, 113, 114, 115
    migration into peripheral nerves, 98
    neoplastic-type, 97, 98
    neuropathy, 109
  lymphoma B-type (bursa-derived), 116, 122
    Marek's disease infection of, 70
    origin, 116
    T-type (thymus-derived), 116, 122
  Marek's disease, 94
  mediation of demyelination, in Marek's disease, 105
  melanoma, inhibition by melanocyte chalone, 197
  mesenchymal, primitive, in lymphoma of Marek's disease, 116
  production centers, 160
  quantitative aspects, 159
  proliferation, controlling factors, 157
    density-dependent inhibition, 192–194
    influence of chemical substances, 189
    negative feedback in. See Chalones
    regulation by nonchalone factors, 189
  rejuvenation hypothesis of Sheldrake, 161
  total number, in mammals, 159
  in transfer amyloidosis. See Amyloidosis: cells
  types, 159
Cell-mediated immunity, 291
  in Marek's disease, 132, 137, 143
Cell-to-cell contact, in density-dependent inhibition of proliferation, 192
Central nervous system, Marek's disease infection, microscopic lesions, 110
Cervical cancer, herpes simplex virus, 6
Chalones, 155–206
  biochemical mechanisms, 167
  and cAMP cycle, 168

and cancer, 194–198
"cascade," 167
and the cell cycle, 165
cell membrane level of activity, 167
definition, 156, 187
epidermal, specificity, 184–185, 187
erythrocyte, specificity of action, 182, 184–185
G_1 and G_2 inhibitors, 184–185, 187
granulocyte, isolation, 169
  of marrow, 164, 198
  specificity of action, 182, 184–185
impurities of preparations, 168–173
  cytotoxic physiological, 170
  nonphysiological contaminants, 169
  physiological, 171
lymphocyte, prevention of graft-v-host reaction, in bone marrow transplants, 198
  specificity of action, 184–185
mechanism, theory, 162–168
protection of bone marrow cells, 164, 198
putative, 186, 187–189
receptor theory, 167
release, 162
synthesis, 162
tissue specificity of action, 179–187
  absence of inhibitors, 180
  degree, 179
  epidermal, 184–185, 187
  experimental evidence, 181
  granulocyte, 182, 184–185
  lymphocyte, 184–185
transport, 162
Chediak–Higashi syndrome, phagocytosis, 255, 265
Chemotaxis, 252–253
  altered, in decreased resistance to infection, 264
  chambers, 253
  generating factors *in vitro,* 253
Chick embryo, chorioallantoic membrane, tumor angiogenesis, 220
Chloramines, amino acid, 257, 258
Chlorination and decarboxylation, in MPO–H_2O_2–Cl⁻ antimicrobial system, 257
Chloroma cells, inhibition by chalone, 197
Chorioallantoic membrane, chick, TAF activity in, 226–227, 230
  tumor angiogenesis, 220
  vascularization of grafted tumor, 222, 224

C_0t, definition, 32
"Cold" thymidine, in chalone studies, 172
  inhibition of ³H-labeled thymidine incorporation, 176
Colony-stimulating factor, 190
Column fractionation of cells, in experimental amyloidosis transfer, 303
  in transfer of amyloid-enhancing factor, 320
Complement, in altered chemotaxis, 264
  in chalone preparations, 170
  serum, generation of chemotaxis, 253
Complement-fixing antibody, in Marek's disease, 131
Copenhagen model, of experimental transfer amyloidosis, 302
Cornea, rabbit, inhibitory effect of cartilage on angiogenesis, 239, 240, 241, 243
  irradiated tumor graft, induction of angiogenesis, 224
  in TAF bioassay, 230
  tumor growth and neovascularization, 218
Cortisone acetate, effect on Marek's disease, 116
Cs_2SO_4 density gradient centrifugation, method of hybridization assay, 29
Cuffing, in Marek's disease, 110, 126
Cyclophosphamide, effect on Marek's disease, 116

D

Decarboxylation, and chlorination, in MPO–H_2O_2–Cl⁻ antimicrobial system, 257
  in mouse spleen cell, 261
Decin mouse, in amyloid-enhancing factor experiments, 326
Degranulation, in phagocytosis, 254
Demyelination of neurites, in Marek's disease, 103
Density-dependent inhibition of cell proliferation, 192–194
  in human umbilical vein endothelium, 213
[1,7-¹⁴C] Diaminopimelic acid, 258
Digestion, S1 nuclease, hybridization assay, 27
DNA
  cDNA, hybridization to excess RNA, 30
  density analysis, 18, 19
  Epstein–Barr virus-specific, 3

DNA—*Continued*
  human cellular, related to tumor virus RNA: RNA tumor virus-related nucleotide sequences, 32
  polymerase, 21–25
    antiviral, specific inhibition, 24
    endogenous human AML pellet, density gradient analysis, 18, 20
    from mammalian type-C viruses, properties, 21
    virus-related, serologic relationships, 24, 25
  protein, splenic, in transfer amyloidosis, 308, 312, 313
  synthesis, endothelial cell, 216
    inhibition by crude leukocyte extracts, 178
    quantitative determination of cells, 172
  transcription, imbalance, 29
  transcripts, of tumor virus RNA, preparation, 27
  viruses in human cancer, molecular probes, 2–6
    transformation of cells in tissue culture, 6
Dorsal air sac, rat, in TAF bioassay, 230

E

Endothelial cells
  proliferation, 210
    relation to tumor growth, 207–247
  turnover, and capillary regeneration, 208–213
    normal, 208
    pathological stimuli, 210
    physiological stimuli, 209
    studies *in vitro*, 211
Endothelial mitosis, in immunological reactions, 237
Endothelium, traumatic injury, and cell proliferation, 210, 211
Enzymes, contaminating, in chalone preparations, 170, 171
  lysosomal, extracellular release, 254
    of monocytes, 252
    in polymorphonuclear leukocyte granules, 251
Epidermal growth factor, 190
Epithelial cells, in nasopharyngeal carcinoma, Epstein–Barr-specific DNA, 4
Epstein–Barr virus, molecular probes, 2
Equilibrium fractionation, in transfer amyloidosis experiments, 309
Erythropoietin, 189
  inhibitors, 190
Escherichia coli RNA polymerase, in detection of Epstein–Barr virus-specific DNA, 3
Eye changes, in lymphomatosis, 126
  lesion, in Marek's disease, 74
  rabbit, tumor growth and neovascularization, 218

F

Feather follicle epithelium, inclusion bodies, 65, 68
  Marek's disease virus infection, 87, 89, 90, 91
Fluorescence polarization, in demonstration of chalone tissue-specificity, 183
Fluorescing antibody, in Marek's disease, 130
Fluorochromasia monitoring of cell proliferation, 172

G

Genotype of host, in pathogenesis of Marek's disease, 141
Gibbon ape lymphosarcoma virus, 10, 11, 12
Globulin, serum, and amyloidosis, 287
Glucose-6-phosphate dehydrogenase deficiency of red cells, 265
Glycolysis, in metabolism of polymorphonuclear leukocytes, 255
Glycopeptide, in amyloid-enhancing factor, 329
Golgi complex, in polymorphonuclear leukocyte production, 251
Graft-versus-host reaction, in experimental amyloidosis, 281, 283
Granulocytes, chalone, isolation, 169
  of marrow, 164
  specificity of action, 182, 184–185
  maturation, stages, 250
Granulocytic "anti-chalone," 190
Granulomatous disease, chronic, phagocytosis, 265
Granulopoietin, 190

SUBJECT INDEX

Guinea pigs, in transfer amyloidosis experiments, 321

H

Heat-stable macromolecule, inhibition of bactericidal function, in mouse spleen cells, 262
HeLa cells, nature, 161
"Helper" virus, 10
Hemagglutinating antibody, in Marek's disease, 131
Hemopoietic cell lines, influence of chemical substances on division, 189
Hepatic lymphoma, in Marek's disease, 76
Herpes virus(es)
  in etiology of neoplastic disease, 60
  of Marek's disease, 62
    particles, 115
    and turkey, serological subtypes, 131
  molecular probes, 5
  simplex, in etiology of human cancers, 6
  turkey (HVT), vaccine, 134
  virus-cell relationships, 69
H_2O_2, in phagocytosis, 256
Hodgkin's disease, Epstein–Barr virus, 3
  extra virus-specific nucleotide sequences, 35
Homogenate, whole spleen, in transfer amyloidosis, 308, 323
Hormones, stress, and chalone G inhibitors, 188
  tissue-specific stimulation of cell proliferation, 191
Host, age of, in pathogenesis of Marek's disease, 144
  genotype, in pathogenesis of Marek's disease, 141
  susceptibility, in lymphomagenesis of Marek's disease, 111
HPRS
  immunofluorescent identification, 122
  -16 strain of MDV, lymphomagenicity, 112
  ultrastructure, 67, 120, 120, 121
Human vector, of primate type-C RNA tumor viruses, 11
Humoral regulation of cell proliferation, 190, 191
Hybridization
  assay, methods, 27, 28
  base mispairing, 33

C_0t, 32
DNA–RNA, in endogenous reverse transcriptase activity, 17
recycling, 35, 36
techniques of molecular probe, 3–5
Hydroxyapatite chromatography, 4, 28

I

IgM, in chalone preparations, 170
Immune disorders, in amyloidogenesis, 291
Immune functional characteristics, of experimental amyloidosis, 281
Immune response, in amyloid formation, 322
  cell mediation, 291
  cellular, reduced, in experimental amyloidosis, 283
  cyclic, in amyloidosis, 318
  impaired, in Marek's disease, 138
Immunity
  in Marek's disease, 126–140
    actively acquired, 129
    cell-mediated, 132, 143
    humoral, 129
    passively acquired, 126
    vaccinal, 133
  in transfer amyloidosis, 329
  vaccinal, effect of maternal antibody to HVT, 129
Immunoglobulin, and nonimmunoglobulin, possible precursors of amyloid, 314
  in Marek's disease, 139
Immunology
  concepts, in origin of lymphoma cells of Marek's disease, 116
  reactions, endothelial proliferation, 237
  relationships, in Marek's disease, 131
  technique of molecular probe, for Epstein–Barr virus, 3
Immunosuppression, in Marek's disease, 138
  and susceptibility to other diseases, 140
Immunosuppressives, in experimental amyloidosis, 282
Inclusion bodies, in Marek's disease, 65, 83, 85, 87, 89, 90
Infection
  in amyloidogenesis, 290
  definition, 2
  in Marek's disease, progress of, 85
  types, 69

Infection—*Continued*
  resistance to, alteration and decrease, 263–269
Infectious mononucleosis, Epstein–Barr virus, 3
Infiltrating cells, in demyelination of Marek's disease, 104, 108
Inflammation, absence of, in dorsal air sac of rat in tumor angiogenesis, 216
  ocular, absence of, in tumor angiogenesis, 219
  and tumor neovascularization, 236
Inflammatory concept, of Marek's disease, 61
Ingestion, in phagocytosis, 254
Injury, immune, types, 291
Interferon, in Marek's disease, 132, 142
Iodination, in phagocytosis, 257
Iris, implanted tumor, vascularization, 219, 220, 221
Irradiation, effect on capacity of tumors to induce angiogenesis, 224

K

Kidney, spleen graft amyloid in, 318, 319, 323
Kirsten sarcoma virus, 13
Kwashiorkor, phagocytosis, 266

L

Lactoferrin, of polymorphonuclear leukocyte granules, 251
Landry–Guillain–Barré syndrome (acute infective polyneuritis), relationship with Marek's disease neuropathy, 109
Leukemic cells, human, DNA polymerase activity, 18
  isolation of type-C virus from, 36
  myelogenous, endogenous reaction, 18–21
Leukemic disorders, acute, phagocytosis, 265
  chronic, phagocytosis, 265
  extra virus-specific nucleotide sequences, 35
Leukemic mice, spleen cells, bactericidal and metabolic properties, 261
Leukemogenesis, hematology, 125

Leukocytes
  extracts, crude, in chalone experiments: composition, 173, 174
  migration test, 284
  movement, in recurrent infection, 264
  phagocytic activity, and susceptibility to infection, 263–269
"Leukocytosis-inducing factor," 190
Lymphoblastoid cell lines derived from lymphomas, in Marek's disease, 118
Lymphoblasts, of Wight's type III lesion of Marek's disease, 97
Lymphocyte chalone. *See* Chalones, lymphocyte.
Lymphocytes, leukemic and PHA-stimulated, RNA, hybridization, 30
  normal, absence of reverse transcriptase, 21
  sensitized, in induction of amyloid, 317
Lymphoid cells. *See* Cells, lymphoid
Lymphoid proliferation, in Marek's disease, correlation with feather follicle antigen, 92
Lymphoid regression and reticulum cell hyperplasia, in Marek's disease, 85, 88
Lymphoid tissues, acute cytolytic infection of Marek's disease, 78
  Epstein–Barr virus tropism, 4
  in experimental amyloidosis, 275
Lymphokines, 284
Lymphoma
  cells. *See* Cells, lymphoma
  of Marek's disease
    effect of maternal antibody, 128
    site of formation, 72, 74, 77
    stimulation, extrinsic, 123
      intrinsic, 123
    ultrastructure, 113
Lymphomagenesis, in Marek's disease, pathology, 111
Lymphomatosis, 61, 126
Lymphopenia, in amyloidogenesis, 281
Lymphosarcoma, extra virus-specific nucleotide sequences, 35

M

Macromolecule, heat-stable, inhibition of bactericidal function, in mouse spleen cells, 262

SUBJECT INDEX

Macrophage alveolar, 252, 260
  in experimental amyloidosis, 288
  in Marek's disease, 81, 85
    in demyelination, 104
    in immunity, 133
  in phagocytosis, 259
  production and maturation, 252
Marek's disease
  acute cytolytic infection of nonlymphoid tissues, 86
  age of host, in pathogenesis, 144
  cells. See under Cells
  definition, 59
  environmental contamination, 87
  experimental model, 60
  experimental transmission, 71
  flock and individual characteristics, 71
  genetic resistance, 142
  gross lesions, 72
  hematological changes, 125
  historical concepts, 61
  humoral responses, suppression, 131
  immunity, 126–140
    influencing factors, 140–145
    vaccinal, mechanism, 136
  immunosuppressive effects, 138
  microscopic lesions, 76–126
  natural occurrence, 70
  neuropathy
    classifications, 93
    nature, 93
    pathogenesis, 106
  nomenclature, 61–62
  pathogenesis, 59–154
    influencing factors, 140–145
    neurological, 106
  pathology, 70–126.
  peripheral nervous system. See Peripheral nervous system in Marek's disease
  replication of virions, 63
  resistance to, correlation with regression of Rous sarcoma virus tumor, 143
  sex, influencing pathogenesis, 144
  vaccinal immunity, mechanism, 136
  virus-cell relationships, 62–70
Marek's disease virus
  different expressions of infection, 69
  envelopment, 65, 68
  infection of cell, 63
  serotypes, 140

  strains, 72
  pathogenicity, 140
  vaccines, 133
    apathogenic, 134
    choice of, influencing factors, 135
    horizontal transmission, in mutation, 135
    interference with vaccination, 135
    killed, 136
    modified, 133
    turkey herpesvirus, 134
Mason–Pfizer monkey virus, 11, 12, 13
MATSA. See Antigen, surface, MD tumor-associated
Melanoma, cells, inhibition by melanocyte chalone, 197
  RNA sequences, 31
6-Mercaptopurine, effect on Marek's disease, 116
Mesenchymal cell, primitive, in lymphoma of Marek's disease, 116
Mitogenic response, impaired, in MDV-infected birds, 139
Molecular probes, for tumor viruses, in human cancer, 1–58
Molecular weights, of cellular DNA polymerases, 22
Moloney murine leukemia virus, 13
Monocytes, production and maturation, 252
Mouse mutant "nude," in experimental amyloidosis, 282, 303, 320
Mouse spleen cells, bactericidal activity, 260
MPO deficiency, hereditary, phagocytosis, 265
$MPO-H_2O_2-Cl^-$ antimicrobial system, chlorination and decarboxylation, 257
Muscular atrophy, in Marek's disease, 75
Myelin. See Demyelination
Myeloperoxidase activity, of granulocytes, 251
Myeloproliferative disorders, phagocytosis, 266

N

NADPH oxidase activity, 265, 269
Nasopharyngeal carcinoma, Epstein–Barr virus-specific DNA, 4
Negative feedback, in cell proliferation. See Chalone concept

Neoplasia, in amyloidogenesis, 290
 human, virogene expression, 27
 of Marek's disease, 61, 62
Neovascularization, 210
 TAF-induced, 216
 and tumor growth, in rabbit eye, 218
Nerve growth factor, 190
Nerves, peripheral, in Marek's disease. *See* Peripheral nervous system in Marek's disease
Neurites, degenerative changes in, in Marek's disease, 101
Neurolymphomatosis, 61
Neuropathic change, in Marek's disease, 92
Nitrogen mustard, in transfer amyloidosis, 297, 298, 314
Nuclear projections, of Marek's disease lymphoma, 114, 120
Nucleic acid hybridization technique, of molecular probes, 3
 ^{3}H-labeled, 4
Nucleocapsids, of Marek's disease virus, 64, 68–69
Nucleosides, contamination of crude tissue extracts, effect on low molecular weight chalones, 175
Nucleotides, contamination of crude tissue extracts, effect on low molecular weight chalones, 175
 sequences, RNA tumor virus-related, in human cellular DNA related to tumor virus RNA, 32
Nucleus, irregular, chromatin-containing, of Marek's disease cell, 97, 99
Nude mouse mutant (nu/nu mouse), in experimental amyloidosis, 282, 303, 320

O

Ocular changes, in lymphomatosis, 126
 in Marek's disease, 74
Oncogenic viruses, formation, 7, 8, 9
 RNA, reverse transcriptase, immunologic groups, 24
 tumor, as models for oncogenesis, 9
"Onion bulbs" in demyelination of Marek's disease, 104, 106
Opsonins, 253, 264
Ovarian lymphoma, in Marek's disease, 74
Oxygen, singlet, mediator of PMN bactericidal activity, 258, 262

P

Parabiosis, syngeneic mouse, 304
Paralysis, transient, of Marek's disease, 111
Particle, viruslike, definition, 2
P component, in pathogenesis of amyloidosis, 315
Peripheral nervous system in Marek's disease, 72, 73
 A-type lesion, 94, 95, 96
 relationship with B-type, 101
 B-type lesion, 99, 100
 relationship with A-type, 101
 C-type lesion, 101
 infection, microscopic lesions, 92–110
Peroxidase activity, of macrophage, 260
 of mouse spleen cells, 260
 of polymorphonuclear leukocytes, 256
pH drop, in human cells, 257
Phagocytes, altered biochemical and microbicidal activity, 265
Phagocytosis
 antimicrobial activities of cells, 255–263
 biochemical activities of cells, 255–263
 biochemical, functional, and structural aspects, 249–271
 morphological events, 254–255
 of murine macrophage during experimental amyloidosis, 288
 receptor mechanism, 254
 recognition factors, 253–254
 altered activity, 264
Phenylbutazone, in phagocytosis, 256
Phosphocellulose chromatography, 21
 paper disc method of hybridization assay, 29
Phytohemagglutinin, in HPRS cell lines, 122
 -stimulated normal human lymphocytes, RNA, hybridization, 30
Plasma cells, in amyloidosis, 285
Poietins, 189
Polykaryocytes, in Marek's disease, 63
Polymerase, DNA, 21–25
 antiviral, specific inhibition, 24
 endogenous human AML pellet, density gradient analysis, 18, 20
 from mammalian type-C viruses, properties, 21
 virus-related, 24, 25

SUBJECT INDEX

Polymorphonuclear leukocytes, metabolic activities, 255, 262
  peroxidase, 256
  production and maturation, 250
Polyneuritis, acute infective. *See* Landry–Guillain–Barré syndrome
Precipitating antibody, in Marek's disease, 129
Prednisolone, effect on Marek's disease, 116
Prednisone therapy, effect on phagocytosis in leukemia, 266
Primate type-C RNA tumor viruses. *See under* RNA tumor viruses
Promine, in control of cell proliferation, 191
Protein, synthesis, inhibition by crude leukocyte extracts, 177
  viral, nomenclature, 25
Pulse cytophotometry, 172
Putrescine, 191
Pyroninophilic phase, of experimental amyloidosis, 277

R

Radioimmune competition assay, of viral antigens, 26
Rat dorsal air sac, tumor angiogenesis in, 216, 217
Rauscher murine leukemia virus, 13
Reassociation rate of Epstein–Barr virus-specific DNA, measurement, 3
Respiratory tract, in Marek's disease, 77
Restrictive infection, of Marek's disease virus, 69
Reticular tissue, in experimental amyloid transfer, 302
Reticuloendothelial tissue, in experimental amyloidosis, 278, 279, 280
Reticulum cell hyperplasia, in Marek's disease, 80, 81, 83, 84
Retine, in control of cell proliferation, 191
Reverse transcriptase, 9, 11, 13
  endogenous, detection, 16
  human, as viral marker enzyme, 24
  immunological characteristics, 23
  of type-C virus, 37
  inhibition of activity by antisera, 24
  of oncogenic RNA viruses, immunologic groups, 24

purified, biochemical and physical properties, 21
Rhesus placenta-embryo, viral reverse transcriptase, 23
RNA
  in amyloidosis transfer with subcellular fractions, 309
  cellular, human, RNA tumor virus-related nucleotide sequences, 27
  hybridization from Rauscher leukemia virus to infected and uninfected cell DNA, 33
  70 S, detection in human neoplasias, 14
  synthesis, inhibition by crude leukocyte extracts, 177
  tumor, avian (ART), interaction with Marek's disease virus infection *in vivo*, 125
  tumor virus, genome, constituents, 14
    in human cancer, molecular probes, 7–38
    molecular relationships to human cells: studies and techniques, 13
    origins, 7
    primate type-C, 10
    -related nucleotide sequences in human cellular DNA related to tumor virus RNA, 32
    in human cellular RNA, 27
  viral, excess labeled, hybridization to infected cell DNA, 31
RNA–DNA transcription, in carcinogenesis, 9
Rous sarcoma virus tumor regression, correlation with resistance to Marek's disease, 143

S

Schwann cells in Marek's disease, 104 *et. seq.*
  in peripheral nervous system, 99, 101, 102
Sciatic nerves, in Marek's disease, 72, 73
  infected with HPRS-16 MDV, sequential study, 105, 106, 107
Seroepidemiological studies, of herpes simplex virus in human cancer, 6
Serum factor, in neovascularization in inflammation, 236
Sex, in pathogenesis of Marek's disease, 144

Sickle-cell anemia, phagocytosis, 264
Simian sarcoma virus, 10, 12
  genetic relation to gibbon ape lymphosarcoma virus, 11
Simultaneous detection test, in reverse transcriptase activity in human leukemias, 17
  of 70 S RNA in human neoplasia, 15, 16
Singlet oxygen, mediator of PMN bactericidal activity, 258, 262
Skin, endothelial proliferation, and the inflammatory process, 237
Skin graft rejection time, in Marek's disease, 138
"Skin window," study of chemotaxis, 252
Soft agar suspension culture, 225
Spleen
  cells, mouse, bactericidal and metabolic activity, 260
  in experimental amyloidosis, 275, 276–277, 279
    transfer amyloidosis, 296, 329
    whole grafts, 302, 317, 318, 319, 323
  extracts, lymphocyte chalones, 180
  in Marek's disease, 78, 79, 139
Splenoperoxidase, 261
Steroid therapy, effect on phagocytic bactericidal activity in leukemia, 266
Stratum transivativum cells, Marek's disease virus-specific changes, 89
Stress hormones, and chalone G inhibitors, 188
Subcellular fractions, in experimental amyloid transfer, 304, 306–307
  of virus-like components, 14
Surface properties, in density-dependent inhibition of cells, 193
Syncytia, reticulum cell, in Marek's disease, 81, 86

T

T cells, in experimental amyloidosis, 281
  splenic, 278
Testicular lymphoma, in Marek's disease, 75
Thrombopoietin, 190
Thymectomy, effect of Marek's disease, 117
Thymidine, in chalone studies of cell proliferation, 171
Thymus, in Marek's disease, 75, 78, 79, 80
  origin of lymphoma cells, 116

Tissues, classification, 158
  normal, angiogenetic properties, 234–235
  transplanted, normal and neoplastic, vascularization, 222
T lymphocytes, in amyloid pathogenesis, 320, 321
Toxins, in neuropathogenesis of Marek's disease, 107
Transformation, in genetic resistance to Marek's disease, 142
Transforming virus, 119
Transient paralysis (Marek's disease), 111
Tumor angiogenesis
  on chorioallantoic membrane, 220
  in dorsal air sac of rat, 216, 217
  and the inflammatory process, 236
  specificity, 233, 244
  therapeutic implications, 244
Tumor angiogenesis factor (TAF), 216, 228–230, 244
  bioassay, 230
  relationship to other tumor factors, 238
  purification, 228
  in tissue cultured cells, 226–227
Tumor(s)
  cells, aberrant properties, 194
    to chick embryo chorioallantoic membrane, vascularization, 222, 224
  graft, irradiated, induction of angiogenesis, 224
  growth, and neovascularization, in rabbit eye, 218, 220
  avascular stage, 231
  in isolated perfused organ, 215
  relation of endothelial proliferation, 207–247
  vascular phase, 232
  inducing neovascularization, 233
Turkey herpes virus. See Herpes virus, turkey

U

Umbilical vein endothelium, human, cell turnover in vitro, 212

V

Vaccinal immunity, to Marek's disease, effect of maternal antibody to HVT, 129
Vaccines, Marek's disease, classification, 133

SUBJECT INDEX

Vascularization, in suppression of non-malignant disease, 245
  of transplanted tissue, normal and neoplastic, 222
Vertical transmission of viruses, 7
Viral antigens
  in human cells, 25
  of Marek's disease, 80, 83, 85
    in CNS neuropathy, 110
    in feather follicle, 91
Viral genome, stimulus for lymphoma formation in Marek's disease, 124
Viral proteins, nomenclature, 25
Virions, in Marek's disease, replication, 63
  unenveloped, 83, 85
Virus(es),
  "classes," 7 et seq.
    interspecies infection, 13
    definition, 2
    endogenous unrelated pairs, in animal systems, 33
    Epstein-Barr, 2, 3, 4–5
    Gibbon ape lymphosarcoma, 10, 11, 12
    "helper," 10
    horizontal transmission, 7, 9

  interspecies pathogenicity, 34
  strain of, in lymphomagenesis of Marek's disease, 111
  tumor, abbreviations, 2
    in human cancer, molecular probes for, 1–58
    type-C, in studies of human leukemias, 10
    isolation, 36
    vertical transmission of, 7
Virus neutralizing antibody, in Marek's disease, 130
Visceral lymphomatosis, 61

W

Woolly monkey sarcoma virus. *See* Simian sarcoma virus
Wound healing, neovascularization in, 236
"Wound hormones," 191

X

Xenogeneic transfer of amyloid-enhancing factor, 327

64493